Baillière's
CLINICAL
HAEMATOLOGY
INTERNATIONAL PRACTICE AND RESEARCH

Baillière's

CLINICAL HAEMATOLOGY

INTERNATIONAL PRACTICE AND RESEARCH

Volume 4/Number 2
April 1991

Paediatric Haematology

I. M. HANN MD, MRCPath, FRCP
B. E. S. GIBSON MB ChB, FRCP, MRCPath, DFM
Guest Editors

Baillière Tindall
London Philadelphia Sydney Tokyo Toronto

This book is printed on acid-free paper.

Baillière Tindall 24–28 Oval Road,
W.B. Saunders London NW1 7DX

The Curtis Center, Independence Square West,
Philadelphia, PA 19106–3399, USA

55 Horner Avenue
Toronto, Ontario M8Z 4X6, Canada

Harcourt Brace Jovanovich Group (Australia) Pty Ltd,
30–52 Smidmore Street, Marrickville, NSW 2204, Australia

Harcourt Brace Jovanovich Japan, Inc
Ichibancho Central Building, 22–1
Ichibancho, Chiyoda-ku, Tokyo 102, Japan

ISSN 0950-3536

ISBN 0-7020-1532–6 (single copy)

Baillière's Clinical Haematology is published four times each year by Baillière Tindall.
Annual subscription prices are:

TERRITORY	ANNUAL SUBSCRIPTION	SINGLE ISSUE
1. UK	£55.00 post free	£27.50 post free
2. Europe	£61.00 post free	£27.50 post free
3. All other countries	Consult your local Harcourt Brace Jovanovich office for dollar price	

The editor of this publication is Stephen Handley, Baillière Tindall,
24–28 Oval Road, London NW1 7DX.

Baillière's Clinical Haematology was published from 1972 to 1986 as
Clinics in Haematology.

Typeset by Phoenix Photosetting, Chatham.
Printed and bound in Great Britain by Mackays of Chatham PLC, Chatham, Kent.

Contributors to this issue

ELAINE J. ABRAMS MD, Assistant Professor of Clinical Pediatrics, College of Physicians & Surgeons of Columbia University; Director, Pediatric AIDS Program, Harlem Hospital Center, 506 Lenox Avenue, New York, New York 10037, USA.

MAUREEN ANDREW MD, FRCP(C), Associate Professor, Pediatrics and Pathology, Director, Coagulation Laboratory, McMaster University Medical Centre, Room 3N27, 1200 Main Street West, Hamilton, Ontario L8N 3Z5, Canada.

VICTOR S. BLANCHETTE MA, MB, BChir(Cantab), MRCP(UK), FRCP(C), Associate Professor, Department of Pediatrics, University of Toronto; Staff Hematologist, The Hospital for Sick Children, 555 University Avenue, Toronto, Ontario M5G 1X8, Canada.

ELIO CASTAGNOLA MD, Grant Holder, G. Gaslini Children's Hospital, Largo G. Gaslini 5, 16147 Genova, Italy.

JUDITH M. CHESSELLS MD, FRCP, MRCPath, Professor of Haematology and Oncology, Institute of Child Health, London WC1N 1EH; Honorary Consultant, Hospital for Sick Children, Great Ormond Street, London WC1N 3JH, UK.

SALLY C. DAVIES MB, MSc, MRCP, MRCPath, Consultant Haematologist, Central Middlesex Hospital, Acton Lane, London NW10 7NS, UK.

STELLA DAVIES MBBS, PhD, Medical Fellow, Pediatric Hematology–Oncology and Bone Marrow Transplant, Box 366 University of Minnesota Hospital and Clinics, 420 Delaware Street, Minneapolis, MN 55455, USA.

BRENDA E. S. GIBSON, MBChB, FRCP, MRCPath, DFM, Consultant Paediatric Haematologist and Honorary Senior Lecturer, Royal Hospital for Sick Children, Yorkhill, Glasgow G3 8SJ, UK.

IAN MALCOLM HANN MD, MRCPath, FRCP, Consultant Haematologist, Hospitals for Sick Children, Great Ormond Street, London WC1N 3JH, UK.

DEREK JOHN KING BMedBiol, MBChB, MRCP(UK), MRCPath, Consultant Haematologist, Royal Aberdeen Children's Hospital, Cornhill Road, Aberdeen AB9 2ZG; Clinical Senior Lecturer, University of Aberdeen Medical School, Polwarth Building, Foresterhill, Aberdeen, AB9 2ZD, UK.

C. A. LUDLAM PhD, FRCP, FRCPath, Director Haemophilia Centre and Consultant Haematologist, Royal Infirmary, Lauriston Place, Edinburgh, Scotland EH3 9YW, UK.

JOHN MICHAEL OLD BSc, PhD, Clinical Molecular Geneticist, C Grade National Haemoglobinopathy Reference Service, Institute of Molecular Medicine, John Radcliffe Hospital, Oxford OX3 9DU, UK.

NORMA K. C. RAMSAY MD, Professor of Pediatrics, Director of Pediatric Bone Marrow Transplantation, Box 366 University of Minnesota Hospital and Clinics, 420 Delaware Street, Minneapolis, MN 55455, USA.

DAVID WATSON ROGERS DM, MRCP, DCH, Clinical Research Physician, Wellcome Research Laboratories, Langley Court, Beckenham, Kent BR3 3BS; and Honorary Consultant Paediatrician, Queen Elizabeth Hospital for Children, Hackney Road, London E2 8PS, UK.

MARTHA F. ROGERS MD, Chief, Epidemiology Branch, Division of HIV/AIDS Center for Infectious Diseases, Centers for Disease, 1600 Clifton Road, Mailstop E4, Atlanta, GA 30333, USA.

CATHERINE R. SPARLING, Advanced Registered Technologist—Hematology, Charge Technologist—Coagulation Laboratory, Hospital for Sick Children, 555 University Avenue, Toronto, Ontario, M5G 1X8, Canada.

RICHARD F. STEVENS BSc, MB ChB, MRCP, MRCPath, Consultant Haematologist/ Oncologist, Royal Manchester Children's Hospital, Pendlebury, Manchester M27 1HA, UK.

CHRISTOPHER TURNER BSc, MD, FRCPC, FAAP, Clinical Lecturer, Dept of Paediatrics, Children's Hospital of Eastern Ontario, University of Ottawa, 401 Smyth Road, Ottawa, K1H 8L1; Section Head, Blood Banks, Bureau of Biologics, Health Protection Branch, Dept of Health and Welfare, Tunney's Pasture, Ottawa, Ontario, K1A 0L2, Canada.

CLAUDIO VISCOLI MD, Associate Professor of Infectious Disease, University of Genova, G. Gaslini Children's Hospital, Largo G. Gaslini, 5, 16147, Genova, Italy.

BEATRIX WONKE MD, FRCPath, Consultant Haematologist, Whittington Hospital, Highgate Hill, London N19; Honorary Senior Lecturer, Royal Free School of Medicine, London NW3, UK.

Table of contents

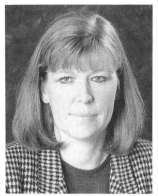
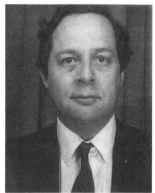

Foreword

Although paediatric haematology is closely affiliated with its adult counterpart, major differences exist and should be appreciated. Many inherited and acquired disorders are peculiar to childhood and where disorders affect all age groups there are striking differences in both the incidence and management, not only between children and adults, but between infants and older children. This issue aims to discuss in an authoritative manner a number of topics from the field of paediatric haematology, selected for their current interest and, in some instances, controversial issues.

The volume is principally clinical in nature and does not set out to discuss in depth new laboratory technologies and diagnostic advances, which often have equal application in the paediatric and adult field. However, these are discussed in detail where an appreciation of recent molecular and biological advances aids the reader in his/her further understanding of disease diagnosis or classification. Major emphasis is placed on management issues which the reader might often find divergent from those in adult practice.

The major differences in the infant's haemostatic system when compared with that of older children or adults complicates the investigation of the newborn with haemorrhagic or thrombotic problems. Management decisions are often based on therapeutic regimens used in adults with similar disorders and may be inappropriate when applied to the newborn's haemostatic mechanism. Reference ranges make the diagnosis of congenital coagulation factor deficiencies in the neonate possible. Inherited bleeding disorders, particularly platelet disorders, are rare. Management issues, which are understandably influenced by the HIV epidemic which has devastated the haemophiliac community, are presently very controversial.

An overview of HIV infection in children, including the epidemiology of the disease, modes of transmission, diagnosis and management, is information that is becoming increasingly valuable to the paediatric haematologist. As our society becomes more cosmopolitan it is encumbent that we recognize the needs of children with haemoglobinopathies, the commonest inherited genetic disorder worldwide, particularly as techniques for antenatal diagnosis and therapeutic strategies improve. Antenatal diagnosis with the possibility of subsequent termination should be available for all families affected by a serious inherited haematological disorder and this is becoming increasingly possible with recent advances in molecular biological techniques.

Although overall cure rates for acute leukaemia in children continue to improve and surpass those of adults, relapse after chemotherapy remains a problem and for such children bone marrow transplantation offers the possibility of cure. An improved understanding of disease pathophysiology and classification by recognition of the significance of prognostic factors should make possible the appropriate selection of treatment choices. Paediatric myelodysplasia, an extremely rare and poorly defined entity, remains a management challenge. The need to minimize late effects from chemotherapy/radiotherapy is now deservedly a major consideration in treatment options. Our improved understanding of the risks of immunosuppression and our ability to manage the resulting infections have allowed the use of chemotherapy protocols of ever-increasing intensity. A proliferation of antibacterials, antivirals and antifungals flow from the pharmaceutical industry making it important that the paediatric haematologist be as familiar with the armamentarium of pharmacological agents against infection as with chemotherapeutic agents. In no other field of medicine has infection and its devastating consequences had such an impact as HIV infection on transfusion practice. Despite concerns about the transmission of infectious agents by blood products, the ready availability of blood and, in particular, blood component therapy has not just revolutionized the lives of children with inherited haemostatic disorders but, in a similar manner to modern antibiotic therapy, has dramatically contributed to the improved survival of children requiring intensive chemotherapy.

B. E. S. GIBSON
I. M. HANN

1

An approach to the management of infants with impaired haemostasis

M. ANDREW

Impaired haemostasis occurs with greater frequency in infancy than during any other time in childhood. This reflects the many pathological complications that may occur in the perinatal period, as well as the early presentation of children with congenital coagulation factor deficiencies. The approach to infants with impaired haemostasis is similar to adults. The clinical history, physical examination, use of coagulation screening tests, and at times more specific testing are necessary to come to the correct diagnosis. However, the evaluation of infants for haemostatic complications presents the following problems not present in older children or adults.

1. The physiological state of the haemostatic system is immature with low concentrations of many coagulation proteins making the diagnosis of some inherited and/or acquired haemostatic problems difficult. Indeed, infants along with the fetus, pregnant women and children can be considered to exist in an alternative physiological state compared to adults.
2. Multiple reference ranges reflecting the gestational and postnatal age of the infant are necessary because the haemostatic system is dynamic and rapidly maturing towards the adult system (Andrew et al, 1987a, 1988a, 1990a).
3. Only small amounts of blood are available for laboratory testing which necessitates the use of microtechniques.
4. The difficulty of obtaining samples from newborns has resulted in extensive evaluation of cord blood which is readily available in large amounts. The latter does not necessarily reflect the physiological state of newborns in the first hours of life.

After confirming the nature of the haemostatic defect present, the clinician is faced with the problem of providing safe and effective therapy. Ideally decisions for specific therapeutic interventions are based on results from clinical trials with strong study designs. Unfortunately, most forms of therapy for infants are based on case reports, case series or extrapolated conclusions from the management of adults with similar disorders. One of the challenges in newborn haemostasis is to devise study designs that can test therapeutic options available for sick neonates. In this review, greater

Baillière's Clinical Haematology—
Vol. 4, No. 2, April 1991
ISBN 0–7020–1532–6

weight is given to conclusions of studies with strong designs than to those with weaker designs. When clinical data from newborn infants is not available, extrapolations are made from adults in combination with studies on newborn plasma and animal models.

HAEMOSTASIS: GENERAL

Blood is normally maintained in a fluid phase. However, in response to damage to the vessel wall, processes are initiated whereby platelets, plasma proteins and the damaged vessel contribute to the formation and regulation of a haemostatic plug. The following is a brief review of this physiological process which will facilitate the discussion of physiological differences in infants (Colman et al, 1987).

Specific plasma proteins, factors XII, XI, prekallikrein (PK) and high molecular weight kininogen (HMWK) initiate the 'contract' or 'intrinsic' phase of coagulation, whereas exposed tissue factor initiates the 'extrinsic' phase of coagulation. The assembly of factors, XI, IX and VIII on a phospholipid surface, or VII bound to tissue factor, in the presence of calcium results in the formation of complexes that generate the enzyme Xa from surface bound factor X. Factor Xa in turn converts prothrombin to thrombin in the presence of factor Va, calcium, and a phospholipid surface.

Thrombin, a key enzyme in haemostasis, has many functions. On the procoagulant side of haemostasis it activates factors V and VIII, thereby augmenting its own formation; it cleaves fibrinopeptides A and B from fibrinogen, which results in fibrin formation; and it activates platelets. Besides functioning as a procoagulant, thrombin functions as an anti-coagulant by binding to thrombomodulin on endothelial cell surfaces, resulting in activation of protein C. Activated protein C, in the presence of protein S (both proteins are vitamin K-dependent inhibitors) cleaves factors Va and VIIIa leading to their inactivation and decreased thrombin generation. The generation of thrombin and activities of thrombin are further regulated by the inhibitors antithrombin III (ATIII), α_2-macroglobulin (α_2M) and heparin cofactor II (HCII) (Shapiro SS et al, 1977) and incorporation into the fibrin clot. ATIII inhibits several serine proteases in the haemostatic system and is considered the major inhibitor of thrombin in adults. HCII is a specific inhibitor of thrombin, but based on in vitro tests, it inhibits only small amounts of thrombin. α_2M inhibits most serine proteases, including thrombin, but has a relatively minor role compared to ATIII in adults.

The components of the human fibrinolytic system include plasminogen, several types of plasminogen activators, and inhibitors of plasmin as well as inhibitors of plasminogen activators (Collen and Lijnen, 1987). Plasminogen binds to fibrin through lysine binding sites on a specific triple-loop structure called a 'Kringle'. Native plasminogen has a NH_2-terminal glutamic acid residue (Glu-plasminogen) which can be converted to a lysine residue (Lys-plasminogen) by limited degradation. The Lys-plasminogen has a higher affinity and activity for fibrin than the Glu-plasminogen. Plasmin cleaves both fibrinogen or fibrin in sequential steps resulting in fibrinogen/ fibrin degradation products. α_2-Antiplasmin (α_2AP) is the major inhibitor of plasmin. It binds to the active site of plasmin forming a 1 : 1 stoichiometric complex which has no further activity against fibrin. α_2M is a less important inhibitor of plasmin in adults. Tissue plasminogen activator (TPA) is a serine protease which functions as a physiological activator of plasminogen. TPA also binds to fibrin through lysine binding sites. Single-chain urokinase is a serine protease produced by kidney cells and found in the urine. Single-chain urokinase has relatively low thrombolytic activity until it is activated to its double-chain form by limited cleavage by plasmin. There are three plasminogen activator inhibitors described (PAI-1, PAI-2, PAI-3). PAI-1 is the major inhibitor of TPA in adults. PAI-2 is found during pregnancy and may have an important physiological role in suppressing fibrinolysis at that time. PAI-3 appears to be a protein C inhibitor.

When the endothelial lining of blood vessels is damaged or removed, one of the first steps in haemostasis is platelet adherence to the subendothelial layers. Platelets then undergo shape change and spread over the surface. This process requires that a plasma factor bind to a specific component of the platelet membrane, glycoprotein Ib (Nachman et al, 1971). von Willebrand factor (vWF) is the plasma component required for adhesion and acts as a bridge between the subendothelial surface and glycoprotein Ib (Jenkins et al, 1976). Following activation by several potential platelet agonists, platelets expose fibrinogen binding sites that are located on glycoproteins IIb/IIIa (Gogstad et al, 1982). Platelet aggregation is mediated by fibrinogen binding to glycoprotein IIb/IIIa.

The process of haemostatic plug formation is complex. There is no evidence that the overall process of haemostatic plug formation/regulation is different in infants. All components are present at birth in viable infants and appear to have similar physiological functions compared to adults. However, there are important physiological differences in the concentration, structure and interaction of components of haemostasis in newborns compared to adults.

HAEMOSTASIS: NEWBORN

Coagulation

Coagulation proteins do not cross the placental barrier from mothers to fetuses (Cade et al, 1969; Forestier et al, 1985, 1986a, 1986b; Toulon et al, 1986). They are synthesized by the fetus and begin to appear by 10 weeks gestational age. The concentration of most coagulation proteins gradually increases with increasing gestational age. True reference ranges for extremely premature infants (less than 30 weeks gestation) are not available in large part because the majority of these infants have postnatal complications and are not normal (Barnard et al, 1979). Recent studies provide reference ranges (Tables 1–4) for the components of fluid phase haemostasis in newborns of 30 to 40 weeks gestational age (Andrew et al, 1987a, 1988a, 1990a).

Table 1. Reference values for coagulation tests in the healthy full-term infant during the first 6 months of life. From Andrew et al (1987a, 1988a, 1990a), with permission.

	Day 1		Day 5		Day 30		Day 90		Day 180		Adult	
	M	B	M	B	M	B	M	B	M	B	M	B
PT (s)	13.0	(10.1–15.9)*	12.4	(10.0–15.3)*	11.8	(10.0–14.3)*	11.9	(10.0–14.2)*	12.3	(10.7–13.9)*	12.4	(10.8–13.9)
INR	1.00	(0.53–1.62)	0.89	(0.53–1.48)	0.79	(0.53–1.26)	0.81	(0.53–1.26)	0.88	(0.61–1.17)	0.89	(0.64–1.17)
APTT (s)	42.9	(31.3–54.5)	42.6	(25.4–59.8)	40.4	(32.0–55.2)	37.1	(29.0–50.1)*	35.5	(28.1–42.9)*	33.5	(26.6–40.3)
TCT (s)	23.5	(19.0–28.3)*	23.1	(18.0–29.2)	24.3	(19.4–29.2)*	25.1	(20.5–29.7)*	25.5	(19.8–31.2)*	25.0	(19.7–30.3)
Fibrinogen (g/l)	2.83	(1.67–3.99)*	3.12	(1.62–4.62)*	2.70	(1.62–3.78)*	2.43	(1.50–3.79)*	2.51	(1.50–3.87)*	2.78	(1.56–4.00)
II (U ml⁻¹)	0.48	(0.26–0.70)	0.63	(0.33–0.93)	0.68	(0.34–1.02)	0.75	(0.45–1.05)	0.88	(0.60–1.16)	1.08	(0.70–1.46)
V (U ml⁻¹)	0.72	(0.34–1.08)	0.95	(0.45–1.45)	0.98	(0.62–1.34)	0.90	(0.48–1.32)	0.91	(0.55–1.27)	1.06	(0.62–1.50)
VII (U ml⁻¹)	0.66	(0.28–1.04)	0.89	(0.35–1.43)	0.90	(0.42–1.38)	0.91	(0.39–1.43)	0.87	(0.47–1.27)	1.05	(0.67–1.43)
VIII (U ml⁻¹)	1.00	(0.50–1.78)*	0.88	(0.50–1.54)*	0.91	(0.50–1.57)*	0.79	(0.50–1.25)*	0.73	(0.50–1.09)	0.99	(0.50–1.49)
vWF (U ml⁻¹)	1.53	(0.50–2.87)	1.40	(0.50–2.54)	1.28	(0.50–2.46)	1.18	(0.50–2.06)	1.07	(0.50–1.97)	0.92	(0.50–1.58)
IX (U ml⁻¹)	0.53	(0.15–0.91)	0.53	(0.15–0.91)	0.51	(0.21–0.81)	0.67	(0.21–1.13)	0.86	(0.36–1.36)	1.09	(0.55–1.63)
X (U ml⁻¹)	0.40	(0.12–0.68)	0.49	(0.19–0.79)	0.59	(0.31–0.87)	0.71	(0.35–1.07)	0.78	(0.38–1.18)	1.06	(0.70–1.52)
XI (U ml⁻¹)	0.38	(0.10–0.66)	0.55	(0.23–0.87)	0.53	(0.27–0.79)	0.69	(0.41–0.97)	0.86	(0.49–1.34)	0.97	(0.67–1.27)
XII (U ml⁻¹)	0.53	(0.13–0.93)	0.47	(0.11–0.83)	0.49	(0.17–0.81)	0.67	(0.25–1.09)	0.77	(0.39–1.15)	1.08	(0.52–1.64)
PK (U ml⁻¹)	0.37	(0.18–0.69)	0.48	(0.20–0.76)	0.57	(0.23–0.91)	0.73	(0.41–1.05)	0.86	(0.56–1.16)	1.12	(0.62–1.62)
HMW-K (U ml⁻¹)	0.54	(0.06–1.02)	0.74	(0.16–1.32)	0.77	(0.33–1.21)	0.82	(0.30–1.46)*	0.82	(0.36–1.28)*	0.92	(0.50–1.36)
XIIIa (U ml⁻¹)	0.79	(0.27–1.31)	0.94	(0.44–1.44)*	0.93	(0.39–1.47)*	1.04	(0.36–1.72)*	1.04	(0.46–1.62)*	1.05	(0.55–1.55)
XIIIb (U ml⁻¹)	0.76	(0.30–1.22)	1.06	(0.32–1.80)	1.11	(0.39–1.73)*	1.16	(0.48–1.84)*	1.10	(0.50–1.70)*	0.97	(0.57–1.37)

PT, prothrombin time; APTT, activated partial thromboplastin time; TCT, thrombin clotting time; VIII, factor VIII procoagulant; vWF, von Willebrand factor; PK, prekallikrein; HMW-K, high molecular weight kininogen; INR, international normalized ratio.
All factors except fibrinogen are expressed as units per millilitre (U ml⁻¹) where pooled plasma contains 1.0 U ml⁻¹. All values are expressed as mean (M) followed by the lower and upper boundary encompassing 95% of the population (B). Between 40 and 77 samples were assayed for each value for the newborn. Some measurements were skewed due to a disproportionate number of high values. The lower limit which excludes the lower 2.5% of the population has been given.

Table 2. Reference values for coagulation tests in the healthy premature infant (30–36 weeks gestation) during the first 6 months of life. From Andrew et al (1987a, 1988a, 1990a), with permission.

	Day 1		Day 5		Day 30		Day 90		Day 180		Adult	
	M	B	M	B	M	B	M	B	M	B	M	B
PT (s)	13.0	(10.6–16.2)*	12.5	(10.0–15.3)*	11.8	(10.0–13.6)*	12.3	(10.0–14.6)*	12.5	(10.0–15.0)*	12.4	(10.8–13.9)
INR	1.00	(0.61–1.70)	0.91	(0.53–1.48)	0.79	(0.53–1.11)	0.88	(0.53–1.32)	0.91	(0.53–1.48)	0.89	(0.64–1.17)
APTT (s)	53.6	(27.5–79.4)†	50.5	(26.9–74.1)	44.7	(26.9–62.5)	39.5	(28.3–50.7)	37.5	(27.1–53.3)*	33.5	(26.6–40.3)
TCT (s)	24.8	(19.2–30.4)*	24.1	(18.8–29.4)*	24.4	(18.8–29.9)*	25.1	(19.4–30.8)*	25.2	(18.9–31.5)*	25.0	(19.7–30.3)
Fibrinogen (g/l)	2.43	(1.50–3.73)*†	2.80	(1.60–4.18)*†	2.54	(1.50–4.14)*	2.46	(1.50–3.52)*	2.28	(1.50–3.60)	2.78	(1.56–4.00)
II (U ml^{-1})	0.45	(0.20–0.77)	0.57	(0.29–0.85)†	0.57	(0.36–0.95)†	0.68	(0.30–1.06)	0.87	(0.51–1.23)	1.08	(0.70–1.46)
V (U ml^{-1})	0.88	(0.41–1.44)*†	1.00	(0.46–1.54)*	1.02	(0.48–1.56)*	0.99	(0.59–1.39)*	1.02	(0.58–1.46)*	1.06	(0.62–1.50)
VII (U ml^{-1})	0.67	(0.21–1.13)	0.84	(0.30–1.38)	0.83	(0.21–1.45)	0.87	(0.31–1.43)	0.99	(0.47–1.51)*	1.05	(0.67–1.43)
VIII (U ml^{-1})	1.11	(0.50–2.13)	1.15	(0.53–2.05)*†	1.11	(0.50–1.99)*†	1.06	(0.58–1.88)*†	0.99	(0.50–1.87)*†	0.99	(0.50–1.49)
vWF (U ml^{-1})	1.36	(0.78–2.10)	1.33	(0.72–2.19)	1.36	(0.66–2.16)	1.12	(0.75–1.84)*	0.98	(0.54–1.58)*	0.92	(0.50–1.58)
IX (U ml^{-1})	0.35	(0.19–0.65)†	0.42	(0.14–0.74)†	0.44	(0.13–0.80)	0.59	(0.25–0.93)	0.81	(0.50–1.20)	1.09	(0.55–1.63)
X (U ml^{-1})	0.41	(0.11–0.71)	0.51	(0.19–0.83)	0.56	(0.20–0.92)	0.67	(0.35–0.99)	0.77	(0.35–1.19)	1.06	(0.70–1.52)
XI (U ml^{-1})	0.30	(0.08–0.52)†	0.41	(0.13–0.69)†	0.43	(0.15–0.71)†	0.59	(0.25–0.93)†	0.78	(0.46–1.10)	0.97	(0.67–1.27)
XII (U ml^{-1})	0.38	(0.10–0.66)†	0.39	(0.09–0.69)†	0.43	(0.11–0.75)	0.61	(0.15–1.07)	0.82	(0.22–1.42)	1.08	(0.52–1.64)
PK (U ml^{-1})	0.33	(0.09–0.57)	0.45	(0.25–0.75)	0.59	(0.31–0.87)	0.79	(0.37–1.21)	0.78	(0.40–1.16)	1.12	(0.62–1.62)
HMW-K (U ml^{-1})	0.49	(0.09–0.89)	0.62	(0.24–1.00)†	0.64	(0.16–1.12)†	0.78	(0.32–1.24)	0.83	(0.41–1.25)*	0.92	(0.50–1.36)
XIII$_a$ (U ml^{-1})	0.70	(0.32–1.08)	1.01	(0.57–1.45)*	0.99	(0.51–1.47)*	1.13	(0.71–1.55)*	1.13	(0.65–1.61)*	1.05	(0.55–1.55)
XIII$_b$ (U ml^{-1})	0.81	(0.35–1.27)	1.10	(0.68–1.58)*	1.07	(0.57–1.57)*	1.21	(0.75–1.67)	1.15	(0.67–1.63)	0.97	(0.57–1.37)

PT, prothrombin time; APTT, activated partial thromboplastin time; TCT, thrombin clotting time; VIII, factor VIII procoagulant; vWF, von Willebrand factor; PK, prekallikrein; HMW-K, high molecular weight kininogen; INR, international normalized ratio.

All factors except fibrinogen are expressed as units per millilitre (U ml^{-1}) where pooled plasma contains 1.0 U ml^{-1}. All values are given as a mean (M) followed by the lower and upper boundary encompassing 95% of the population (B). Between 40 and 96 samples were assayed for each value for the newborn. Some measurements were skewed due to a disproportionate number of high values. The lower limits which excludes the lower 2.5% of the population has been given (B).

* Values that are indistinguishable from the adult.

† Values different from those of the full-term infants.

Table 3. Reference values for the inhibitors of coagulation in the healthy full-term infant during the first 6 months of life. From Andrew et al (1987a, 1988b, 1990c), with permission.

	Day 1		Day 5		Day 30		Day 90		Day 180		Adult	
	M	B	M	B	M	B	M	B	M	B	M	B
ATIII (U ml⁻¹)	0.63 (0.39–0.87)		0.67 (0.41–0.93)		0.78 (0.48–1.08)		0.97 (0.73–1.21)*		1.04 (0.84–1.24)*		1.05 (0.79–1.31)	
α_2M (U ml⁻¹)	1.39 (0.95–1.83)		1.48 (0.98–1.98)		1.50 (1.06–1.94)		1.76 (1.26–2.26)		1.91 (1.49–2.33)		0.86 (0.52–1.20)	
C₁E-INH (U ml⁻¹)	0.72 (0.36–1.08)		0.90 (0.60–1.20)*		0.89 (0.47–1.31)		1.15 (0.71–1.59)		1.41 (0.89–1.93)		1.01 (0.71–1.31)	
α_1AT (U ml⁻¹)	0.93 (0.49–1.37)*		0.89 (0.49–1.29)*		0.62 (0.36–0.88)		0.72 (0.42–1.02)		0.77 (0.47–1.07)		0.93 (0.55–1.31)	
HCII (U ml⁻¹)	0.43 (0.10–0.93)		0.48 (0.01–0.96)		0.47 (0.10–0.87)		0.72 (0.10–1.46)		1.20 (0.50–1.90)		0.96 (0.66–1.26)	
Protein C (U ml⁻¹)	0.35 (0.17–0.53)		0.42 (0.20–0.64)		0.43 (0.21–0.65)		0.54 (0.28–0.80)		0.59 (0.37–0.81)		0.96 (0.64–1.28)	
Protein S (U ml⁻¹)	0.36 (0.12–0.60)		0.50 (0.22–0.78)		0.63 (0.33–0.93)		0.86 (0.54–1.18)*		0.87 (0.55–1.19)*		0.92 (0.60–1.24)	

ATIII, antithrombin III; α_2M, α_2-macroglobulin; C₁E-INH, C₁-esterase inhibitor; α_1-AT, α_1-antitrypsin; HCII, heparin cofactor II.
All values are expressed in units per millilitre (U ml⁻¹) where pooled plasma contains 1.0 (U ml⁻¹). All values are given as a mean (M) followed by the lower and upper boundary encompassing 95% of the population (B). Between 40 and 75 samples were assayed for each value for the newborn. Some measurements were skewed due to a disproportionate number of high values. The lower limits which excludes the lower 2.5% of the population has been given (B).
* Values that are indistinguishable from those of the adult.

Table 4. Reference values for the inhibitors of coagulation in the healthy premature infant (30–36 weeks gestation) during the first 6 months of life. From Andrew et al (1987a, 1988b, 1990c), with permission.

	Day 1		Day 5		Day 30		Day 90		Day 180		Adult	
	M	B	M	B	M	B	M	B	M	B	M	B
ATIII (U ml⁻¹)	0.38 (0.14–0.62)†		0.56 (0.30–0.82)		0.59 (0.37–0.81)†		0.83 (0.45–1.21)†		0.90 (0.52–1.28)†		1.05 (0.79–1.31)	
α_2M (U ml⁻¹)	1.10 (0.56–1.82)†		1.25 (0.71–1.77)		1.38 (0.72–2.04)		1.80 (1.20–2.66)		2.09 (1.10–3.21)		0.86 (0.52–1.20)	
C₁E-INH (U ml⁻¹)	0.65 (0.31–0.99)		0.83 (0.45–1.21)		0.74 (0.40–1.24)†		1.14 (0.60–1.68)*		1.40 (0.96–2.04)		1.01 (0.71–1.31)	
α_1AT (U ml⁻¹)	0.90 (0.36–1.44)*		0.94 (0.42–1.46)*		0.76 (0.38–1.12)†		0.81 (0.49–1.13)*†		0.82 (0.48–1.16)*		0.93 (0.55–1.31)	
HCII (U ml⁻¹)	0.32 (0.10–0.60)†		0.34 (0.10–0.69)		0.43 (0.15–0.71)		0.61 (0.20–1.11)		0.89 (0.45–1.40)*†		0.96 (0.66–1.26)	
Protein C (U ml⁻¹)	0.28 (0.12–0.44)†		0.31 (0.11–0.51)		0.37 (0.15–0.59)†		0.45 (0.23–0.67)†		0.57 (0.31–0.83)		0.96 (0.64–1.28)	
Protein S (U ml⁻¹)	0.26 (0.14–0.38)†		0.37 (0.13–0.61)		0.56 (0.22–0.90)		0.76 (0.40–1.12)†		0.82 (0.44–1.20)		0.92 (0.60–1.24)	

ATIII, antithrombin III; α_2M, α_2-macroglobulin; C₁E-INH, C₁-esterase inhibitor; α_1-AT, α_1-antitrypsin; HCII, heparin cofactor II.
All values are expressed in units per millilitre (U ml⁻¹) where pooled plasma contains 1.0 (U ml⁻¹). All values are given as a mean (M) followed by the lower and upper boundary encompassing 95% of the population (B). Between 40 and 75 samples were assayed for each value for the newborn. Some measurements were skewed due to a disproportionate number of high values. The lower limits which excludes the lower 2.5% of the population has been given (B).
* Values that are indistinguishable from those of the adult.
† Values different from those of the full-term infant.

The prothrombin time (PT), activated partial thromboplastin time (APTT), thrombin clotting time (TCT) and fibrinogen levels are screening tests used in patients with a suspected coagulopathy. The PT and APTT are frequently prolonged in newborns reflecting low levels of the vitamin K-dependent and contact factors (Andrew and Karpatkin, 1982). Differences between studies for some of these tests reflect a combination of parameters including: use of cord blood instead of samples from infants, differing ethnic populations and different reagents (Hirsh et al, 1986; Koepke, 1986). TCT's in Tables 1 and 2 were measured with calcium present in the buffering system so that the normally present 'fetal' fibrinogen would not prolong the TCT (Witt et al, 1969; Galanakis and Mosesson, 1976). Both heparin and low fibrinogen levels will prolong the TCT.

Concentrations of both vitamin K-dependent coagulant proteins and contact factors are approximately half adult values at birth and gradually increase to concentrations approaching adult values by 6 months of life (Aballi and de Lamerens, 1962; Andrew et al, 1987a, 1988a). In contrast, the concentrations of factor VIII and von Willebrand factor are higher in infants than in adults. Furthermore, the high molecular weight multimeric forms of vWF are disproportionately increased (Katz et al, 1989; Weinstein et al, 1989). The fibrinogen concentration is similar to adults and continues to increase over the first week of life.

Concentrations of the inhibitors—C_1-esterase inhibitor, α_2-macroglobulin and α_1-antitrypsin—are near or above adult values at birth. Both α_2M and C_1-esterase inhibitor levels increase to values well above adult levels by 6 months of age (Tables 3 and 4). In contrast, concentrations of ATIII, protein C, protein S and HCII, are low in the first weeks of life with mean values less than $0.70\,\text{U ml}^{-1}$ (Tables 3 and 4) (Aballi and de Lamerens, 1962; Peters et al, 1984a; Karpatkin et al, 1986; Andersson et al, 1988). Although protein S circulates in decreased total amounts in newborns compared to adults, it is only present in the active free form due to an absence of C4b binding protein at birth (Moalic et al, 1988; Schwarz et al, 1988). Only protein C levels remain low at 6 months of age and do not reach adult values until later childhood (Karpatkin et al, 1986).

The net result of differences in concentrations of coagulation proteins in newborns is that the generation of thrombin is both delayed and decreased compared to adults (Figure 1) (Schmidt et al, 1989a). The degree of impairment is similar to plasma from adults receiving therapeutic amounts of coumadin or heparin. The amount of thrombin generated is directly proportional to the prothrombin concentration (Andrew et al, 1990b), whereas the rate at which thrombin is generated is dependent upon all procoagulants. α_2M is a more important inhibitor of thrombin in newborns than adults (Schmidt et al, 1989b) and compensates in part for low concentrations of ATIII in newborns (Levine et al, 1987; Schmidt et al, 1989b). The presence of a glycosaminoglycan dermatan sulphate in newborn plasma may provide another alternative mechanism by which newborns compensate for physiologically low concentrations of ATIII (Andrew et al, 1990c). The net result is that the inhibition of thrombin in the physiological state is slower in newborns compared to adults (Figure 2) (Schmidt et al, 1989b). In the

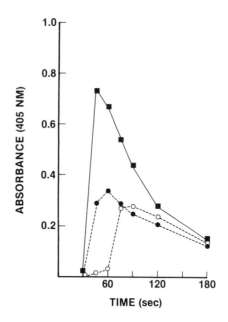

Figure 1. Thrombin generation following activation in the APTT system in plasma from adults (■), full-term infants on day 1 of life (●), and premature infants on day 1 of life (○). The amount of thrombin generated was determined by its ability to cleave a chromogenic substrate resulting in a change in the absorbance reading at 405 nm. From Andrew et al (1990a), with permission.

presence of pathological insults, sick newborns may well be at greater risk for thromboembolic complications compared to adults.

Mechanisms potentially responsible for the 'alternative' physiological state of the haemostatic system in newborns include decreased synthesis of coagulation proteins (Klisker et al, 1988), accelerated clearance of coagulation proteins (Karitsky et al, 1971; Feusner et al, 1983; Schmidt et al, 1984; Suarez et al, 1985; Andrew et al, 1988b), consumption of components at the time of birth (Suarez et al, 1984, 1985; Yuen et al, 1989), and synthesis of proteins with decreased functional activity (Gordon et al, 1980; Andrew et al, 1981; Greffe et al, 1989).

Plasma concentrations of components of the fibrinolytic system also differ in infants compared to adults (Aballi and de Lamerens, 1962; Corrigan, 1988; Corrigan et al, 1989; Runnebaum et al, 1989; Andrew et al, 1990a) (Tables 5 and 6). Plasminogen is only half adult concentrations, α_2AP is 80% adult values and both TPA and PAI are elevated to almost twice adult values. Levels of TPA and PAI are higher in plasma from newborns than cord blood, likely reflecting release from endothelial cells. Plasminogen exists in a 'fetal' form with an increased concentration of sialic acid (Summarian, 1989; Edelberg et al, 1990). The net result of these differences is decreased plasmin generation in infants (Andrew et al, 1989b; Corrigan et al, 1989).

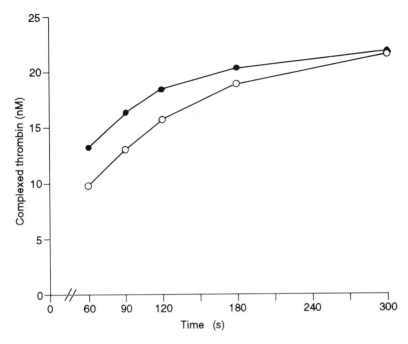

Figure 2. Inhibition of ^{125}I-thrombin (25 nM) in adult (●——●), and neonatal (○——○) plasma is dependent on incubation time ($p < 0.0001$) and differs significantly between the two age groups ($p = 0.0021$). From Schmidt et al (1989b), with permission.

Platelet and vessel wall

Very little is known about differences in vessel wall function between infants and adults. In contrast, the functions of platelets from cord blood have been extensively studied. Both glycoprotein Ib and glycoproteins IIb/IIIa are present on cord platelets in adult amounts from early fetal life (Gruel et al, 1986). The bridging proteins are present in increased (vWF) or similar (fibrinogen) concentrations compared to adults. Thus, the components necessary for normal adhesion and aggregation are present in newborns.

Physiological differences in cord platelets from adult platelets are: (i) decreased aggregation in response to adrenalin (Corby and O'Barr, 1981; Stuart et al, 1984; Jones et al, 1985), (ii) enhanced platelet aggregation to ristocetin (Ts'ao et al, 1976), and (iii) a variable response to ADP, collagen, thrombin and arachidonic acid (Ahlsten et al, 1985; Barradas and Mikharilidis, 1986; Gader et al, 1988). Possible explanations for variable results are: the speed with which samples are processed, the influence of labour, the use of different concentrations and compositions of platelet agonists, and platelet activation during collection. Neither a 'classic' storage pool deficiency nor an 'aspirin-like' platelet defect adequately explain the functional deficits of cord platelets. The poor response to adrenalin appears to be due to decreased surface binding sites for adrenalin which may be due

Table 5. Reference values for the components of the fibrinolytic system in the healthy full-term infant during the first 6 months of life. From Andrew et al (1987a, 1988a, 1990a), with permission.

	Day 1		Day 5		Day 30		Day 90		Day 180		Adult	
	M	B	M	B	M	B	M	B	M	B	M	B
Plasminogen (U ml⁻¹)	1.95	(1.25– 2.65)	2.17	(1.41– 2.93)	1.98	(1.26–2.70)	2.48	(1.74– 3.22)	3.01	(2.21– 3.81)	3.36	(2.48– 4.24)
TPA (ng/ml)	9.6	(5.0–18.9)	5.6	(4.0–10.0)*	4.1	(1.0–6.0)*	2.1	(1.0– 5.0)*	2.8	(1.0– 6.0)*	4.9	(1.4– 8.4)
α₂AP (U ml⁻¹)	0.85	(0.55– 1.15)	1.00	(0.70– 1.30)*	1.00	(0.76–1.24)*	1.08	(0.76– 1.40)*	1.11	(0.83– 1.39)*	1.02	(0.68– 1.36)
PAI (U ml⁻¹)	6.4	(2.0–15.1)	2.3	(0.0– 8.1)*	3.4	(0.0–8.8)*	7.2	(1.0–15.3)	8.1	(6.0–13.0)	3.6	(0.0–11.0)

TPA, tissue plasminogen activator; α₂AP, α₂-antiplasmin; PAI, plasminogen activator inhibitor.
For α₂AP, values are expressed as units per millilitre (U ml⁻¹) where pooled plasma contains 1.0 U ml⁻¹. Plasminogen units are those recommended by the Committee on Thrombolytic Agents. Values for TPA are given as nanograms per millilitre. Values for PAI are given as units per ml where one unit of PAI activity is defined as the amount of PAI that inhibits the one international unit of human single chain TPA. All values are given as a mean (M) followed by the lower and upper boundary encompassing 95% of the population (B).
* Values that are indistinguishable from those of the adult.

Table 6. Reference values for the components of the fibrinolytic system in the healthy premature infant during the first 6 months of life. From Andrew et al (1987a, 1988a, 1990a), with permission.

	Day 1		Day 5		Day 30		Day 90		Day 180		Adult	
	M	B	M	B	M	B	M	B	M	B	M	B
Plasminogen (U ml⁻¹)	1.70	(1.12– 2.48)†	1.91	(1.21–2.61)†	1.81	(1.09– 2.53)	2.38	(1.58– 3.18)	2.75	(1.91– 3.59)†	3.36	(2.48– 4.24)
TPA (ng/ml)	8.48	(3.00–16.70)	3.97	(2.00–6.93)*	4.13	(2.00– 7.79)*	3.31	(2.00– 5.07)*	3.48	(2.00– 5.85)*	4.96	(1.46– 8.46)
α₂AP (U ml⁻¹)	0.78	(0.40– 1.16)	0.81	(0.49–1.13)†	0.89	(0.55– 1.23)†	1.06	(0.64– 1.48)*	1.15	(0.77– 1.53)	1.02	(0.68– 1.36)
PAI (U ml⁻¹)	5.4	(0.0–12.2)*†	2.5	(0.0–7.1)*	4.3	(0.0–10.9)*	4.8	(1.0–11.8)*†	4.9	(1.0–10.2)*†	3.6	(0.0–11.0)

TPA, tissue plasminogen activator; α₂AP, α₂-antiplasmin; PAI, plasminogen activator inhibitor.
For α₂AP, values are expressed as units per millilitre (U ml⁻¹) where pooled plasma contains 1.0 U ml⁻¹. Plasminogen units are those recommended by the Committee on Thrombolytic Agents. Values for TPA are given as nanograms per millilitre. Values for PAI are given as units per ml where one unit of PAI activity is defined as the amount of PAI that inhibits the one international unit of human single chain TPA. All values are given as a mean (M) followed by the lower and upper boundary encompassing 95% of the population (B).
* Values that are indistinguishable from those of the adult.
† Values that are different from those of the full-term infant.

to receptor occupation. The enhanced response to ristocetin likely reflects the increased amounts of the reactive high molecular weight forms of vWF. Both adult and newborn clots have similar platelet mediated clot retraction (Israels et al, 1987). The physiological significance of differences described in cord platelet function compared to adults is still unclear.

Activation of haemostasis (including platelets) with thrombin generation occurs during birth as evidenced by elevated levels of thromboxane B_2, β-thromboglobulin, platelet factor IV, and fibrinopeptide A in cord blood (suarez et al, 1984, 1988). The mechanisms by which cord platelets are activated during birth are multifaceted and likely related to thermal changes, stress with adrenogenic stimulation, acidosis, hypoxia and liberation of tissue factor.

Probably, the most important in vivo test of platelet interaction with the vessel wall is the bleeding time. Bleeding times are performed either with modified template or Ivy bleeding time devices and more recently with automated bleeding time devices designed for newborns (Feusner, 1980; Andrew et al, 1989a, 1990d). The latter devices make reproducible, small cuts that are only 2.5–3.0 mm in length by 0.5 mm in depth. The bleeding time in newborns is similar or shorter than adults (upper limit of 135 seconds) suggesting that platelet vessel wall interaction is at least comparable to adults. The shortened bleeding time likely reflects increased concentrations of vWF (Tables 1 and 2), enhanced vWF function (Katz et al, 1989; Weinstein et al, 1989), high haematocrits (Fernandez et al, 1985) and large size of red cells (Aarts et al, 1983).

HAEMOSTASIS: CONGENITAL DEFICIENCIES

Infants with congenital deficiencies of specific coagulation factors may present symptomatically in the first days of life with spontaneous bleeding or excessive bleeding from minor trauma (Girolami et al, 1985). Unfortunately the first clinical presentation can be intracranial haemorrhage (Mariani and Mazzucconi, 1983; Girolami et al, 1985; Abbondanzo et al, 1988; Yoffe and Buchanan, 1988). The correct diagnosis can be difficult if the physiological level of the coagulation protein in question is low or if the infant has an additional acquired coagulopathy (Schmidt and Zipursky, 1986).

Haemophilia A (factor VIII : C deficiency) and haemophilia B (factor IX deficiency) are the most common congenital defects to present in newborns (Baehner and Strauss, 1966; Girolami et al, 1985; Yoffe and Buchanan, 1988). Severe, moderate and mild forms of haemophilia A can be diagnosed at birth because the lower limit for factor VIII : C, 0.50 U ml^{-1}, is similar to adults. The severe and moderate forms of haemophilia B can also be diagnosed in newborns. However, mild forms may require repeat testing in later infancy because the lower limit of normal for infants at birth is 0.15 U ml^{-1}. Most infants with haemophilia do not develop haemorrhagic manifestations until later in the first year of life when their mobility increases. Von Willebrand's disease is the commonest inherited haemostatic defect in children and adults. However, vWF levels are elevated at birth and early infancy masking the presence of some types of vWD. Infants with vWD rarely present with haemorrhagic complications suggesting that the physiological enhancement of vWF function at birth is protective. The rarer forms of vWD with concomitant factor VIII deficiency may present with bleeding on occasion (Donner et al, 1987).

Other congenital coagulation factor deficiencies that may cause bleeding in newborns include factors II, V, VII, X and XI. The homozygous forms of these deficiencies are rare and usually distinguishable at birth by the very low concentrations of the factor involved (values $<0.10\,\mathrm{U\,ml^{-1}}$). The concentration of these factors in the heterozygote state overlap with physiological levels (Rapaport et al, 1961; Mammen 1983b, 1983c, 1983d; Mariani and Mazzucconi, 1983; Girolami et al, 1985). Treatment of bleeding complications of elective haemostatic insults in infants with homozygous deficiencies of factors II, V, VII, X and XI require factor replacement with either stored plasma (except for factor V), fresh frozen plasma and less commonly factor concentrates. Administering $10\,\mathrm{ml\,kg^{-1}}$ of a plasma product should raise the factor level by approximately $0.10\,\mathrm{U\,ml^{-1}}$; however, the recovery of factors infused has not been measured during infancy and may be lower than for adults due to a faster clearance. The target replacement level depends upon the underlying disorder and should be directly measured.

Abnormalities in fibrinogen (hypofibrinogenaemia, afibrinogenaemia, dysfibrinogenaemia) and homozygous factor XIII deficiency often present in newborns with persistent umbilical bleeding (Lorand et al, 1980; Mammen, 1983e; Girolami et al, 1985; Abbondanzo et al, 1988). The identification of infants with factor XIII deficiency is important because as many as a third of these patients have spontaneous intracranial haemorrhage at some time during their lives. In the homozygous state, factor XIII activity is less than $0.01\,\mathrm{U\,ml^{-1}}$ and therefore easily distinguished from the physiological state. Because the half-life of factor XIII is long, and only very low levels of factor XIII are required for haemostasis, these patients are best treated prophylactically with either fresh frozen plasma, cryoprecipitate or factor XIII concentrates. Patients with the severe forms of fibrinogen defects are easily treated with cryoprecipitate.

Similar to procoagulants, physiological anticoagulants are autosomally inherited. Heterozygote deficiencies produce complications in adults but rarely during infancy and childhood in the absence of a second insult (Bjarke et al, 1974; Shapiro ME et al, 1981; De Stefano et al, 1987; Israels and Seshia, 1987). In contrast, the homozygote form of protein C deficiency presents in newborns with extensive life-threatening thrombotic complications (Marlar et al, 1989). The clinical features include purpura fulminans, severe DIC, central nervous system thrombi, blindness and venous thrombi. Diagnosis of homozygote protein C deficiency depends upon the clinical presentation, a protein C level below the reference range for infants and confirmation of the heterozygote state in the parents. The presence of a low concentration of protein C in the absence of clinical manifestations and family history cannot be considered diagnostic since physiological levels may be as low as $0.12\,\mathrm{U\,ml^{-1}}$. The level of protein C in heterozygotes at birth is not known, but may be lower than the physiological levels. The initial treatment of affected infants is plasma replacement therapy. The long-term treatment includes several options: oral anticoagulant therapy, protein C replacement with plasma products, and liver transplantation (Marlar et al, 1989). The homozygote forms of ATIII, HCII, or protein S deficiency have not been confirmed in newborns but one would anticipate that they would present with severe life-threatening thromboembolic complications.

ACQUIRED HAEMOSTATIC DISORDERS

Thrombocytopenia

General

Healthy infants have the same platelet count as adults ($150–450 \times 10^9$ litre^{-1}) (Mehta, 1980; Gill, 1983; Andrew and Kelton, 1984). A stable mean platelet count of approximately 250×10^9 litre^{-1} is present between 18 to 30 weeks gestation (Forestier et al, 1986a). The mean platelet volume in newborns is also similar to adults with values averaging 7–9 fl (Arad et al, 1986; Castle et al, 1986).

Thrombocytopenia is perhaps the most common haemostatic abnormality in newborns. The definition of thrombocytopenia in newborns is the same as in adults: a platelet count less than 150×10^9 litre^{-1}. A single prospective cohort study (Castle et al, 1986; Andrew et al, 1987b) and five retrospective reviews (Mehta et al, 1980; Feusner et al, 1983; Samuels et al, 1987; Austen and Darlow, 1988; Lupton et al, 1988) provide the most reliable information on the frequency, natural history, mechanisms and clinical impact of thrombocytopenia in newborns. There is general agreement that thrombocytopenia is indicative of an underlying pathological process, however, the clinical relevance of mild thrombocytopenia remains to be proven.

Approximately 22% of infants admitted to a tertiary care neonatal intensive care unit develop thrombocytopenia. For over half of affected infants the platelet count falls below 100×10^9 litre^{-1} with 20% of thrombocytopenic infants having at least one platelet count less than 50×10^9 litre^{-1}. The natural history of the thrombocytopenia is remarkably consistent. It is present by day 2 of life, reaches a nadir by day 4 of life and recovers to values above 150×10^9 litre^{-1} by about day 10 of life.

Mechanisms responsible for thrombocytopenia include increased platelet destruction, decreased platelet production, platelet pooling in an enlarged spleen, or a combination of these mechanisms (Table 7). Increased platelet destruction causes thrombocytopenia in most infants (Castle et al, 1986, 1987). This conclusion is based on the following: mean increased platelet volume during the first week of life, megakaryocytes present in the bone marrow, and platelet survivals performed with [111]Indium oxine uniformly shorter in thrombocytopenia infants. A reduced recovery of labelled platelets suggest the presence of hypersplenism in some infants. Although platelet survivals have not been measured in healthy full-term infants, platelet survivals in newborn rabbits are similar to adult rabbits (Castle et al, 1988).

Increased platelet destruction in newborns is due to both immune and non-immune events. Almost half of infants with platelet counts less than 100×10^9 litre^{-1} have elevated amounts of PAIgG, which is likely maternal in origin, on their platelets. The non-immune causes of thrombocytopenia include disseminated intravascular coagulation (DIC) and thrombocytopenia secondary to exchange transfusions.

Thrombocytopenia in newborns due to decreased platelet production is very rare and accounts for less than 5% of neonatal thrombocytopenia (Table 7). This group includes disorders characterized by bone marrow replacement with malignant cells or various forms of aplasia. Infants with

Table 7. Disease states associated with neonatal thrombocytopenia. From Andrew (1991a), with permission.

1. Increased destruction
   (a) Immune-mediated
       Maternal ITP
       Maternal SLE
       Maternal hyperthyroidism
       Maternal drugs
       Maternal pre-Eclampsia
       Neonatal alloimmune thrombocytopenia
   (b) Non-immune—probably related to DIC
       Asphyxia
       Perinatal aspiration
       Necrotizing enterocolitis
       Haemangiomas
       Neonatal thrombosis
       Respiratory distress syndrome
   (c) Unknown
       Hyperbilirubinaemia
       Phototherapy
       Polycythaemia
       Rh haemolytic disease
       Congenital thrombotic thrombocytopenic purpura
       Total parenteral nutrition
       Inborn errors of metabolism
       Wiskott–Aldrich syndrome
       Multiple congenital anomalies

2. Hypersplenism

3. Decreased production of platelets
   (a) Bone marrow replacement disorders
       Congenital leukaemia
       Congenital leukaemoid reactions
       Neuroblastoma
       Histiocytosis
       Osteopetrosis
   (b) Bone marrow aplasia
       Thrombocytopenia absent radii
       Amegakaryocytic thrombocytopenia
       Fanconi's anaemia
       Other marrow hypoplastic or aplastic disorders

aplastic disorders are at risk of intracranial haemorrhage in the first months of life (Hedberg and Lipton, 1988). Platelet transfusions are highly effective in these disorders, but should be reserved for symptomatic infants because frequent platelet transfusions may result in refractoriness due to allo-immunization. By several months of age some disorders of decreased platelet production improve as evidenced by increased platelet counts.

At any given platelet count, bleeding is less likely to occur in patients with thrombocytopenia caused by increased platelet consumption rather than regenerative thrombocytopenia. In addition, bleeding is more likely to occur in patients with both thrombocytopenia and a defect in platelet function. Choosing a platelet count at which one should intervene is simplistic. However, there are no better predictors of bleeding. In general, a platelet count less than 30×10^9 litre^{-1} places otherwise healthy full-term infants at risk of serious bleeding (Hegde, 1985; Hedberg and Lipton, 1988). In contrast, a platelet count greater than 50×10^9 litre^{-1} in otherwise well full-term infants presents very little risk of bleeding. The importance of 'moderate' thrombo-cytopenia (platelet counts between 50 and 100×10^9 litre^{-1}) in sick premature infants is not certain. Some studies have linked 'moderate thrombocytopenia' to haemorrhagic complications. The bleeding time, which reflects both platelet number and function, is prolonged in approximately 60% of premature infants with 'moderate' thrombocytopenia and shortens when the platelet count increases above 100×10^9 litre^{-1}.

The management of thrombocytopenic infants depends upon the underlying disorder. If the infant is bleeding a trial of platelet concentrates ($10-15$ ml kg^{-1}) is indicated. The increased platelet count usually shortens the bleeding time and is frequently clinically effective. Infants with auto-immune or alloimmune thrombocytopenia require specialized therapy as discussed subsequently.

Alloimmune thrombocytopenia

Neonatal alloimmune thrombocytopenia is characterized by the presence of severe thrombocytopenia, usually in otherwise healthy full-term infants. Mothers of infants with alloimmune thrombocytopenia characteristically have normal platelet counts and no bleeding history although they may have previously delivered thrombocytopenic newborns (Blanchette, 1988; Mueller-Eckhardt et al, 1989). Maternal IgG alloantibodies are directed against specific paternally-derived antigens on the infant's platelets which are absent from the mother's platelets. The most frequently implicated alloantigen is the Pl^{A1} antigen that is present on the platelets of 98% of the general population. Other alloantigens include Br^a (Zav^{a}Hc^a), Pl^{A2} (Zw^6), Bak^a (LeK^a), BaK^b, Pen^a (YuK^b), PeN^b (YUK^a), Pl^{E2}, and Ko^a.

The frequency of neonatal alloimmune thrombocytopenia is approximately 1:2000 newborns. Minor bleeding in the form of gastrointestinal tract haemorrhage, haematuria and purpura occur frequently. Intracranial haemorrhage may occur in as many as 15% of infants and may occur prenatally as well as postnatally. Hydrocephalus, porencephalic cysts and seizures are a few of the outcomes (Herman et al, 1986; Burrows et al, 1988).

The severity of bleeding in infants with alloimmune thrombocytopenia may reflect the presence of additional platelet dysfunction due to an antiplatelet alloantibody that impairs platelet aggregation by binding to glycoproteins IIb/IIIa.

The diagnosis of alloimmune thrombocytopenia is based on the clinical presentation and laboratory confirmation of severe thrombocytopenia. Specific therapy should be instituted immediately followed by serological testing for confirmation of the diagnosis (McFarland et al, 1989). The most effective therapy is the transfusion of washed, irradiated, compatible platelets as illustrated in Figure 3. The most readily available source of compatible platelets is usually the mother. If the delivery is planned, maternal platelets can be prepared prior to the delivery of the infant. The maternal platelets must be washed to remove maternal alloantibody and irradiated to prevent graft vs. host disease caused by maternal lymphocytes (Martin et al, 1983). Frozen maternal platelets have also been successfully used (McGill et al, 1982). Intravenous IgG will effectively raise the platelet count in some infants when compatible platelets are not available. Other forms of therapy are probably not effective. Random donor platelets should be used if the infant has significant haemorrhage and compatible platelets are not yet available.

There is a high probability that subsequent infants will be affected. Because of the risk of intracranial haemorrhaging in utero, therapeutic interventions now begin prenatally. All affected infants should be monitored by ultrasound after approximately 20 weeks gestational age looking for evidence of intracranial haemorrhage. One approach is to perform cordiocentesis to

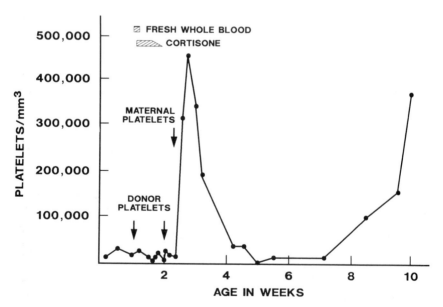

Figure 3. The response in the platelet count to washed, irradiated maternal platelets in an infant with alloimmune thrombocytopenia. From Andrew (1991b), with permission.

confirm the presence of thrombocytopenia and to administer compatible platelets to treat affected fetuses (Kaplan et al, 1988). A less invasive approach is to administer intravenous IgG (IVIgG) with or without dextramethasone to the mother in the latter part of pregnancy (Bussel et al, 1988). The last approach may not be effective for all fetuses. Elective caesarean section is recommended at the time of fetal maturity in order to facilitate the postnatal management of the infant. The necessity of caesarean section to prevent intracranial haemorrhage has not been shown.

Autoimmune thrombocytopenia

Newborns with thrombocytopenia secondary to maternal autoimmune disorders usually present with a milder clinical course than newborns affected with alloimmune thrombocytopenia. The mother frequently has ITP but may have other immune disorders including systemic lupus erythematosus, lymphoproliferative disorders and hypothyroidism (Karpatkin et al, 1972; de Swiet, 1985). The maternal antibodies are directed against antigens common to both maternal and neonatal platelets (Dixon and Rosse, 1975). Maternal thrombocytopenia secondary to ITP must be distinguished from the frequent occurrence of thrombocytopenia in healthy pregnant women at term. The latter does not appear to have any significance to the mother or fetus (Burrows and Kelton, 1988).

Based on case reports of intracranial haemorrhage in infants affected by maternal ITP, recommendations for delivery by caesarean section (Territo et al, 1973) and prenatal platelet count monitoring have been made in the hope of lowering infant morbidity and mortality (Daffos et al, 1988). However, recent information from a large consecutive case study has drawn these recommendations into question (Burrows and Kelton, 1991). Historically, the lowest platelet count was reported not the cord platelet count. Based on this information caesarean sections were recommended for the presumed benefit to the fetus. However, fetal platelet counts at birth are rarely below $50 \times 10^9 \text{litre}^{-1}$ and intracranial haemorrhage rarely if ever occurs prenatally nor is it clearly related to the birth processes. Following birth the platelet count falls in affected newborns over subsequent days (Karpatkin et al, 1981). Although some infants may develop an intracranial haemorrhage from thrombocytopenia in the first days of life, the risk of such an event is unclear.

Based on current information, pregnant women with ITP should be treated according to their own platelet count and not the haemostatic risk to the fetus because of the rarity of platelet counts $< 50 \times 10^9 \text{litre}^{-1}$ at birth. There are no reliable predictors of severe thrombocytopenia in affected infants except for direct determination of the platelet count by cordocentesis which would be rarely if ever indicated in ITP (Barbui et al, 1985). The risk of the procedure is similar or perhaps greater than the risk of ITP to the fetus. Fetal scalp sampling should not be used because the technical failure rate is high and falsely low platelet counts occur, resulting in unnecessary caesarean sections (Scott et al, 1980). Neither the maternal platelet count, the value of maternal platelet associated IgG, nor serum platelet bindable

IgG provide accurate predictors of thrombocytopenia in infants (Blanchette et al, 1989a). Prenatal treatment of mothers with either corticosteroids or IVIgG is for the benefit of the mother not the fetus.

Infants born to mothers with ITP should be monitored closely because the platelet count falls in the postnatal period. A platelet count less than 50×10^9 litre^{-1} is a guide for institution of therapy. Usually the infants are healthy, full-term with minor manifestations of thrombocytopenia. The diagnosis is based on the clinical presentation and confirmed by laboratory evidence of elevated platelet-associated IgG. Therapeutic options in the past included platelet transfusions, exchange transfusions followed by platelet transfusions and corticosteroids (Karpatkin, 1984). More recently IVIgG has been used (Ballin et al, 1988) and appears to be a safe and effective form of therapy. Approximately 80% of infants respond to IVIgG used alone or in combination with steroids (Ballin et al, 1988). Based on currently available information, the response rate to IVIgG appears faster than to corticosteroids. IVIgG may be administered at a dose of 0.4 g kg^{-1} daily for 5 days or as 1 g kg^{-1} of IVIgG on two consecutive days (Figure 4). If there is no response to IVIgG, corticosteroids at a dose of at least 2 mg kg^{-1} should be instituted. If the infant is bleeding, random donor platelet transfusions should be given. If there is no response methylprednisolone in high doses (3 mg kg^{-1}) may be substituted for prednisone.

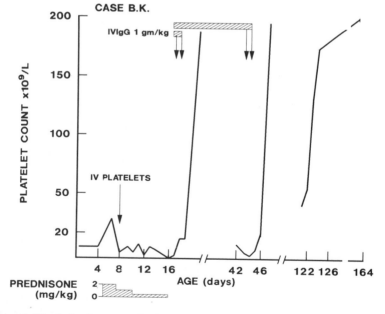

Figure 4. The lack of response in the platelet count to prednisone and the response to intravenous IgG in an infant born to a mother with idiopathic thrombocytopenia purpura. From Blanchette (1989b), with permission.

Coagulopathy

Disseminated intravascular coagulation (DIC)

Clinical presentation of DIC. Disseminated intravascular coagulation is characterized by the pathological finding of diffuse fibrin deposition in the microvasculature, haemorrhagic and thrombotic complications, and decreased concentrations of coagulation factors secondary to consumption. DIC is a process that is secondary to a variety of underlying diseases. In newborns, DIC is usually secondary to adverse events related to the fetal–placental unit that result in asphyxia and shock and disorders related to prematurity, such as RDS, viral or bacterial infections, hypothermia, meconium or amniotic fluid aspiration syndromes (Corrigan, 1979). The clinical spectrum of DIC is changing, reflecting the ever-improving perinatal care of sick infants.

Laboratory diagnosis of DIC. The diagnosis of DIC is based upon compatible clinical features in conjunction with prolongation of screening tests (PT, APTT), low levels of specific coagulation factors (fibrinogen, factor V and VIII) and inhibitors (antithrombin III, heparin cofactor II, protein C), elevated fibrinogen/fibrin split products, thrombocytopenia and red cell fragmentation. The physiological concentrations of fibrinogen, factors V and VIII are similar in newborns to adults, therefore, pathological decreases, are readily identified. The laboratory diagnosis of DIC, particularly milder forms, is facilitated by performing paracoagulation tests that measure the subtle effects of very small amounts of thrombin and/or plasmin. These tests include measurements of fibrin monomer, thrombin–antithrombin III complexes, fibrinogen/fibrin degradation products and D-dimer. The precise relationship of depleted coagulation factors, and positive paracoagulation tests, to fibrin deposition in the microvasculature and haemorrhage is unclear. For example, many paracoagulation tests are positive in cord plasma from healthy infants likely reflecting activation of coagulation during the normal birth process. Infants with large haematomas may have a positive D-dimer test secondary to fibrin degradation. In the latter examples sensitive measurements of thrombin and plasmin generation do not indicate the presence of DIC nor the need to intervene. In practice, no single laboratory test can be used to confirm or exclude DIC.

Treatment of DIC. The cornerstone for management of DIC remains the successful treatment of the underlying disease state. The decision to treat the haemostatic disorder can be difficult. Infants with thrombotic or haemorrhagic complications plus laboratory confirmation of DIC, should be treated to control the secondary haemostatic problem pending resolution of the primary problem that initiated the DIC. In contrast, infants without clinical manifestations of impaired haemostasis probably do not require therapy for the haemostatic disorder itself. For infants between these two ends of the spectrum, haemostatic management is dictated by the severity of the clinical and laboratory impairment and the underlying problem.

Available forms of treatment include coagulation factor replacement, platelet transfusions, and anticoagulant drugs. The argument that replacement therapy may 'fuel the fire' is theoretical and not proven. Some case studies have reported improved laboratory tests and clinical outcome when coagulation factor replacement was given for the treatment of DIC (Hambleton and Appleyard, 1968; Waltl et al, 1973; Turner et al, 1981; Yamada et al, 1983). One controlled study did not show a benefit, but had a small sample size (Gross et al, 1982).

Fresh frozen plasma is used extensively in the management of DIC because it contains all coagulation proteins present in normal adult concentrations. Cryoprecipitate is used because of the high concentration per unit volume of fibrinogen and factor VIII; two coagulation proteins that are frequently depleted in DIC. In more severe cases of DIC, exchange transfusions can be used to improve haemostasis. However they are not without risk and the effects are transient unless the underlying problem resolves. Although factor IX concentrates have been used in newborns, they are not generally recommended because of potential complicating side-effects (Waltl et al, 1973). A reasonable therapeutic goal is to maintain the platelet count above 50×10^9 litre^{-1}, the fibrinogen level above 1.0 g litre^{-1}, and the PT at normal levels for age.

There is one randomized controlled trial and several case series evaluating the use of heparin in DIC. There is no conclusive evidence that heparin is beneficial (Yamada et al, 1983; Gobel et al, 1980). ATIII concentrates have been tested with the goal of decreasing the morbidity from DIC (Hanada et al, 1985; von Kries et al, 1985). To date, these products are of unproven benefit and clinical trials are needed to clarify their role, if any, in the management of DIC.

Vitamin K deficiency

The discovery of vitamin K and its important role in haemostasis is intertwined with the therapeutic and prophylactic role of vitamin K in the treatment and prevention of haemorrhagic disease of the newborn (HDN). The debate over the benefits of prophylactic vitamin K has spanned the 20th century. The controversy underscores the need for carefully controlled, epidemiologically sound clinical trials when a potentially helpful form of therapy is being evaluated.

Haemolytic disease of the newborn (HDN) as first described by Townsend consisted of bleeding from multiple sites in otherwise healthy infants, in the absence of trauma, asphyxia, or infection on days 1 to 5 of life (Townsend, 1894). This report was followed by the recognition that newborn blood takes a longer time to clot than adult blood. Subsequently, a causal link between HDN and abnormal blood clotting was made. The association between vitamin K deficiency and HDN quickly followed (Aballi and de Lamerens, 1962). The identification of vitamin K was followed by the successful treatment of infants with HDN with vitamin K (Aballi and de Lamerens, 1962).

Clinical presentation of vitamin K deficiency. Vitamin K deficient infants are at greater risk of haemorrhagic complications than similarly affected adults probably because their levels of the four vitamin K-dependent factors—II, VII, IX, X—are already physiologically low. Thus infants have little reserve capacity and the additive insult of vitamin K deficiency rapidly places neonates at risk of serious haemorrhagic complications.

The clinical presentation of vitamin K deficiency can be classified into three patterns based on the timing and type of complications (Aballi and de Lamerens, 1962; Lane and Hathaway, 1985; Shapiro et al, 1986; Hathaway, 1987; Fetus and Newborn Committee, 1988; von Kries, 1988). As discussed previously, the classic form of vitamin K deficiency was first described by Townsend. These infants are usually breast-fed, full-term and otherwise healthy. The contributing features to this form of vitamin K deficiency are the low placental transfer of vitamin K (Hiraike et al, 1988; Mandelbrot et al, 1988), low concentration of vitamin K in breast milk (less than $20 \, \mu g \, ml^{-1}$), the low intake of milk in the first days of life, and a sterile gut (Haroon et al, 1982; von Kries, 1987; Greer et al, 1988). Vitamin K deficiency does not occur as frequently in formula-fed infants because of the increased concentrations of vitamin K in commercially available formula (approximately 830 mg/l). The frequency of HDN, in the absence of vitamin K prophylaxis, depends upon the population studied, the frequency of breast-feeding and the use of supplemental formula; in some populations the frequency is as high as 1.7% (Sutherland and Glueck, 1967).

Vitamin K deficiency may also present in the first 24 hours of life with serious bleeding in infants born to mothers taking drugs such as warfarin, anticonvulsants, rifampicin and isoniazid. These drugs interfere with either vitamin K stores or function in newborns. Occasionally no underlying predisposing factor is identified.

A third, late pattern of vitamin K deficiency occurs beyond the first weeks of life in breast-fed infants (Motohara, 1987). Not infrequently these infants present with an intracranial haemorrhage. This delayed form is usually associated with underlying diseases which compromise the supply of vitamin K. These diseases include chronic diarrhoea, diarrhoea in breast-fed infants, infants with cystic fibrosis, α_1-antitrypsin deficiency, hepatitis, coeliac disease and other rare disorders.

Laboratory diagnosis of vitamin K deficiency. Patients with vitamin K deficiency produce decarboxylated forms of the vitamin K dependent factors (PIVKA) which can be measured directly or as a discrepancy between the coagulant activity and immunological concentrations (Corrigan and Earnst, 1980a; Widdershoven et al, 1988). The laboratory tests available for detection of vitamin K deficiency include: (i) screening tests as well as specific factor assays; (ii) assays for the decarboxylated forms of the vitamin K dependent factors and; (iii) direct measurements of vitamin K. The results of these tests must always be compared to values from age-matched, healthy, non vitamin K-deficient infants in order to distinguish physiological from pathological values.

Prophylactic vitamin K therapy. Vitamin K exists in three forms, (i) vitamin K1 (phytomenadione), which is present in green leafy vegetables (ii) vitamin K2 (menaquinone), which is synthesized by intestinal bacterial flora, and (iii) vitamin K3 a synthetic, water-soluble form (menadione). Vitamin K3 is rarely used in newborns because, in high doses, it causes haemolytic anaemia, resulting in jaundice and potential morbidity (Committee on Nutrition, 1961). Newborn stores of vitamin K are low as evidenced by low levels of vitamin K in cord blood and in livers of aborted fetuses. Recent studies in animals and in pregnant women, using very sensitive measures of placental transport of vitamin K, show that only 10% of maternally administered vitamin K, reaches the fetus (Hiraike et al, 1988).

The controversy over the use of prophylactic vitamin K in newborns reflects, in part, the confusion that results from large numbers of different studies reporting apparently conflicting results. There are two randomized controlled trials assessing the benefits of vitamin K prophylaxis using clinical bleeding as the outcome measure (Table 8) (Vietti et al, 1960; Sutherland and Glueck, 1967). In the first study, 3338 full-term infants were randomized to receive either placebo, 100 µg of menadione or 5 mg menadione intramuscularly. Minor and major bleeding outcomes were assessed by healthcare personnel who were unaware of which therapy the infants had received.

Table 8. Prophylactic vitamin K-randomized controlled trials. From Andrew (1991b), with permission.

Author	All bleeding†			Significant bleeding‡		Coagulation studies§	
	N	N	%	N	%	N	Abnormal
Sutherland (1967)							
Vitamin K	2195	121	5.5	7	0.3	76	1
Control	1143	86	7.5	19	1.7*	60	18*
Vietti (1960)							
Vitamin K	240	6	2.5	1	0.4	22	1
Control	230	32	13.9*	14	6.0*	25	11*

* P value less than 0.01.
† Sutherland—bleeding from any site; Vietti—any bleeding post-circumcision.
‡ Sutherland—bleeding in a significant site (CNS, adrenal), causing anaemia, resuturing a circumcision; Vietti—bleeding requiring resuturing of a circumcision.
§ Prothrombin time in both studies.

There was a significantly higher risk of intracranial haemorrhage as well as minor bleeding in the placebo group compared to both treatment arms. This clinical result was supported by laboratory tests which showed that the PT was prolonged in infants with haemorrhagic complications. The PT corrected following the administration of vitamin K. A later study randomized 470 infants to receive vitamin K or nothing (Vietti et al, 1960). The study population consisted of male infants who were undergoing circumcision. Thirty-two of the 230 infants who did not receive vitamin K, compared to 6 of 240 vitamin K tested infants, bled following circumcision—a highly significant difference. The same group produced similar results in a subsequent, smaller, non-blinded trial (Vietti et al, 1961).

A second and lower level of evidence supporting the use of vitamin K prophylaxis comes from numerous studies in which groups of infants treated with prophylactic vitamin K at birth were compared to concurrent untreated control groups (Aballi and de Lamerens, 1962; O'Connor and Addiego, 1986; Ogata et al, 1988). These studies consistently indicate that biochemical evidence of vitamin K deficiency is less frequently observed in infants who received vitamin K prophylaxis.

A third level of evidence of the value of vitamin K prophylaxis comes from studies reporting biochemical indices of vitamin K deficiency at birth (Greer et al, 1988; Hiraike et al, 1988) and from large population studies in which vitamin K prophylaxis was instituted and then withdrawn or never instituted (Aballi and de Lamerens, 1962; Hanawa et al, 1988). A fourth level of evidence comes from numerous studies reporting a beneficial effect (either clinically or biochemically) following administration of vitamin K to the mother (Aballi and de Lamerens, 1962; Lane and Hathaway, 1985). The weakest supportive data comes from comparing the higher frequency of HDN in countries where vitamin K is not administered to countries administering vitamin K prophylaxis. Finally there are numerous case reports of infants with HDN who for a variety of reasons did not receive vitamin K at birth, and responded to vitamin K therapy.

There are no randomized controlled trials reporting the failure of vitamin K prophylaxis in preventing HDN. Some investigators, studying cord blood only, could not find biochemical evidence of vitamin K deficiency (Corrigan and Kryc, 1980; Malia et al, 1980). In some studies mothers rather than infants received vitamin K prophylaxis which introduced the confounding variable of placental transport of vitamin K. Some studies reporting failure of vitamin K prophylaxis were flawed because of small sample sizes, sequential rather than concurrent controls, and absence of information on feeding practices. In summary, the information currently available supports a recommendation for vitamin K prophylaxis in all newborn infants.

The recommendations for vitamin K prophylaxis from many countries are reasonably similar (Aballi and de Lamerens, 1962; Lane and Hathaway, 1985; von Kries et al, 1988; Fetus and Newborn Committee, 1988; Hathaway, 1986). Daily vitamin K requirements for newborns are approximately $1–5 \mu g \, kg^{-1}$ body weight^{-1}. Most groups recommend a single dose of 0.5–1.0 mg intramuscularly or an oral dose of 2–4 mg at birth. Recent studies show that the oral route of administration of vitamin K is probably as effective, and less expensive and less traumatic than intramuscular administration. Occasionally vitamin K deficiency is observed in infants who have received oral vitamin K. The absorption of oral vitamin K varies widely among infants and some infants do not swallow all of an administered dose. It is possible that oral vitamin K may not be as efficacious as intramuscular vitamin K, but the magnitude of the problem, if it exists, is unclear.

In addition to general prophylaxis at birth, certain high-risk groups require additional vitamin K prophylaxis (i.e. infants with α_1-antitrypsin deficiency, chronic diarrhoea, cystic fibrosis, coeliac disease). Pregnant women receiving oral anticonvulsant therapy should receive supplemental vitamin K1 in the third trimester to prevent overt vitamin K deficiency in their infants. Although concerns regarding potential adverse effects of vitamin K prophylaxis have been raised, currently the benefits of vitamin K prophylaxis outweigh the still speculative negative effects.

Treatment of vitamin K deficiency. An infant suspected of having vitamin K deficiency should be treated immediately with vitamin K while awaiting laboratory confirmation. All infants with HDN should receive vitamin K either subcutaneously or intravenously dependent upon the clinical problem. Vitamin K should not be given intramuscularly to infants with HDN as a large haematoma may occur at the site of the injection. Intravenous vitamin K is the preferred route but it should be given slowly; vitamin K given rapidly by the intravenous route has caused, on rare occasion, an anaphylactoid reaction in adults. Infants with non life-threatening bleeding secondary to vitamin K deficiency should also be treated with plasma to increase the plasma concentrations of the vitamin K-dependent proteins immediately. Intracranial haemorrhage or other forms of life-threatening bleeding may require treatment with factor IX concentrates which immediately increase the levels of the vitamin K-dependent factor to haemostatic values. There is, however the potential risk of hepatitis and DIC from these products; infants receiving factor IX concentrates should also receive both hepatitis B immunoglobulin and hepatitis B vaccination.

Liver disease

Impaired haemostasis secondary to liver disease is similar in newborns to adults. It is due to: (i) the failure of hepatic synthetic functions, (ii) activation of the coagulation and fibrinolytic systems, (iii) poor clearance of the products of haemostasis, (iv) loss of haemostatic proteins into ascitic fluid; and (v) abnormally glycosylated proteins. In newborns, hepatic dysfunction occurs secondary to many disorders: including viral hepatitis, hypoxic liver damage, shock, inherited inborn errors of metabolism, fetal hydrops and cirrhosis. The management goals for these infants is to sustain them until the liver recovers normal function. The latter frequently necessitates the replacement of coagulation proteins, either by simple transfusion or in severe cases, by exchange transfusions.

Intracranial haemorrhage

In full-term infants intracranial haemorrhage may occur spontaneously in the absence of identifiable haemostatic defects (Hayden, 1985), although case reports indicate an association with perinatal insults such as birth asphyxia or trauma. Intracranial haemorrhages are most frequently subependymal in location although subdural haemorrhages also occur. Some infants require surgical intervention and suffer long-term neurological morbidity. Although there is no convincing data that the immature coagulation system in full-term infants places them at risk for spontaneous intracranial haemorrhage, all infants with an intracranial haemorrhage should be carefully evaluated for an underlying haemostatic deficit.

Premature infants are at considerable risk for intraventricular haemorrhage (IVH) (Volpe, 1983; Goddard-Finegold, 1984; Ment et al, 1987). Initially IVH was a pathological diagnosis, however, with the availability of ultrasonography, IVH is diagnosed with accuracy in sick, premature infants. These diagnostic manoeuvres have provided information regarding the natural history of IVH and the potential benefits of therapeutic intervention.

IVH is characterized by bleeding from the fragile microvasculature of the subependymal germinal matrix. The bleeding can extend into the lateral ventricles or into the brain parenchyma (Levene and de Vries, 1984). Approximately 40% of premature infants with a birth weight less than 1500 g develop an IVH. Most occur in the first 24 hours following birth, with almost all developing in the first 72 hours. Approximately 10–20% of IVH will extend following the initial bleed. IVH is associated with perinatal asphyxia, assisted ventilation, hypercarbia, acidosis, hypoxia, pneumothorax, and prematurity (Ment et al, 1984; Cooke, 1981).

The aetiology of IVH in premature infants is incompletely understood and probably multifactorial. Abnormal regulation of cerebral blood flow with eventual decreased perfusion of brain tissue is probably the mechanism of primary importance to IVH and to the subsequent long-term morbidity. Other potential contributing mechanisms include an abnormal fragility of the germinal matrix capillaries, oxidative damage to the endothelium and concurrent impairment of the haemostatic system (Ackerman and Fraser, 1968; Gray et al, 1968; Gilles et al, 1971; Beverley et al, 1984, 1985; McDonald et al, 1984).

Whether the physiological immaturity of the newborn's coagulation system contributes to the occurrence and extent of IVH is unknown. One randomized, controlled trial compared the use of (FFP) (10 ml kg^{-1} on admission and at 24 hours) to no therapy in 73 infants at risk for IVH, but with no obvious impairment of haemostasis. A beneficial outcome evidenced by decreased IVH in the FFP group was reported although no alteration in screening tests was observed (Beverley et al, 1985). It is possible that the screening tests used were not sensitive enough to detect a subtle but clinically important affect. Because a placebo control was not used it is also possible that the beneficial effect of the FFP was not due to increasing concentration of coagulation proteins.

Pathological alterations of the newborn's haemostatic system are associated with IVH and include both thrombocytopenia (Castle et al, 1986; Andrew et al, 1987b) and decreased concentrations of coagulation proteins (Ackerman and Fraser, 1968; Gray et al, 1968; Gilles et al, 1971; Beverley et al, 1984, 1985; McDonald et al, 1984). Some investigators have suggested that IVH can be caused by an enhanced local fibrinolytic activity (Gilles et al, 1971), but a study treating a group of babies with tranexamic acid, an antifibrinolytic agent, failed to show benefit (Hensey et al, 1984). Three randomized controlled trials evaluated whether vitamin K administered antenatally to the mother could prevent IVH (Morales et al, 1988; Pomerance et al, 1987; Kazzi et al, 1989). The hypothesis tested was that infants are vitamin K deficient and that antenatal administration of vitamin K corrects this problem. Thus, infants are born with higher levels of functional vitamin K-dependent factors and thereby enhanced haemostasis. The results were conflicting with two studies demonstrating benefit and one finding no benefit from vitamin K.

Cerebral blood flow is regulated in part by major prostaglandins such as prostacyclin (PGI_2), a vasodilator that inhibits platelet aggregation, and thromboxane A_2 (TXA_2), a potent vasoconstrictor that promotes platelet aggregation. In an animal model, indomethacin, which blocks cyclo-oxygenase, resulted in decreased serum levels of 6-keto-$PGF_{1\alpha}$ and TXB_2, the stable metabolites of PGI_2 and TXA_2 and decreased the incidence of IVH in the Beagle puppy (Ment et al, 1983). In neonates, several randomized controlled trials have been conducted with indomethacin, some reporting a beneficial effect (Setzer et al, 1984; Ment et al, 1985; Bandstra et al, 1988; Hannigan et al, 1988; Bada et al, 1989) and some not (Rennie et al, 1986).

Because of the long-term morbidity and mortality associated with IVH, a variety of other potentially protective therapeutic interventions have been tested in controlled trials (Ment et al, 1987). Many of the drugs tested are thought to act by decreasing cerebral blood-flow or by preventing tissue damage induced by sudden changes in cerebral blood-flow. The drugs tested include ethamsylate, bicarbonate, phenobarbitol, pancuronium and vitamin E. At this time no firm recommendations can be made for any of these interventions because of a lack of consistent results.

Respiratory distress syndrome

Respiratory distress syndrome (RDS) is an acute lung disorder that primarily affects premature infants. It is characterized by diffuse atelectasis, oedema, hyaline membrane formation and right-to-left shunting of pulmonary blood flow (Strang, 1966). The pathogenesis of RDS is related at least in part to increased pulmonary surface tension secondary to surfactant deficiency (Avery and Mead, 1959). Pathologically, RDS is characterized by fibrin deposition both intra-alveolarly and intravascularly (Gajl-Peczalska, 1964). Because of the abnormal fibrin deposition in RDS, many studies have looked for abnormalities in the coagulation system (Schmidt et al, 1990; Shah et al, 1990). More recently, cell culture techniques in combination with animal studies have elucidated some of the events leading to fibrin deposition in RDS.

The normally intact epithelial cell, similar to the endothelial cell, has anticoagulant properties due to cell surface associated glycosaminoglycans (GAGs) (Berry et al, 1991) and the cell surface receptor thrombomodulin (Maruyama and Majerus, 1987). GAGs produced by epithelial cells may remain associated with the cell surface or be shed into the surrounding environment. GAGs exert an anticoagulant effect by potentiating the antithrombin activity of the physiological inhibitors ATIII and HCII. In addition, thrombin bound to epithelial cell surface thrombomodulin activates protein C to its activated form (APC), which in the presence of protein S inactivates factors Va and VIIIa. This directly decreases thrombin generation. Damage to epithelial cell surfaces may alter the physiologically anticoagulant properties of epithelial cells. Animal and human studies of adult RDS have shown an increase in factor VII procoagulant activity in bronchoalveolar lavage fluid (Idell et al, 1989a, 1989b). There is also decreased fibrinolytic activity due to enhanced inhibition of plasmin and plasminogen activators (Liebermann, 1961).

The haemostatic abnormalities of RDS in newborns include prolongation of screening tests and low levels of coagulation factors and inhibitors of coagulation, such as antithrombin III, protein C and heparin cofactor II (Markarian et al, 1971a; Mahasandana and Hathaway, 1973; Watkins et al, 1980; Andrew et al, 1983, 1985; Peters et al, 1984; Van Den Berg et al, 1989). More recently, thrombin–antithrombin III complexes, a specific marker of increased thrombin formation, were found to be increased in severe neonatal RDS (Schmidt et al, 1990). These abnormalities, in combination with the pathological feature of fibrin deposition, provide the rationale for conducting intervention studies directed at decreasing fibrin deposition. There are four controlled clinical trials assessing the effect of heparin or thrombolytic therapy in RDS (Ambrus et al, 1966, 1977; Markarian et al, 1971b; Gobel et al, 1980). Heparin did not improve the outcome from RDS. However, heparin's antithrombotic effectiveness is mediated through the natural thrombin inhibitor, antithrombin III, which is present in decreased concentrations in infants with RDS. The two clinical trials that enhanced the fibrinolytic system by the infusion of urokinase-activated plasmin or plasminogen both reported a beneficial effect. However, these trials were conducted in 1966 and 1977, and the results cannot be extrapolated to infants receiving current intensive care management. There is one additional study in which infants with RDS were randomized to receive ATIII concentrate or placebo. Beneficial effects from ATIII concentrates could not be demonstrated (Muntean and Rosegger, 1989). Future clinical trials are needed to assess the potential benefits of antithrombotic and/or thrombolytic therapy in RDS.

Thrombotic complications: acquired

Secondary thromboembolic complications occur more frequently in sick newborn infants than at any other time in the paediatric population, reflecting the critically ill state of these infants (Barnard and Hathaway, 1979; Schmidt and Zipursky, 1984; Schmidt and Andrew, 1988a). The three major risk factors for thromboembolic complications in adults also apply to newborns are (i) abnormalities in the vessel wall, (ii) disturbances of blood-flow, and (iii) alterations in blood coagulability. The clinical information describing thromboembolic complications in newborns consists, without exception, of case reports and case series.

Thrombosis associated with indwelling catheters. Seriously ill infants admitted to neonatal intensive care units frequently require indwelling arterial catheters (usually umbilical), and these carry a potential risk of thrombosis regardless of the vessel and type of catheter used (O'Neill et al,

1981). Thrombotic complications in association with arterial catheters occur in essentially all vessels that are accessed including radial, pulmonary, temporal, femoral and most commonly, the aorta.

A catheter-related thrombus may not only occlude catheters with loss of patency, but may also obstruct major arterial vessels leading to serious morbidity or death (Tyson et al, 1976). In a retrospective examination of approximately 4000 infants who underwent umbilical artery catheterization between 1971 and 1980, severe symptomatic vessel obstruction was observed in 38 cases (1%) (O'Neil, 1981). Asymptomatic catheter-related thrombi occur more frequently as evidenced by post mortem identification of catheter related thrombosis (3–59% of cases). In addition, prospective angiographic studies demonstrate the presence of unsuspected thrombi in many patients.

The sequelae of symptomatic catheter-related thrombi can be immediate or long-term. The acute thrombotic symptoms depend on the location of the catheter. They include renal hypertension, intestinal necrosis and peripheral gangrene. The long-term side-effects of a symptomatic thrombosis of major vessels are probably mild, but there are only case series evaluating long-term morbidity.

The high incidence of catheter-associated thrombosis and loss of catheter patency provide the rationale for heparin prophylaxis. Catheter prophylaxis with heparin is used in approximately three quarters of nurseries in the United States (Gilhooly et al, 1987). Randomized controlled trials show that catheter patency is maintained for a longer period of time when heparin prophylaxis is used (Rajani, 1979; David et al, 1981; Alpan et al, 1984; Bosque and Weaver, 1986). However, in one study, prophylactic heparin was linked to a four-fold increase risk of IVH (Lesko et al, 1986). Because this study was retrospective, the evidence linking heparin to IVH is fairly weak. Nevertheless, the potential morbidity of prophylactic heparin for catheter patency needs to be assessed in prospective studies.

Umbilical venous catheters, similar to arterial catheters, are associated with a high risk of thrombosis. The unique feature of umbilical venous catheters is the predisposition to hepatic necrosis when hyperosmolar solutions are injected directly into the portal or hepatic system. Long-term sequelae of umbilical venous catheterization although rare, include portal vein thrombosis with portal hypertension, splenomegaly, and gastric and oesophageal varices.

Spontaneous thromboembolic complications. Spontaneous occlusion of arterial vessels, in the absence of a catheter, is unusual but may occur in ill infants. The clinical presentation reflects the vessel that is occluded. Complete occlusion of a vessel can lead to gangrene and loss of the affected limb or ischaemic organ damage. Other complications include systemic hypertension in newborns related to renal artery thrombosis and pulmonary thromboembolism. The recent availability of ventilation lung scintigrams, in addition to perfusion lung scintigrams, has greatly facilitated the diagnosis of pulmonary embolism in newborns (Arnold et al, 1985).

The important sites of spontaneous venous thrombosis include renal venous thrombosis (Arneil et al, 1973), adrenal vein thrombosis, thrombosis of the vena cava, and thrombosis of the portal and hepatic veins due to omphalitis. The most frequent complication is a renal vein thrombosis. The clinical presentation of renal venous thrombosis includes haematuria, an enlarged kidney and thrombocytopenia. If the inferior vena cava is also involved there may be oedema and cyanosis of the lower limbs. The cornerstone of management is supportive care including dialysis (Duncan et al, 1977). Other forms of therapy are of questionable benefit. Thromboectomy in selected cases of bilateral thrombi may be helpful.

Diagnosis of thromboembolic complications. Because of the infrequency of clinically apparent thrombi and because of the multiple sites of vessel occlusion in newborns, no standard approach to the diagnoses of thrombotic complications has been developed. In most instances, contrast angiography is considered the reference test. Non-invasive techniques such as doppler and ultrasonography offer advantages for newborns, but they have not been adequately evaluated against contrast angiography to determine their sensitivity and specificity (Vailas et al, 1986). In some instances, such as renal vein thrombosis, there is no accepted reference diagnostic technique against which newer diagnostic techniques can be evaluated.

Prophylaxis/treatment of thromboembolic complications. The lack of consensus for the appropriate prophylaxis and management of thromboembolic complications in newborns reflects the difficulty of conducting controlled trials in this area. Guidelines for prevention, diagnosis and treatment of thrombotic disease in adult patients cannot be extrapolated to newborns without further evaluation. Therapeutic options available include supportive care alone, anticoagulant therapy, thrombolytic therapy and surgical removal of thrombi. For most infants who develop a thrombotic complication, it is a catheter-related thrombus and clinically silent. In most nurseries catheters are not routinely screened for associated thrombi, so by exclusion most infants with clinically-silent thrombi receive supportive care alone. For the moment, this appears to be sufficient as the long-term morbidity appears to be small.

Should a clinically apparent thromboembolic complication occur with significant limb or organ impairment, anticoagulant and/or thrombolytic drugs can be used to re-establish patency of the vessel or to prevent extension of the thrombi. When anticoagulant therapy is used, heparin is the drug of choice (McDonald and Hathaway, 1982; Andrew and Schmidt, 1988). Urokinase, streptokinase and tissue plasminogen activator (TPA) have all been used for thromboembolytic therapy. Current protocols for anticoagulant and thrombolytic therapy in adults have been validated in many trials. This approach is hindered in newborns by the relative rarity of symptomatic thrombosis and the lack of data demonstrating the need to treat the more frequent clinically silent thrombi. In vitro studies and studies in newborn animal models provide insights into potential differences in response to anticoagulant or thrombolytic drugs in newborns compared to adults. For example, heparin clearance is accelerated in the young (Andrew

Table 9. Guidelines for initiating anticoagulant and thrombolytic therapy in paediatric patients.

1. Anticoagulant therapy
Heparin
bolus—50–100 U kg^{-1}
infusion—20–30 U kg^{-1} h^{-1}
Coumadin
load—0.2 mg kg^{-1} for 2 days
maintenance—adjust to INR value desired
2. Thrombolytic therapy—systemic
Streptokinase
bolus—4000 U kg^{-1} over 30 minutes
infusion—1500 U kg^{-1} h^{-1}
Urokinase
bolus—4400 U kg^{-1} over 10 minutes
infusion—4400 U kg^{-1} h^{-1}
3. Thrombolytic therapy—local
Streptokinase
infusion—50–70 U kg^{-1} h^{-1}
Urokinase
infusion—200–500 U kg^{-1} h^{-1}

INR, international normalized ratio.

et al, 1988c; McDonald et al, 1981); the effectiveness of heparin is limited by the low ATIII level in piglets and can be corrected by ATIII supplementation (Schmidt et al, 1988a), the measurement of heparin in plasma is affected by the low levels of ATIII (Schmidt, 1988b); plasma from newborns generates less plasmin than adult plasma (Corrigan et al, 1989) resulting in impaired clot lysis in an in vitro system; and increasing the plasminogen concentration in newborn plasma increases clot lysis (Andrew et al, 1989b). These preclinical sources of information help refine the choice of drugs and drug dosages which need to be tested in clinical trials. Table 9 summarizes guidelines for using anticoagulant and thrombolytic therapy in newborns. Future clinical trials with innovative study designs are needed to validate current protocols for anticoagulant and thrombolytic therapy in newborns.

Acknowledgements

The author acknowledges the secretarial assistance of Janice Butera, Barbara Lahie, and Rosemary Phillis in the preparation of this manuscript.

REFERENCES

Aarts PAMM, Bolhuis PA, Sakariassen KS et al (1983) Red blood cell size is important for adherence of blood platelets to artery subendothelium. *Blood* **62:** 214–217.
Aballi AJ & De Lamerens S (1962) Coagulation changes in the neonatal period and in early infancy. *Pediatric Clinics in North America* **9:** 785–817.

Abbondanzo SL, Gootenberg JE, Lofts RS et al (1988) Intracranial hemorrhage in congenital deficiency of factor XIII. *American Journal of Pediatric Hematology and Oncology* **10:** 65–68.

Ahlsten G, Ewald U, Tuvemo T et al (1985) Arachidonic acid induced aggregation of platelets from human cord blood compared with platelets from adults. *Biology of the Neonate* **47:** 199–204.

Alpan G, Eyal F, Springer C et al (1984) Heparinization of alimentation solutions administered through peripheral veins in premature infants. A controlled study. *Pediatrics* **74:** 375–378.

Ambrus CM, Weintraub DH & Ambrus JL (1966) Studies on hyaline membrane disease. III Therapeutic trial of urokinase-activated human plasmin. *Pediatrics* **38:** 231–243.

Ambrus CM, Choi TS, Cunnanan E et al (1977) Prevention of hyaline membrane disease with plasminogen. A cooperative study. *Journal of the American Medical Association* **237:** 1837–1841.

Andersson TR, Bangstad H & Larsen ML (1988) Heparin cofactor II, antithrombin and protein C in plasma from term and preterm infants. *Acta Paediatrica Scandinavica* **77:** 485–488.

Andrew M (1991a) Hemorrhagic and thrombotic complications in children. In Hirsh J & Colman R (eds) *Hemostasis and Thrombosis.* Philadelphia: JB Lippincott (in press).

Andrew M (1991b) Hemorrhagic disorders. In Nathan D & Oski F (eds) *Hematology of Infancy and Childhood,* 4th edn. Boston: WB Saunders (in press).

Andrew M & Karpatkin M (1982) A simple screening test for evaluating prolonged partial thromboplastin times in newborn infants. *Journal of Pediatrics* **101:** 610–612.

Andrew M & Kelton J (1984) Neonatal thrombocytopenia. *Clinics in Perinatology* **11:** 359.

Andrew M & Schmidt B (1988) Use of heparin in newborn infants. *Seminars in Thrombosis and Hemostasis* **14:** 28.

Andrew M, Bhogal M & Karpatkin M (1981) Factors XI and XII and prekallikrein in sick and healthy premature infants. *New England Journal of Medicine* **305:** 1130–1133.

Andrew M, Massicotte-Nolan P & Karpatkin M (1983) Plasma protease inhibitors in premature infants: Influence of gestational age, postnatal age and health status. *Proceedings of the Society of Experimental Biology and Medicine* **173:** 495–500.

Andrew M, Massicotte-Nolan P & Mitchell L (1985) Dysfunctional antithrombin III in sick premature infants. *Pediatric Research* **19:** 237–239.

Andrew M, Paes B, Milner R et al (1987a) The development of the human coagulation system in the fullterm infant. *Blood* **70:** 165–172.

Andrew M, Castle V, Saigal S et al (1987b) Clinical impact of neonatal thrombocytopenia. *Journal of Pediatrics* **110:** 457–464.

Andrew M, Paes B, Milner R et al (1988a) Development of the human coagulation system in the healthy premature infant. *Blood* **72:** 1651–1657.

Andrew M, Mitchell L, Berry L et al (1988b) Fibrinogen has a rapid turnover in the healthy newborn lamb. *Pediatric Research* **23:** 249–252.

Andrew M, Ofosu FA, Schmidt B et al (1988c) Heparin clearance and ex vivo recovery in newborn piglets and adult pigs. *Thrombosis Research* **52:** 517–527.

Andrew M, Castle V, Mitchell L et al (1989a) A modified bleeding time in the infant. *American Journal of Hematology* **30:** 190–191.

Andrew M, Brooker L & Weitz J (1989b) Fibrin clot lysis by thrombolytic agents is impaired in the newborn. *Thrombosis Hemostasis* **62:** 288 (abstract).

Andrew M, Paes B, Johnston M et al (1990a) Development of the hemostatic system in the neonate and young infant. *American Journal of Pediatric Hematology/Oncology* **12:** 95–104.

Andrew M, Schmidt B, Mitchell L et al (1990b) Thrombin generation in newborn plasma is critically dependent on the concentration of prothrombin. *Thrombosis Haemostasis* **63:** 27–30.

Andrew M, Mitchell L, Paes B et al (1990c) A circulating anticoagulant in the fetus and mother. *Pediatric Research* **27:** 262a.

Andrew M, Paes B, Bowker J et al (1990d) Evaluation of an automated bleeding time device in the newborn. *American Journal of Hematology* **35:** 275–277.

Arad ID, Alpan G, Sznajderman SD et al (1986) The mean platelet volume (MPV) in the neonatal period. *American Journal of Perinatology* **3:** 1–3.

Arneil GC, MacDonald AM, Morphy AV et al (1973) Renal venous thrombosis. *Clinical Nephrology* **1:** 119–131.

Arnold J, O'Brodovich H, Whyte R & Coates G (1985) Pulmonary thromboemboli after neonatal asphyxia. *Journal of Pediatrics* **106:** 806–809.

Austin N & Darlow BA (1988) Transfusion-associated fall in platelet count in very low birthweight infants. *Australian Paediatric Journal* **24:** 354–356.

Avery ME & Mead J (1959) Surface properties in relation to atelectasis and hyaline membrane disease. *American Journal of Diseases of Children* **97:** 516–523.

Bada HS, Green RS, Pourcyrous M et al (1989) Indomethacin reduces the risks of severe intraventricular hemorrhage. *Journal of Pediatrics* **115:** 631–637.

Baehner RL & Strauss HS (1966) Hemophilia in the first year of life. *New England Journal of Medicine* **275:** 524–528.

Ballin A, Andrew M, Ling E et al (1988) High-dose intravenous gammaglobulin therapy for neonatal autoimmune thrombocytopenia. *Journal of Pediatrics* **112:** 789–792.

Bandstra ES, Montalvo BM, Goldberg RN et al (1988) Prophylactic indomethacin for prevention of intraventricular hemorrhage in premature infants. *Pediatrics* **82:** 533–542.

Barbui T, Cortelazzo S, Viero P et al (1985) Idiopathic thrombocytopenic purpura and pregnancy. Maternal platelet count and antiplatelet antibodies do not predict the risk of neonatal thrombocytopenia. *Ricerca in Clinica e in Laboratorio* **15:** 139–144.

Barnard DR & Hathaway WE (1979) Neonatal thrombosis. *American Journal of Pediatric Hematology/Oncology* **1:** 235–244.

Barnard DR, Simmons MA & Hathaway WE (1979) Coagulation studies in extremely premature infants. *Pediatric Research* **13:** 1330–1335.

Barradas MA & Mikhailidis DP (1986) An investigation of maternal and neonatal platelet function. *Biological Research Pregnancy Perinatology* **7:** 60–65.

Berry L, Andrew M, Post M et al (1991) A549 lung epithelial cell line synthesize and express anticoagulant molecules on the cell surface and in conditioned medium. *American Journal of Respiratory Cellular and Molecular Biology* (in press).

Beverley DW, Chance GW, Inwood MJ et al (1984) Intraventricular haemorrhage and haemostasis defects. *Archives of Disease in Childhood* **59:** 444–448.

Beverley DW, Pitts-Tucker TJ, Congdon J et al (1985) Prevention of intraventricular haemorrhage by fresh frozen plasma. *Archives of Disease in Childhood* **60:** 710–713.

Bjorke B, Herin P & Blomback M (1974) Neonatal aortic thrombosis. A possible clinical manifestation of congenital antithrombin III deficiency. *Acta Paediatrica Scandinavica* **63:** 297–301.

Blanchette VS (1988) Neonatal alloimmune thrombocytopenia: A clinical perspective. *Current Studies in Hematology Blood Transfusion* **54:** 112–126.

Blanchette VS, Sacher RA, Ballem PJ et al (1989a) Commentary on the management of autoimmune thrombocytopenia during pregnancy and in the neonatal period. *Blut* **59:** 121–123.

Blanchette VS, Andrew M, Perlman M et al (1989b) Neonatal autoimmune thrombocytopenia: Role of high-dose intravenous immunoglobulin G therapy. *Blut* **59:** 139–144.

Bosque E & Weaver L (1986) Continuous versus intermittent heparin infusion of umbilical artery catheters in the newborn infant. *Journal of Pediatrics* **108:** 141–143.

Burrows RF & Kelton JG (1988) Incidentally detected thrombocytopenia in healthy mothers and their infants. *New England Journal of Medicine* **319:** 142–145.

Burrows RF & Kelton JG (1991) Low fetal risks in pregnancies associated with idiopathic thrombocytopenic purpura do not justify obstetrical interventions. *American Journal of Obstetrics and Gynecology* (in press).

Burrows RF, Caco CC, Kelton JG et al (1988) Neonatal alloimmune thrombocytopenia: Spontaneous in utero intracranial hemorrhage. *American Journal of Hematology* **28:** 98–102.

Bussel JP, Berkowitz RL, McFarland JG et al (1988) Antenatal treatment of neonatal alloimmune thrombocytopenia. *New England Journal of Medicine* **319:** 1374–1378.

Cade JF, Hirsh J & Martin M (1969) Placental barrier to coagulation factors: Its relevance to the coagulation defect at birth and to haemorrhage in the newborn. *British Medical Journal* **2:** 281–283.

Castle V, Andrew M, Kelton J et al (1986) Frequency and mechanism of neonatal thrombocytopenia. *Journal of Pediatrics* **108:** 749–755.

Castle V, Coates G, Kelton J et al (1987) [111]Indium oxine platelet survivals in the thrombocytopenic infant. *Blood* **70:** 652–656.

Castle V, Coates G, Mitchell L et al (1988) The effect of hypoxia on platelet survival and site of sequestration in the newborn rabbit. *Thrombosis Haemostasis* **59:** 45–48.

Collen D & Lijnen HR (1987) Fibrinolysis and the control of hemostasis. In Stamatoyamopoulos G, Nienhuis AW, Leder P & Jaerus PW (eds) *The Molecular Basis of Blood Diseases*, pp 662–688. Philadelphia: WB Saunders.

Colman RW, Marder VJ, Salzman EW & Hirsh J (1987) In Colman RW, Hirsh J, Marder VJ & Salzman EW (eds) *Hemostasis and Thrombosis; basic principles and clinical practice*, pp 3–18. Philadelphia: JB Lippincott.

Committee on Nutrition, Academy of Pediatrics (1961) Vitamin K compounds and water-soluble analogues: Use in therapy and prophylaxis in pediatrics. *Pediatrics* **28:** 501–507.

Cooke RWI (1981) Factors associated with periventricular haemorrhage in very low birthweight infants. *Archives of Disease in Childhood* **56:** 425–431.

Corby DG & O'Barr TP (1981) Decreased alpha-adrenergic receptors in newborn platelets. Cause of abnormal response to epinephrine. *Developmental Pharmacology and Therapeutics* **2:** 215–225.

Corrigan JJ (1979) Activation of coagulation and disseminated intravascular coagulation in the newborn. *American Journal of Pediatric Hematology/Oncology* **1:** 245–249.

Corrigan JJ (1988) Neonatal thrombosis and the thrombolytic system. Pathophysiology and therapy. *American Journal of Pediatric Hematology/Oncology* **10:** 83–91.

Corrigan JJ & Earnst D (1980) Factor II antigen in liver disease and warfarin induced vitamin K deficiency: Correlation with coagulation activity using echis venom. *American Journal of Hematology* **8:** 249–255.

Corrigan JJ & Kryc JJ (1980) Factor II (prothrombin) levels in cord blood. Correlation of coagulant activity with immunoreactive protein. *Journal of Pediatrics* **97:** 979–983.

Corrigan JJ, Sluth JJ, Jeter M et al (1989) Newborn's fibrinolytic mechanism: Components and plasmin generation. *American Journal of Hematology* **32:** 273–278.

Daffos F, Forestier F, Kaplan C et al (1988) Prenatal diagnosis and management of bleeding disorders with fetal blood sampling. *American Journal of Obstetrics and Gynecology* **158:** 939–946.

David RJ, Merten DF, Anderson JC et al (1981) Prevention of umbilical artery catheter clots with heparinized infusates. *Developmental Pharmacology and Therapeutics* **12:** 117–126.

De Stefano V, Leone G & Carolis MP (1987) Antithrombin III in fullterm and preterm newborn infants: Three cases of neonatal diagnosis of ATIII congenital defect. *Thrombosis Haemostasis* **57:** 329–331.

de Swiet M (1985) Maternal autoimmune disease and the fetus. *Archives of Disease in Childhood* **60:** 794–797.

Dixon RH & Rosse WF (1975) Platelet antibody in autoimmune thrombocytopenia. *British Journal of Haematology* **31:** 129–134.

Donner M, Holmberg L & Nilsson IM (1987) Type IIB von Willebrand's disease with probable autosomal recessive inheritance and presenting as thrombocytopenia in infancy. *British Journal of Haematology* **66:** 349–354.

Duncan RE, Evans AT & Martin LW (1977) Natural history and treatment of renal vein thrombosis in children. *Journal of Pediatric Surgery* **12:** 639–645.

Edelberg JM, Enghild JJ, Pizzo SV & Gonzalez-Gronow M (1990) Neonatal plasminogen displays altered cell surface binding and activation kinetics. Correlation with increased glycosylation of the protein. *Journal of Clinical Investigation* **86:** 107–112.

Fernandez F, Gaudable C, Sie P et al (1985) Low hematocrit and prolonged bleeding time in uraemic patients: Effect of red cell transfusions. *British Journal of Haematology* **59:** 139–148.

Fetus and Newborn Committee (1988) Canadian Pediatric Society: The use of vitamin K in the perinatal period. *Canadian Medical Association Journal* **139:** 127–130.

Feusner JH (1980) Normal and abnormal bleeding times in neonates and young children utilizing a fully standardized template technique. *American Journal of Clinical Pathology* **74:** 73–77.

Feusner JH, Slichter SJ & Harker LA (1983) Acquired haemostatic defects in the ill newborn. *British Journal of Haematology* **53:** 73–84.

Forestier F, Daffos F, Daffos F et al (1985) Vitamin K dependent proteins in fetal hemostasis at mid trimester pregnancy. *Thrombosis Haemostasis* **53:** 401–403.

Forestier F, Daffos F, Galacteros F et al (1986a) Hematological values of 163 normal fetuses between 18 and 30 weeks of gestation. *Pediatric Research* **20**: 342–346.

Forestier F, Daffos E, Rainaut M et al (1986b) Prenatal diagnosis of hemophilia by fetal blood sampling under ultrasound guidance. *Haemostasis* **16**: 346–351.

Gader AMA, Bahakim H, Jabber FA et al (1988) Dose-response aggregometry in maternal/ neonatal platelets. *Thrombosis Haemostasis* **60**: 314–318.

Gajl-Peczalska K (1964) Plasma protein composition of hyaline membrane in the newborn as studied by immunofluorescence. *Archives of Disease in Childhood* **39**: 226–231.

Galanakis DK & Mosesson MW (1976) Evaluation of the role of in vivo proteolysis (fibrinogenolysis) in prolonging the thrombin time of human umbilical cord fibrinogen. *Blood* **48**: 109–118.

Gilhooly JT, Lindenberg JA & Reynold JW (1987) Survey of umbilical catheter practices. *Clinical Res* **34**: 142A.

Gill FM (1983) Thrombocytopenia in the newborn. *Seminars in Perinatology* **7**: 201–212.

Gilles FH, Price RA, Kevy SV & Berenberg W (1971) Fibrinolytic activity in the ganglionic eminence of the premature human brain. *Biology of the Neonate* **18**: 426–432.

Girolami A, De Marco L, Dal Bo Zanon R et al (1985) Rarer quantitative and qualitative abnormalities of coagulation. *Clinics in Haematology* **14**: 385–411.

Gobel U, von Voss H, Jurgens H et al (1980) Efficiency of heparin in the treatment of newborn infants with respiratory distress syndrome and disseminated intravascular coagulation. *European Journal of Pediatrics* **133**: 47.

Goddard-Finegold J (1984) Periventricular, intraventricular hemorrhages in the premature newborn: Update on pathologic features, pathogenesis and possible means of prevention. *Archives of Neurology* **41**: 766–771.

Gogstad GO, Brostad F, Krutnes MB et al (1982) Fibrinogen-binding properties of the human platelet glycoprotein IIb–IIIa complex: A study using cross-radioimmunoelectrophoresis. *Blood* **60**: 663–671.

Gordon EM, Ratnoff OD, Saito H et al (1980) Studies on some coagulation factors (Hageman factor, plasma prekallikrein, and high molecular weight kininogen) in the normal newborn. *American Journal of Pediatric Hematology/Oncology* **2**: 213–216.

Gray OP, Ackerman A & Fraser AJ (1968) Intracranial hemorrhage and clotting defects in low birth weight infants. *Lancet* **i**: 545–551.

Greer FR, Mummah-Schendel LL, Marshall S et al (1988) Vitamin K_1 (phylloquinone) and vitamin K_2 (menaquinone) status in newborns during the first week of life. *Pediatrics* **81**: 137–140.

Greffe BS, Marlar RA & Manco-Johnson M (1989) Neonatal protein C: Molecular composition and distribution in normal term infants. *Thrombosis Research* **56**: 91–98.

Gross SJ, Filston HC & Anderson JC (1982) Controlled study of treatment for disseminated intravascular coagulation in the neonate. *Journal of Pediatrics* **100**: 445–448.

Gruel Y, Boizard B, Daffos F et al (1986) Determinations of platelet antigens and glycoproteins in the human fetus. *Blood* **68**: 488–492.

Hambleton G & Appleyard W (1968) Controlled trial of fresh frozen plasma in asphyxiated low birthweight infants. *Lancet* **i**: 545.

Hanada T, Abe T & Takita H (1985) Antithrombin III concentrates for treatment of disseminated intravascular coagulation in children. *American Journal of Pediatric Hematology/ Oncology* **7**: 3–8.

Hanawa Y, Maki M, Murata B et al (1988) The second nation-wide survey in Japan of vitamin K deficiency in infants. *European Journal of Pediatrics* **147**: 472–477.

Hanigan WC, Kennedy G, Roemisch F et al (1988) Administration of indomethacin for the prevention of periventricular intraventricular hemorrhage in high risk neonates. *Journal of Pediatrics* **112**: 941–947.

Haroon Y, Shearer MJ, Rahim S et al (1982) The content of phylloquinone (vitamin K_1) in human milk, cow's milk and infant formula foods determined by high-performance liquid chromatography. *Journal of Nutrition* **112**: 1105–1117.

Hathaway WE (1986) ICTH Subcommittee on Neonatal Hemostasis. *Thrombosis Haemostasis* **55**: 145.

Hathaway WE (1987) New insights on vitamin K. *Hematology/Oncology Clinics of North America* **1**: 367–379.

Hayden CK, Shattuck KE, Richardson CJ et al (1985) Subependymal germinal matrix

hemorrhage in fullterm neonates. *Pediatrics* **75:** 714–718.
Hedberg VA & Lipton JM (1988) Thrombocytopenia with absent radii. A review of 100 cases. *American Journal of Pediatric Hematology/Oncology* **10:** 51–64.
Hegde UM (1985) Immune thrombocytopenia in pregnancy and the newborn. *British Journal of Obstetrics and Gynaecology* **92:** 657–659.
Hensey OJ, Morgan MEI & Cooke RWI (1984) Tranexamic acid in the prevention of peri-ventricular haemorrhage. *Archives of Disease in Childhood* **59:** 719–721.
Herman JH, Jumbelic MI, Ancona RJ et al (1986) In utero cerebral hemorrhage in alloimmune thrombocytopenia. *American Journal of Pediatric Hematology/Oncology* **8:** 312–317.
Hiraike H, Kimura M & Itokawa Y (1988) Determination of K vitamins (phylloquinone and menaquinones) in umbilical cord plasma by a platinum-reduction column. *Journal of Chromatography* **430:** 143–148.
Hirsh J, Ofosu F & Cairns J (1986) Advances in antithrombotic therapy. In Hoffbrand AV (ed.) *Recent Advances in Haematology*, pp 333–367. New York: Churchill-Livingstone.
Idell S, James KK, Levin EG et al (1989a) Local abnormalities in coagulation and fibrinolytic pathways predispose to alveolar fibrin deposition in the adult respiratory distress syndrome. *Journal of Clinical Investigation* **84:** 695–705.
Idell S, Peters J, James KK, Fair DS & Coalson JJ (1989b) Local abnormalities of coagulation and fibrinolytic pathways that promote alveolar fibrin deposition in the lungs of baboons with diffuse alveolar damage. *Journal of Clinical Investigation* **84:** 181–193.
Israels SJ & Seshia SS (1987) Childhood stroke associated with protein C or S deficiency. *Journal of Pediatrics* **111:** 562–564.
Israels SJ, Gowen B & Gerrard JM (1987) Contractile activity of neonatal platelets. *Pediatric Research* **21:** 293–295.
Jenkins CS, Phillips DR, Clemetson KJ et al (1976) Platelet membrane glycoproteins implicated in ristocetin-induced aggregation. *Journal of Clinical Investigation* **57:** 112–124.
Jones CR, McCabe R, Hamilton CA et al (1985) Maternal and fetal platelet responses and adrenoreceptor binding characteristics. *Thrombosis Haemostasis* **53:** 95–98.
Kaplan C, Daffos F, Forestier F et al (1988) Management of alloimmune thrombocytopenia. Antenatal diagnosis and in utero transfusion of maternal platelets. *Blood* **72:** 340–343.
Karitsky D, Kleine N, Pringsheim W et al (1971) Fibrinogen turnover in the premature infant with and without idiopathic respiratory distress syndrome. *Acta Paediatrica Scandinavica* **60:** 465–470.
Karpatkin M (1984) Corticosteroid therapy in thrombocytopenic infants of women with autoimmune thrombocytopenia. *Journal of Pediatrics* **105:** 623–625.
Karpatkin M, Porges RF & Karpatkin S (1981) Platelet counts in infants of women with autoimmune thrombocytopenia: Effects of steroid administration to the mother. *New England Journal of Medicine* **305:** 936–939.
Karpatkin M, Mannucci PM, Mannuccio P et al (1986) Low protein C in the neonatal period. *British Journal of Haematology* **62:** 137–142.
Karpatkin S, Strick N, Karpatkin MG et al (1972) Cumulative experience in the detection of antiplatelet antibody in 234 patients with idiopathic thrombocytopenic purpura, systemic lupus erythematosus and other clinic disorders. *American Journal of Medicine* **52:** 776–785.
Katz JA, Moake JL, McPherson PD et al (1989) Relationship between human development and disappearance of unusually large von Willebrand factor multimers from plasma. *Blood* **73:** 1851–1858.
Kazzi NJ, Ilagen MB et al (1989) Maternal administration of vitamin K does not improve the coagulation profile of preterm infants. *Pediatrics* **84:** 1045.
Kisker CT, Perlman S, Bohlken D et al (1988) Measurement of prothrombin mRNA during gestation and early neonatal development. *Journal of Laboratory and Clinical Medicine* **112:** 407–412.
Koepke JA (1986) Partial thromboplastin time test-proposed performance guidelines. ICSH Panel on the APTT. *Thrombosis Haemostasis* **55:** 143–144.
Lane PA & Hathaway WE (1985) Medical progress: Vitamin K in infancy. *Journal of Pediatrics* **106:** 351–359.
Lesko SM, Mitchell AA, Eopstein MF et al (1986) Heparin use as a risk factor for intra-ventricular hemorrhage in low birth weight infants. *New England Journal of Medicine* **314:** 1156–1160.

Levene MI & de Vries L (1984) Extension of neonatal intraventricular haemorrhage. *Archives of Disease in Childhood* **59**: 631–636.

Levine JJ, Udall JN, Evernden BA et al (1987) Elevated levels of α_2-macroglobulin-protease complexes in infants. *Biology of the Neonate* **51**: 149–155.

Liebermann J (1961) The nature of the fibrinolytic enzyme defect in hyaline membrane disease. *New England Journal of Medicine* **265**: 363–369.

Lorand L, Losowsky MS & Miloszewski KJM (1980) Human factor XIII: Fibrin stabilizing factor. *Progress in Hemostasis and Thrombosis* **5**: 245–290.

Lupton BA, Hill A, Whitfield MF et al (1988) Reduced platelet count as a risk factor for intraventricular hemorrhage. *American Journal of Diseases of Childhood* **142**: 1222–1224.

McDonald MM & Hathaway WE (1982) Anticoagulant therapy by continuous heparinization in newborn and older infants. *Journal of Pediatrics* **101**: 451–457.

McDonald MM, Jacobson LJ, Hay WW et al (1981) Heparin clearance in the newborn. *Pediatric Research* **15**: 1015–1018.

McDonald MM, Johnson ML, Rumack CM et al (1984) Role of coagulopathy in newborn intracranial hemorrhage. *Pediatrics* **74**: 26–31.

McFarland JG, Frenzke M & Aster RH (1989) Testing of maternal sera in pregnancies at risk for neonatal alloimmune thrombocytopenia. *Transfusion* **29**: 128–133.

McGill M, Mayhaus C, Hoff R et al (1982) Frozen maternal platelets for neonatal thrombocytopenia. *Transfusion* **27**: 347–349.

Mahasandana C & Hathaway WE (1973) Circulating anticoagulants in the newborn: relation to hypercoagulability and the idiopathic respiratory distress syndrome. *Pediatric Research* **7**: 670–673.

Malia RG, Preston FE & Mitchell VE (1980) Evidence against vitamin K deficiency in normal neonates. *Thrombosis Haemostasis* **44**: 159–160.

Mammen EF (1983a) Factor V deficiency. *Seminars in Thrombosis and Hemostasis* **9**: 17–18.

Mammen EF (1983b) Factor II abnormalities. *Seminars in Thrombosis and Hemostasis* **9**: 13–16.

Mammen EF (1983c) Factor X abnormalities. *Seminars in Thrombosis and Hemostasis* **9**: 31–33.

Mammen EF (1983d) Fibrinogen abnormalities. *Seminars in Thrombosis and Hemostasis* **9**: 1–9.

Mandelbrot L, Guillaumont M, Forestier F et al (1988) Placental transfer of vitamin K_1 and its implications in fetal hemostasis. *Thrombosis Haemostasis* **60**: 39–43.

Mariani G & Mazzucconi MG (1983) Factor VII congenital deficiency. *Haemostasis* **13**: 169–177.

Markarian M, Githens JW, Rosenblut E et al (1971a) Hypercoagulability in premature infants with special reference to the respiratory distress syndrome and hemorrhage. 1. Coagulation studies. *Biology of the Neonate* **17**: 84.

Markarian M, Lubchenco LO, Rosenblut E et al (1971b) Hypercoagulability in premature infants with special reference to the respiratory distress syndrome and hemorrhage. II. The effect of heparin. *Biology of the Neonate* **17**: 98–111.

Marlar RA, Montgomery RR, Broekmans AW et al (1989) Diagnosis and treatment of homozygous protein C deficiency. *Journal of Pediatrics* **114**: 528–534.

Martin B, Robin H, Williams R et al (1983) Neonatal graft vs host disease following transfusion of maternal platelets. *Transfusion* **23**: 417.

Maruyama I & Majerus PW (1987) Protein C inhibits endocytosis of thrombin–thrombomodulin complexes in A549 lung cancer cells and human umbilican vein endothelial cells. *Blood* **69**: 1481–1484.

Mehta P, Vasa R, Newman L et al (1980) Thrombocytopenia in the high-risk infant. *Journal of Pediatrics* **97**: 791–794.

Ment LR, Stewart WB & Duncan CC (1983) Beagle puppy model of intraventricular hemorrhage. Effect of superoxide dismutase on cerebral blood flow and prostaglandins. *Journal of Neurosurgery* **62**: 563–569.

Ment LR, Duncan CC, Ehrenkranz RA et al (1984) Intraventricular hemorrhage in the preterm neonate: Timing and cerebral blood flow changes. *Journal of Pediatrics* **104**: 419–425.

Ment LR, Duncan CC, Ehrenkranz RA et al (1985) Randomized indomethacin trial for the prevention of intraventricular hemorrhage in very low birth weight infants. *Journal of Pediatrics* **107**: 937–943.

Ment LR, Duncan CC, Ehrenkranz RA et al (1987a) Randomized low dose indomethacin trial for prevention of intraventricular hemorrhage in very low birth weight neonates. *Journal of Pediatrics* 112: 948–955.

Ment LR, Duncan CC et al (1987b) Intraventricular hemorrhage of the preterm neonate. *Seminars in Perinatology* 11: 132–141.

Moalic P, Gruel Y & Body G (1988) Levels and plasma distribution of free and C_4b-BP-bound protein S in human fetuses and fullterm newborns. *Thrombosis Research* 49: 471–480.

Morales WJ, Angel JL, O'Brien WF et al (1988) The use of antenatal vitamin K in the prevention of early neonatal intraventricular hemorrhage. *American Journal of Obstetrics and Gynecology* 159: 774–778.

Motohara K, Endo F & Matsuda I (1987) Screening for late neonatal vitamin K deficiency by acarboxyprothrombin in dried blood spots. *Archives of Disease in Childhood* 62: 370–375.

Mueller-Eckhardt C, Kiefel V, Grubert A et al (1989) 348 cases of suspected neonatal alloimmune thrombocytopenia. *Lancet* i: 363–366.

Muntean W & Rosegger H (1989) Antithrombin III concentrate in preterm infants with IRDS: An open, controlled randomized clinical trial. *Thrombosis and Haemostasis* 62: 288 (abstract).

Nachman RL, Jaffe EA & Weksler BB (1971) Immuno-inhibition of ristocetin induced aggregation. *Journal of Clinical Investigation* 59: 143–158.

O'Connor ME & Addiego JE (1986) Use of oral vitamin K to prevent hemorrhagic disease of the newborn infant. *Journal of Pediatrics* 108: 616–619.

O'Neill JA, Neblett WW III & Born ML (1981) Management of major thromboembolic complications of umbilical artery catheters. *Journal of Pediatric Surgery* 16: 972–978.

Ogata T, Motohara K, Endo F et al (1988) Vitamin K effect in low birth weight infants. *Pediatrics* 81: 423–427.

Peters M, Jansen E, ten Cate JW et al (1984a) Neonatal antithrombin III. *British Journal of Haematology* 58: 579–587.

Peters M, ten Cate JW, Breederveld C et al (1984b) Low antithrombin III levels in neonates with idiopathic respiratory distress syndrome: poor prognosis. *Pediatric Research* 18: 273–276.

Pomerance JJ, Teal JG, Gogdok JF et al (1987) Maternally administered antenatal vitamin K_1: effect on neonatal prothrombin activity, partial thromboplastin time, and intraventricular hemorrhage. *Obstetrics and Gynecology* 70: 235–241.

Rajani K, Goetzman BW, Wennberg RP et al (1979) Effect of heparinization of fluids infused through an umbilical artery catheter on catheter patency and frequency of complications. *Pediatrics* 63: 552–556.

Rapaport SI, Proctor RR, Patch JJ et al (1961) The mode of inheritance of PTA deficiency: Evidence for the existence of major PTA deficiency and minor PTA deficiency. *Blood* 128: 149–165.

Rennie JM, Doyle J & Cooke RWI (1986) Early administration of indomethacin to preterm infants. *Archives of Diseases in Childhood* 61: 233–238.

Runnebaum IB, Maurer SM, Daly L & Bonnar J (1989) Inhibitors and activators of fibrinolysis during and after childbirth in maternal and cord blood. *Journal of Perinatal Medicine* 17: 113–119.

Samuels P, Main EK, Tomaski A et al (1987) Abnormalities in platelet antiglobulin tests in preeclamptic mothers and their neonates. *American Journal of Obstetrics and Gynecology* 157: 109–113.

Schmidt B & Andrew M (1988) Neonatal thrombotic disease: Prevention, diagnosis and treatment. *Journal of Pediatrics* 113: 407–410.

Schmidt B & Zipursky A (1984) Thrombotic disease in newborn infants. *Clinics in Perinatology* 11: 461–488.

Schmidt B & Zipursky A (1986) Disseminated intravascular coagulation masking neonatal hemophilia. *Journal of Pediatrics* 109: 886–888.

Schmidt B, Wais U, Pringsheim W et al (1984) Plasma elimination of antithrombin III is accelerated in term newborn infants. *European Journal of Pediatrics* 141: 225–227.

Schmidt B, Buchanan MR, Ofosu F et al (1988a) Antithrombotic properties of heparin in a neonatal piglet model of thrombin induced thrombosis. *Thrombosis Haemostasis* 60: 289–292.

Schmidt B, Mitchell L, Ofosu F et al (1988b) Standard assays underestimate the concentration of heparin in neonatal plasma. *Journal of Laboratory and Clinical Medicine* **112:** 641–643.

Schmidt B, Ofosu FA, Mitchell L et al (1989a) Anticoagulant effects of heparin in neonatal plasma. *Pediatric Research* **25:** 405–408.

Schmidt B, Mitchell L, Ofosu F et al (1989b) Alpha-2-macroglobulin is an important progressive inhibitor of thrombin in neonatal and infant plasma. *Thrombosis Haemostasis* **62:** 1074–1077.

Schmidt B, Shah J, Andrew M & Weitz J (1990) Thrombin formation is increased in severe neonatal respiratory distress syndrome (RDS). *Pediatric Research* **27:** 224A (abstract).

Schwarz HP, Muntean W, Watzke H et al (1988) Low total protein S antigen but high protein S activity due to decreased C_4b-binding protein in neonates. *Blood* **71:** 562–565.

Scott JR, Cruikshank DP, Kochenouri NK et al (1980) Fetal platelet counts in the obstetric management of immunologic purpura. *American Journal of Obstetrics and Gynecology* **136:** 495–499.

Setzer ES, Morse BM, Goldberg RN et al (1984) Prophylactic indomethacin and intraventricular hemorrhage in the premature. *Pediatric Research* **18:** 345 (abstract).

Shah J, Mitchell L, Paes B, Andrew M (1989) Thrombin inhibition is impaired in the sick newborn. *Pediatric Research* **25:** 273A.

Shapiro AD, Jacobson LJ & Aranson ME (1986) Vitamin K deficiency in the newborn infant: Prevalence and perinatal risk factors. *Journal of Pediatrics* **109:** 675–680.

Shapiro ME, Riodvien R, Bauer KA et al (1981) Acute aortic thrombosis in antithrombin III deficiency. *Journal of the American Medical Association* **245:** 1759–1761.

Shapiro SS & Anderson DB (1977) Thrombin inhibitor in normal plasma. In Lundblad RL, Fenton JW & Mann KG (eds) *Chemistry and Biology of Thrombin*, pp 361–374. Ann Arbor, MI: Ann Arbor Science Publishing.

Strang LB (1966) The pulmonary circulation in the respiratory distress syndrome. *Pediatric Clinics of North America* **13:** 693–730.

Stuart MJ, Dusse J, Clark DA et al (1984) Differences in thromboxane production between neonatal and adult platelets in response to arachidonic acid and epinephrine. *Pediatric Research* **18:** 823–826.

Suarez CR, Menendez CE, Walenga JM et al (1984) Neonatal and maternal hemostasis. Value of molecular markers in the assessment of hemostatic status. *Seminars in Thrombosis and Hemostasis* **10:** 280–284.

Suarez CR, Walenga J, Mangogna LC et al (1985) Neonatal and maternal fibrinolysis: Activation at time of birth. *American Journal of Hematology* **19:** 365–372.

Suarez CR, Gonzalez J, Menendez C et al (1988) Neonatal and maternal platelets: Activation at time of birth. *American Journal of Hematology* **29:** 18–21.

Summarian L (1989) Comparison of human normal, fullterm, fetal and adult plasminogen by physical and chemical analyses. *Haemostasis* **19:** 266–273.

Sutherland JM & Glueck HI (1967) Hemorrhagic disease of the newborn. Breast feeding as a necessary factor in the pathogenesis. *American Journal of Diseases of Childhood* **113:** 524–533.

Territo M, Finklestein J, Oh W et al (1973) Management of autoimmune thrombocytopenia in pregnancy and in the neonate. *Obstetrics and Gynecology* **41:** 579–584.

Toulon P, Rainaut M, Aiach M et al (1986) Antithrombin III (ATIII) and heparin cofactor II (HCII) in normal fetuses (21st–27th week) (letter). *Thrombosis Haemostasis* **56:** 237.

Townsend CW (1884) The haemorrhagic disease of the newborn. *Archives of Paediatrics* **11:** 559.

Ts'ao CH, Green D, Schultz K et al (1976) Function and ultrastructure of platelets of neonates; enhanced ristocetin aggregation of neonatal platelets. *British Journal of Haematology* **32:** 225–233.

Turner T, Prouse CV, Prescott RJ et al (1981) A clinical trial on the early detection and correction of haemostatic defects in selected high-risk neonates. *British Journal of Haematology* **47:** 65–75.

Tyson JE, deSa DJ & Moore S (1976) Thromboatheromatous complications of umbilical arterial catheterization in the newborn period. Clinicopathological study. *Archives of Disease in Childhood* **51:** 774–784.

Vailas GN, Brouillette RT, Scott JP et al (1986) Neonatal aortic thrombosis: Recent experience. *Journal of Pediatrics* **109:** 101–108.

Van Den Berg W, Breederveld C et al (1989) Low antithrombin III: accurate predictor of idiopathic respiratory distress syndrome in premature neonates. European Journal of Pediatrics 148: 445.

Vietti TJ, Murphy TP, James JA & Pritchard JA (1960) Observation on the prophylactic use of vitamin K in the newborn. Journal of Pediatrics 56: 343–346.

Vietti TJ, Stephens JC & Bennett KR (1961) Vitamin K prophylaxis in the newborn. Journal of the American Medical Association 176: 791–793.

Volpe JJ (1983) Intraventricular hemorrhage: Incidence, neuropathology, and pathogenesis. Neonatology Letter 1: 1.

von Kries RV, Stannigel H & Gobel U (1985) Anticoagulant therapy by continuous heparin–antithrombin III infusion in newborns with disseminated intravascular coagulation. European Journal of Pediatrics 144: 191–194.

von Kries RV, Becker A & Gobel U (1987) Vitamin K in the newborn: Influence of nutritional factors on acarboxy-prothrombin detectability and factor II and VII clotting activity. European Journal of Pediatrics 146: 123–127.

von Kries RV, Shearer MJ & Gobel U (1988) Vitamin K in infancy. European Journal of Pediatrics 147: 106–112.

Waltl H, Kurz R, Mitterstieler G et al (1973) Intracranial haemorrhage in low birth weight infants and prophylactic administration of coagulation factor concentrates. Lancet i: 1284–1288.

Watkins MN, Swan S, Caprini JA et al (1980) Coagulation changes in the newborn with respiratory failure. Thrombosis Research 17: 153–175.

Weinstein MJ, Blanchard R, Moake JL et al (1989) Fetal and neonatal von Willebrand factor (vWF) is unusually large and similar to the vWF in patients with thrombotic thrombocytopenic purpura. British Journal of Haematology 72: 68–72.

Widdershoven J, Lambert W & Motohara K (1988) Plasma concentrations of vitamin K_1 and PIVKA-II in bottle-fed and breast-fed infants with and without vitamin K prophylaxis at birth. European Journal of Pediatrics 148: 139–142.

Witt I, Muller H, Kunter LJ et al (1969) Evidence for the existence of fetal fibrinogen. Thrombosis et Diathesis Haemorrhasica 22: 101–109.

Yamada K, Shirahata A, Inagaki M et al (1983) Therapy for DIC in newborn infants. Bibliotheca Haematologica 49: 329–341.

Yoffe G & Buchanan GR (1988) Intracranial hemorrhage in newborn and young infants with hemophilia. Journal of Pediatrics 113: 333–336.

Yuen PMP, Yin JA & Lao TTH (1989) Fibrino–peptide A levels in maternal and newborn plasma. European Journal of Obstetrics and Gynecology 30: 239–244.

2

Inherited bleeding disorders

VICTOR S. BLANCHETTE
CATHY SPARLING
CHRISTOPHER TURNER

Cessation of bleeding requires the interaction of a damaged blood vessel with circulating clotting (coagulation) proteins and platelets to form a stable platelet–fibrin plug. Reflecting this physiological process, three elements are essential for normal haemostasis: intact blood vessels, a normally functioning coagulation system (both procoagulant and anticoagulant pathways) and platelets that are adequate in number and function. Abnormalities of any of these elements, either inherited or acquired, can result in clinically significant bleeding. In practice, however, significant haemorrhage almost always reflects abnormalities of the coagulation system or platelets; disorders of blood vessels are an uncommon cause of bleeding. This chapter will review inherited bleeding disorders; the equally important, and perhaps more frequent, acquired haemorrhagic disorders will not be discussed.

CONGENITAL COAGULATION DISORDERS

Consideration of the inherited disorders of coagulation and discussion of their clinical significance requires an understanding of the complex and delicately balanced human blood coagulation system. This system is comprised of a number of coagulation proteins or clotting factors that interact in the presence of the divalent cation Ca^{2+}, and negatively charged surfaces to form fibrin, an essential component of the normal blood clot. The system can be regarded as a 'cascade' in which activation of specific proteins (zymogens) occurs with the formation of active enzymes (Figure 1). At each activation step the process is amplified. In the normal state factors that favour clot formation (procoagulants) are balanced by factors that either inhibit clot formation (anticoagulants) or lead to clot dissolution (fibrinolysins). For convenience the coagulation system is often divided into an intrinsic pathway, an extrinsic pathway and a final common pathway (Figure 1). This schematic approach is useful for descriptive purposes provided it is remembered that, in vivo, the system functions as a single, interactive and highly regulated entity.

Baillière's Clinical Haematology—
Vol. 4, No. 2, April 1991
ISBN 0–7020–1532–6

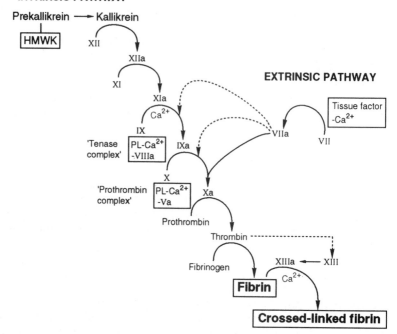

Figure 1. Schematic representation of the human coagulation system. The solid lines indicate major reactions of the intrinsic and extrinsic pathways. The dotted lines indicate the potential activation of factors IX and X by factor VIIa, and are an example of interaction between the intrinsic and extrinsic pathways. For simplicity other important interactions (for example the activation of factors V and VIII by thrombin or factor Xa) are not shown.

Intrinsic pathway

The intrinsic pathway of coagulation (Figure 1) is activated when human plasma is exposed to a negatively charged surface such as collagen. The coagulation protein that mediates contact activation is factor XII (Hageman factor). Factor XII binds to negatively charged surfaces and undergoes a surface-induced conformational change that renders the molecule much more sensitive to proteolytic activation by plasma kallikrein and other plasma proteases. The negatively charged surface also acts to localize high molecular weight kininogen (HMWK)–prekallikrein complexes and thus promotes the HMWK-dependent interaction between factor XII and pre-kallikrein that results in reciprocal activation of each molecule.

The principal action of activated factor XII (factor XIIa) is the activation of factor XI, a glycoprotein that contains two identical polypeptide chains held together by disulfide bonds. Activation of factor XI involves cleavage at a single site. Like prekallikrein, factor XI associates non-covalently to

HMWK in the fluid phase and the HMWK–factor XI complex binds to negatively charged surfaces by a specific receptor on HMWK. Localized factor XI is available for activation by factor XIIa.

The next step in the intrinsic pathway is the activation of factor IX, a single chain glycoprotein, to active factor IXa. This activation step is Ca^{2+}-dependent and requires two proteolytic cleavages of the factor IX zymogen. Factor IX can also be activated by factor VIIa. Activated factor IX serves to catalyse the activation of factor X to factor Xa, a reaction that requires phospholipids (PL), Ca^{2+} and thrombin or Xa-activated factor VIII (VIIIa) as cofactors.

Extrinsic pathway

The sequence of the extrinsic pathway is as follows: tissue factor in the presence of Ca^{2+} activates factor VII to VIIa (Figure 1). Tissue factor is a lipoprotein that is present in many tissues, and is found in high concentration in brain, lung and placental tissue. Human factor VII is a single-chain glycoprotein.

Common pathway

The extrinsic and intrinsic pathways converge at factor Xa (Figure 1), an enzyme that cleaves prothrombin (factor II) to yield thrombin. This reaction requires factor Va, phospholipids and Ca^{2+} as cofactors (prothrombinase complex). Thrombin cleaves negatively charged fibrinopeptides A and B from fibrinogen to yield fibrin monomers which are strengthened and stabilized by lysine to glutamine cross-linking, a reaction that requires the enzyme factor XIIIa (Figure 1).

An important feature of the coagulation process is the localization, containment and mobilization of the participating reactions on negatively charged cell surfaces (endothelial cells or platelets) or polymerizing macromolecular aggregates.

INHERITED COAGULATION DISORDERS

Prekallikrein deficiency

Fletcher factor deficiency was first described by Hathaway and colleagues (1965). Fletcher factor was later identified as prekallikrein (Wuepper, 1973). The abnormality was recognized as a result of routine preoperative coagulation screening in asymptomatic siblings who were born to consanguineous parents. The disorder is inherited in an autosomal recessive manner and the biochemical defect is fully expressed in homozygous individuals (Abildgaard and Harrison, 1974). Individuals with Fletcher factor deficiency are asymptomatic and have no haemorrhagic or thrombotic tendency.

Kininogen deficiencies

Fitzgerald factor deficiency was described by Waldman et al (1975) in a 71-year-old asymptomatic man who was unexpectedly found to have a prolonged activated partial thromboplastin time. Fitzgerald factor deficiency results in plasma lacking high molecular weight kininogen. Similar defects have been independently reported and named after the affected kindreds— Flaujeac factor (Lacombe et al, 1975), Williams factor (Colman et al, 1975) and Reid trait (Lutcher, 1976). The Reid defect appears similar to Fitzgerald factor deficiency, but in both the Williams and Flaujeac traits there is a deficiency of both high and low molecular weight kininogens. In the Fujiwara trait reported in Japan there is a similar deficiency of high and low molecular weight kininogens (Oh-Ishi et al, 1981). Individuals with kininogen deficiencies are symptomless and do not have tendencies to abnormal bleeding or thrombosis.

Factor XII deficiency

Factor XII deficiency was first described by Ratnoff and Colopy (1955) in a patient called Hageman. The patient had no haemorrhagic symptoms and, in fact, he and several other similarly affected persons died from thromboembolic disease (Ratnoff et al, 1968). Factor XII deficiency is transmitted as an autosomal characteristic and is fully expressed only in homozygous individuals. Most affected individuals are asymptomatic, but rarely there may be a mild tendency to bleed and an association with subarachnoid haemorrhage was reported in one case (Kovalainen et al, 1979). More often factor XII deficiency has been associated with arterial or venous thrombosis (Dyerberg and Stoffersen, 1980; Hellstern et al, 1983).

Factor XI deficiency

Factor XI deficiency was first described by Rosenthal et al (1953). The disorder occurs mainly in Jews of Ashkenazi descent (Seligsohn, 1978); in this population the frequency of the heterozygous state may be as high as 10%. Factor XI deficiency is rare in Jews of other origins or in other ethnic groups. Factor XI deficiency is inherited as an autosomal trait and occurs in homozygous and heterozygous forms. The haemorrhagic tendency in individuals with factor XI deficiency is often mild, even in patients with homozygous disease, and symptoms do not always relate to the measured level of factor XI coagulant protein or antigen (Rimon et al, 1976; Bolton-Maggs et al, 1988). The bleeding tendency is also variable within an individual in response to different haemostatic challenges. When present, symptoms include easy bruising, epistaxis, menorrhagia, postoperative and post-extraction bleeding. Haemarthroses and intramuscular bleeding are rare.

Factor X deficiency

Factor X deficiency was originally described in the Prower and Stuart kinships by Telfer et al (1956) and Hougie et al (1957). Other kindreds have since been reported (Girolami et al, 1970a, 1970b, 1983; Lechner et al, 1979; Endo, 1981; Eastman et al, 1983). The bleeding disorder may reflect a reduction in circulating factor X levels or presence of a functionally abnormal molecule (Denson et al, 1970; Fair et al, 1979). Factor X deficiency is inherited as a highly penetrant autosomal recessive trait (Graham et al, 1957) and is extremely rare. Heterozygotes have a mild tendency to bleed, but are generally symptomless. Severe homozygous factor X deficiency may result in a clinically significant bleeding disorder. Haemarthroses may occur, and spontaneous intracerebral or intraspinal haemorrhage has been notable in several reports (Girolami et al, 1970b; Machin et al, 1980; Endo, 1981).

Haemophilia A and B

Haemophilia A and B are the most important inherited coagulation disorders and are due to deficiencies of coagulant factor VIII (factor VIIIC) and factor IX respectively. Although biochemically distinct, they are identical in clinical expression. The more common factor VIII deficiency will be discussed first.

Factor VIII deficiency (haemophilia A)

Factor VIII deficiency (haemophilia A) was recognized as early as the second century, and was apparently first recorded in the medical literature in 1793 (Hynes et al, 1969). Haemophilia A is inherited as an X-linked recessive disorder with a frequency of 1 per 10000 males in a Caucasian population. The biochemical basis of haemophilia A is a deficiency of coagulant factor VIII, a glycoprotein that is synthesized in the liver, possibly in sinusoidal endothelial cells. Factor VIIIC circulates as a complex with von Willebrand factor (vWf); this association is required for the normal survival of factor VIIIC. Deficiency of vWf or presence of a dysfunctional molecule is often associated with a concomitant reduction in factor VIIIC levels.

A diagnosis of haemophilia A often follows laboratory investigation that is prompted by prolonged or unusual bleeding or bruising (Table 1). In some cases laboratory evaluation is initiated because of a positive family history. In approximately one third of cases of newly diagnosed haemophiliacs, however, there is no family history of the disorder. Once diagnosed, haemophilia A may be classified as severe (VIIIC level <2%), moderate (VIIIC level 2–10%) or mild (VIIIC level >10%). This classification is useful since the severity of bleeding in affected individuals relates to the level of circulating factor VIIIC. In our experience greater than 80% of children with severe haemophilia experience clinically significant bleeding during the first year of life (Table 2). Examples of bleeding include excessive bruising and prolonged bleeding following venepuncture or surgical procedures such as circumcision; oral bleeding following injury to the soft tissues of the mouth is also common. Once children with haemophilia begin to walk, those with the severe form of the disorder typically experience recurrent bleeding into muscles and joints (haemarthroses). Patients with

Table 1. Initial reason for laboratory investigation of a cohort of 122 children with haemophilia A and B.*

	Haemophilia A and B	
Reason	Severe	Moderate/mild
Positive family history	26†	31
Excessive bleeding or significant soft tissue haematoma	47	22
Oral haemorrhage	10	31
Excessive bleeding at or after surgery	4	14
Haemarthroses	4	2
Central nervous system haemorrhage	2	0
Other reasons	7	0

* Children ≤ 18 years of age followed in the Comprehensive Care Haemophilia Clinic, the Hospital for Sick Children, Toronto.
† Values shown are percentages, i.e. 26% of children with severe haemophilia were investigated because of a positive family history.

Table 2. Age at diagnosis in a cohort of 122 children with haemophilia A and B.*

	Haemophilia A and B	
Age at diagnosis (yr)	Severe	Moderate/mild
<1	88†	41
1–5	12	36
>5	0	23

* Children ≤ 18 years of age followed in the Comprehensive Care Haemophilia Clinic, the Hospital for Sick Children, Toronto.
† Values shown are percentages, i.e. 88% of children with severe haemophilia were less than 1 year of age at the time of initial diagnosis.

Table 3. Haemorrhagic symptoms in a cohort of 122 children with haemophilia A and B.*

	Haemophilia A and B	
	Severe	Moderate/mild
Haemarthroses	91†	23
Haematuria	11	0
Central nervous system haemorrhage	14	0

* Children ≤ 18 years of age followed in the Comprehensive Care Haemophilia Clinic, the Hospital for Sick Children, Toronto.
† Values shown are percentages, i.e. 91% of haemophiliac children with severe haemophilia had experienced at least one haemarthrosis.

mild to moderate haemophilia experience fewer haemorrhagic symptoms (Table 3) and may not present with abnormal bleeding until much later in life (Table 2). In some patients significant haemorrhage occurs only after major trauma or associated with a surgical procedure such as tonsillectomy (Table 1).

In the older child the clinical hallmark of severe haemophilia is recurrent bleeding into soft tissues and joints (Table 3). Features of acute joint haemorrhage include swelling, warmth of the skin overlying the joint, pain and loss of motion. Many severe haemophiliacs are able to describe an unusual feeling inside the joint associated with the onset of bleeding; if factor VIII is infused promptly the classic signs of an acute haemarthrosis (skin warmth, joint swelling and local pain) may not develop. Recurrent bleeding into a joint results in synovial hypertrophy, an increased tendency

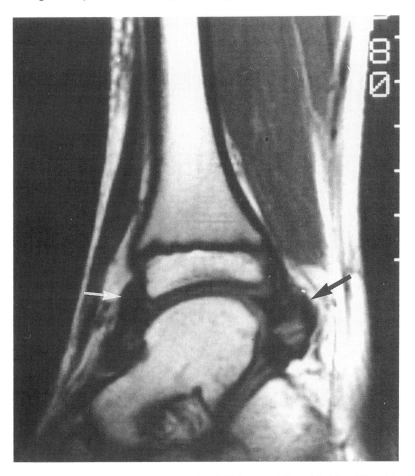

Figure 2. Saggital magnetic resonance imaging (MRI) scan of the ankle joint (T1-weighted) from a boy with severe haemophilia demonstrating synovial proliferation with haemosiderin deposition anterior (white arrow) and posterior (black arrow) to the tibiotalar joint.

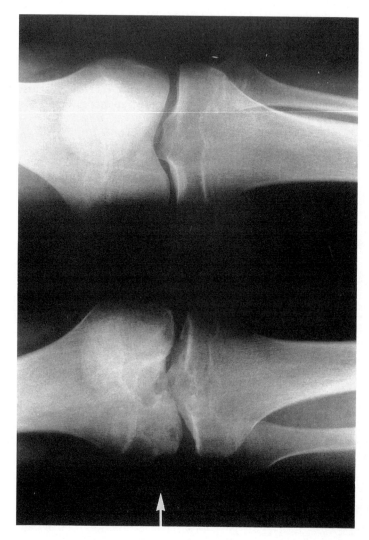

Figure 3. X-ray of the knee (left-hand side) from a boy with severe haemophilia demonstrating chronic arthropathy with multiple subchondral cyst formation and epiphyseal irregularity. The normal contralateral knee from the same patient is shown for comparison on the right-hand side.

to bleed into the 'target' joint and ultimately chronic joint damage. Early features of recurrent bleeding into a target joint include synovial thickening and advanced bone maturation (due to increased blood flow to the joint); soft tissue abnormalities are particularly well demonstrated by magnetic resonance imaging (Figure 2). Late features of chronic haemophilic arthropathy include loss of joint space, subchondral cyst formation and epiphyseal irregularity (Figure 3).

Other important but less frequent haemorrhagic symptoms include haematuria, muscle haematoma and central nervous system (CNS) bleeding (Table 3). Of these, bleeding into closed compartments (for example the iliopsoas muscle or forearm) and CNS bleeding are particularly worrying since they may be limb- or life-threatening. Prompt diagnosis and aggressive replacement therapy is necessary for a good outcome. Ultrasound examination is particularly useful to document the presence and extent of deep soft tissue haematoma (Figure 4), whereas computerized tomography (CT scanning) can be used with confidence to diagnose or exclude bleeding into the CNS. It is important to remember that a history of trauma is not always present in haemophiliacs with CNS bleeding, and that in those cases with a history of trauma symptoms may be delayed for several days.

Factor IX deficiency

Factor IX deficiency (haemophilia B or Christmas disease) is an X-linked bleeding disorder that is associated with a reduced factor IX procoagulant activity. The disorder was first described by Aggeler et al (1952) and Biggs et al (1952). The prevalence of the disorder is approximately 1 per 50 000 males.

Haemophilia B may reflect a true deficiency of coagulation factor IX (approximately 70% of cases) or presence of a dysfunctional protein (approximately 30% of cases). The factor IX variants are named after the place of birth of affected patients, e.g. factor IX Chapel Hill, and have been classified based on Ox-brain prothrombin times (reviewed in Bertina, 1987). Similar to patients with factor VIII deficiency, individuals with factor IX deficiency can be classified as severe (factor level <2%), moderate (factor level 2–10%) and mild (factor levels >10%). The clinical features of factor IX deficiency are identical to those of factor VIII deficiency.

von Willebrand's disease (vWD)

von Willebrand's disease is perhaps the commonest of the inherited bleeding disorders. vWD is due to a quantitative or qualitative abnormality of the coagulation protein von Willebrand factor (vWf). vWf plays a critical role in the adhesion of platelets to damaged subendothelium; as a result abnormalities in vWf result in a bleeding disorder that is typically platelet in type, i.e. bleeding is mucocutaneous rather than into muscles and joints. For this reason vWD will be reviewed under the section Platelet disorders.

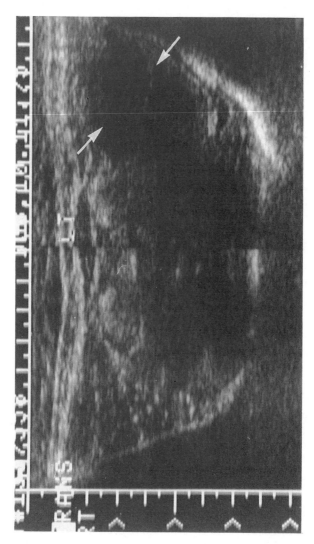

Figure 4. Ultrasound from a boy with severe haemophilia showing a large, left-sided, liquifying iliopsoas haematoma (indicated by arrows). At presentation the patient had neurological findings consistent with femoral nerve compression by the large intramuscular haematoma.

Factor VII deficiency

Factor VII deficiency was first described by Alexander et al (1951). Reviews of large numbers of cases have been reported (Marder and Schulman, 1964; Marianni and Mazzucconi, 1983). In many cases the disorder may reflect a functionally abnormal molecule (Denson et al, 1972; Briet et al, 1976; Girolami et al, 1977, 1978b, 1979; Mazzucconi et al, 1977; Triplett et al, 1985). Factor VII deficiency is a rare bleeding disorder that is inherited as an autosomal recessive characteristic. Most patients with homozygous factor VII deficiency have a life-long tendency to bleed (Marder and Schulman, 1964; Zimmerman et al, 1979), although coincidental thromboembolic complications have been reported (Godal et al, 1962; Gershwin and Gude, 1973; Shifter et al, 1984). Haemorrhagic symptoms are sometimes manifested in the neonatal period or early in life and intracranial haemorrhage at this time is particularly dangerous (Matthay et al, 1979; Ragni et al, 1981). Epistaxis, haemarthrosis and gastrointestinal bleeding may occur as well as menorrhagia in females. The severity in the tendency to bleed is widely different in individuals and the relationship to circulating factor VII levels is not clear (Ragni et al, 1981; Mariani and Mazzucconi, 1983). Greene and McMillan (1982) point out that minimal factor VII replacement therapy was needed to prevent postoperative bleeding in a severely affected patient, so it seems that only a small amount of factor VII is needed to offer considerable haemostatic protection.

Factor V deficiency

Factor V deficiency was first described by Owren (1947). It is an uncommon disorder; Seeler (1972) reviewed the syndrome and defined 58 recorded cases. The inheritance pattern is autosomal. Symptomatic patients are usually homozygous, but a bleeding diathesis is sometimes manifested in heterozygotes in whom levels of factor V may be below the normal range. Haemorrhagic symptoms, if they occur, include easy bruising, epistaxis, oral haemorrhage, bleeding after minor lacerations and menorrhagia. Muscle haematoma and haemarthroses occur but are relatively rare. Excessive bleeding after dental extractions is relatively common; intracranial bleeding is rare but has been recorded.

Prothrombin (factor II) deficiency

Prothrombin deficiency is a rare hereditary coagulation disorder. Affected individuals may have a true deficiency of prothrombin, i.e. hypoprothrombinaemia or may inherit an abnormal molecular variant of prothrombin, i.e. dysprothrombinaemia (Shapiro et al, 1969; 1974; Josso et al, 1971; 1982; Girolami et al, 1974, 1978a; Kahn and Govaerts, 1974; Gill et al, 1978; Owen et al, 1978; Bezeaud et al, 1979; 1984; Shapiro, 1975; Weigner et al, 1980; Board et al, 1982; Board and Shaw, 1983; Rubio et al, 1983; Rabiet, 1984). Some affected individuals are thought to have compound or double heterozygosity for hypo- and dysprothrombinaemia. Patients suffering from homozygous or compound heterozygous familial types of hypo- and dys-prothrombinaemia have manifested a haemorrhagic syndrome with excessive bruising, mucous membrane bleeding, menorrhagia and post-operative bleeding. Muscle haematoma have been reported, but haem-arthroses do not feature in most reports. Heterozygous individuals have been symptomless or have had a mild tendency to bleed.

Fibrinogen disorders

Fibrinogen is composed of three non-identical (α_2, β_2 and γ_2) polypeptide chains. The triggering event in the formation of fibrin is the cleavage of fibrinopeptides A and B from fibrinogen α and β chains. Quantitative (afibrinogenaemia and hypofibrinogenaemia) and qualitative (dysfibrino-genaemia) abnormalities of fibrinogen are recognized (Lane and Southan, 1987). It is likely that hypofibrinogenaemia is the symptomless heterozygous form of afibrinogenaemia. Patients with severe (homozygous) afibrino-genaemia often experience significant clinical bleeding (Mammen, 1974). Symptoms frequently start in the first year of life, and prolonged bleeding from the umbilical cord has been reported. Haematoma, gastrointestinal and mucous membrane bleeding are common. Haemarthroses occur but are less common than in severe haemophilia. Menorrhagia is sometimes a problem, and cerebral haemorrhage has been noted as a common cause of death (Fried and Kaufman, 1980). Patients with dysfibrinogenaemia may or may not have a bleeding diathesis; in some cases a tendency to thrombosis is present. In a review of 120 cases of dysfibrinogenaemia Lane and Southan (1987) reported that 46% of cases were asymptomatic, 43% presented with mild to severe bleeding (including deficient wound healing and spontaneous abortions) and 13% had thrombosis as a problem alone or associated with bleeding. The tendency to thrombosis may be associated with impaired absorption of thrombin to the abnormal fibrinogen molecule or altered interaction with tissue plasminogen activator.

Factor XIII deficiency

The first patient with factor XIII deficiency was reported by Duckert et al (1960). The condition is inherited in an autosomal manner and has been reviewed by Britten (1967) and by Lorand et al (1980). Factor XIII is a zymogen which is activated by thrombin to form a transamidase. In the presence of Ca^{2+}, activated factor XIII catalyses the formation of glutamyl–lysine cross-links between fibrin monomers. Deficiency of factor XIII renders the blood clot less stable than normal and more susceptible to digestion by plasmin. Plasma clots from affected individuals are soluble in 5 M urea and 1% monochloroacetic acid. The homozygous or severe form of factor XIII deficiency often presents with excessive bleeding from the umbilical stump during the first few days of life. There is a life-long history of a bleeding disorder with excessive bruising, haematoma formation and post-traumatic bleeding. There is also a relatively high incidence of intracranial haemorrhage and a tendency to haemorrhagic abortions in females. Although bleeding may occur directly following trauma, it is characteristically delayed for several hours or days. Factor XIII deficiency must be differentiated from congenital afibrinogenaemia, dysfibrinogenaemia and α_2-antiplasmin deficiency.

Combined deficiencies of the coagulation factors

Combined deficiencies of the vitamin K-dependent factors and the combination of factor V and VIII deficiency have been reported. More extensive combined coagulation factor deficiencies have been described, and the combination of coagulation factor deficiencies and platelet abnormalities has also been reported. These rare disorders have been reviewed (Bloom, 1987).

α_2-plasmin inhibitor (antiplasmin) deficiency

Koie and colleagues (1978) reported a patient with severe α_2-antiplasmin deficiency and a severe haemorrhagic defect resembling haemophilia. The disorder is inherited in an autosomal recessive manner (Kluft et al, 1982; Miles et al, 1982). The euglobulin lysis time was abnormally short and bleeding responded to treatment with the antifibrinolytic agent, tranexamic acid (Aoki et al, 1979).

LABORATORY EVALUATION OF THE INHERITED COAGULATION DISORDERS

The presence of a congenital coagulation disorder may be suspected because of a positive family history, occurrence of abnormal or unusual bleeding or the unexpected finding of an abnormal screening coagulation test. The abnormality present in screening coagulation tests may be typical of a specific deficiency, e.g. the isolated prolongation of the activated partial thromboplastin time (APTT) in patients with contact factor deficiencies or of the prothrombin time (PT) in patients with factor VII deficiency. The thrombin time is prolonged in patients with afibrinogenaemia or dysfibrinogenaemia; in these latter patients the reptilase time is generally prolonged. The diagnosis of any congenital coagulation deficiency must be confirmed by specific factor analysis or by tests that reveal the presence of a dysfunctional protein. This is particularly true for patients with factor XIII deficiency in whom all screening coagulation tests are normal and diagnosis depends on demonstrating clot solubility in 5 M urea or 1% monochloroacetic acid.

Inherited deficiencies of many components of the haemostatic system may present with bleeding symptoms in early infancy. A correct diagnosis can be made in some, but not all, disorders (reviewed in Blanchette et al, 1990). Thus the homozygous form of factor II, V, VII, X, XI, XII, HMWK and prekallikrein deficiencies can usually be diagnosed at birth. Factor VIII deficiency (haemophilia A) and the severe and moderate forms of factor IX deficiency (haemophilia B) can also be diagnosed in the newborn period; however, the mild forms of factor IX deficiency may require reinvestigation in later infancy because the lower limit of the reference range for full-term and premature infants at birth is $0.15\,\text{Uml}^{-1}$. Similar to mild factor IX deficiency, most forms of von Willebrand's disease cannot be confidently diagnosed in the newborn. The physiological levels of vWf, as well as the high molecular weight forms of vWf, are elevated at birth and persist into early infancy, thus masking the presence of most forms of the disease. Thrombocytopenia in infancy, as a manifestation of type IIb von Willebrand's disease, has been reported (Donner et al, 1987).

MANAGEMENT OF THE CONGENITAL BLEEDING DISORDERS

Therapy of the inherited bleeding disorders involves replacement, by intravenous infusion, of the deficient or abnormal coagulant factor. The decision to treat should be based on a knowledge of the coagulation disorder plus the clinical circumstance for which therapy is proposed and not solely on the presence of laboratory abnormalities. Thus patients with severe factor XII deficiency and marked abnormalities of in vitro coagulation tests do not bleed excessively at surgery and require no therapy (Ratnoff and Colopy, 1955; Ratnoff et al, 1968). By contrast, congenital deficiencies of factors V and VIII and of the vitamin K-dependent factors (II, VII, IX and X) are often associated with significant clinical bleeding. The severe (homozygous) form of factors XI, XIII and fibrinogen may also be associated with severe bleeding. Once a decision to treat is made, the amount and timing of therapy is dependent on the minimal factor level required to stop or prevent bleeding, and knowledge of the survival of the deficient factor (Table 4).

Table 4. Therapeutic considerations in the management of congenital coagulation disorders.

Coagulation deficiency	Plasma concentration required for haemostasis in surgery (% normal)	Half-life of transfused factor under ideal conditions	Available replacement therapy
Prothrombin	40	3 days	FFP, PCC
Factor V	10–15	12–15 h	FFP
Factor VII	5–10	4–6 h	FFP, PCC, factor VII concentrate
Factor VIII*	>40	8–12 h	Cryoprecipitate, factor VIII concentrate
Factor IX	>40	12–24 h	FFP, PCC, factor IX concentrate
Factor X	10–15	2 days	FFP, PCC
Factor XI	30	2–3 days	FFP
Factor XIII	1–5	6–10 days	FFP, factor XIII concentrate
Fibrinogen	100 mg/dl^{-1}	4–6 days	FFP, Cryoprecipitate

* Recombinant product in clinical trial.
FFP, fresh frozen plasma; PCC, prothrombin complex concentrates.

Thus in patients with severe haemophilia A a factor VIIIC level of 40% is considered adequate to prevent bleeding during surgery or in the immediate postoperative period; because of the short half-life of factor VIIIC, therapy should be given every 8 to 12 hours. In some centres factor VIII has been administered by continuous infusion (Hathaway et al, 1984). By contrast, factor levels of 3% are sufficient to prevent bleeding in patients with severe factor XIII deficiency. Moreover, since the half-life of infused factor XIII is of the order of 6–10 days, replacement therapy need only be given infrequently. Kitchens and Newcombe (1979) have recommended that severely affected subjects receive 500 ml of fresh frozen plasma once every 3 weeks. The level of factor VII required to achieve haemostasis is likewise low; however, since the half-life of factor VII is short, frequent infusions of this product may be necessary in the deficient patient with severe bleeding (Kelleher et al, 1986).

Fresh frozen plasma (FFP) contains all coagulation factors and is used to provide clotting factor cover in situations where a specific factor concentrate is not available (Table 4). The advantage of FFP is the potential to limit donor exposure; the disadvantage is the relatively large volume of product that may be required to treat or prevent haemorrhage (hence a risk of hypervolaemia), and the fact that FFP cannot be treated during preparation to inactivate the hepatitis and human immunodeficiency type I (HIV-I) viruses. By contrast, specific factor concentrates are prepared from very large plasma pools; however, these products can be treated during preparation with one of a number of effective virus-inactivating methods, e.g. wet heat, super dry-heat, pasteurization and solvent–detergent treatment. These virus-inactivating methods significantly reduce, and may possibly eliminate, the risk of transmitting hepatitis or human acquired immuno-deficiency type I (HIV-I) virus infection following clotting factor therapy. These important technological developments have significantly influenced treatment recommendations for patients with congenital bleeding disorders. Virus-inactivated, plasma-derived concentrates are now the product of choice for a number of coagulation factor disorders: factors VII, VIII, IX and XIII (Mariani et al, 1978; Winkelman et al, 1986; Daly and Haddon, 1988; Michalski et al, 1988; Brettler and Levine, 1989; Bray, 1990). The future holds even more promise since factor VIII concentrates prepared by DNA recombinant technology are in advanced clinical trial and should be commercially licensed in the near future (Schwartz et al, 1990). These concentrates will provide a pure product that will carry no risk of trans-mitting the hepatitis or HIV-I virus infections. There remains concern, however, that the risk of forming coagulation factor inhibitors could be increased with use of ultra-pure factor concentrates.

For more detailed information regarding the treatment of individual coagulation disorders, the reader is referred to several excellent reviews (Rizza and Matthews, 1984; Cash, 1987; Lusher, 1987; Hilgartner, 1989). Finally it is important to emphasize the role of 'non-blood products' in the management of patients with congenital bleeding disorders. The vaso-pressin analogue 1-deamino-8-D-arginine-vasopressin (DDAVP) is an important alternative to the use of blood products in the treatment or prevention of bleeding in patients with von Willebrand's disease and mild haemophilia A (Warrier and Lusher, 1983; de la Fuente et al, 1985; Mannucci, 1986). In patients with oral bleeding and those who must undergo dental extractions antifibrinolytic therapy is of value (Walsh et al, 1971; Forbes et al, 1972).

PLATELETS

Platelets are small, contractile cells that circulate as discs in the bloodstream. They are produced from megakaryocytes in the bone marrow under regulation by humoral factors including granulocyte–macrophage colony-stimulating factor (GM-CSF), interleukin 3 (IL-3), and interleukin 6 (IL-6) (reviewed in Gerwitz and Hoffman, 1990). The normal circulating platelet count in healthy individuals is 150 to 400×10^9 litre^{-1} and platelets survive approximately 10 days in the circulation before destruction in the spleen.

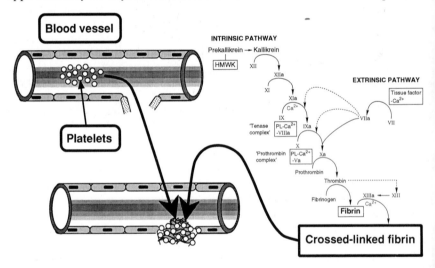

Figure 5. A schematic representation of normal haemostasis indicating the interaction of a damaged blood vessel, platelets and cross-linked fibrin.

Platelets form an integral part of the normal blood clot (Figure 5) and a bleeding tendency may occur because of quantitative and qualitative platelet disorders. Before discussion of the inherited bleeding disorders that are caused by abnormalities of platelets it is useful to review briefly normal platelet ultrastructure and physiology.

Platelet ultrastructure

The ultrastructure of platelets has been reviewed in detail by White (1987). Three zones can be identified in resting platelets (Figure 6): a peripheral zone,

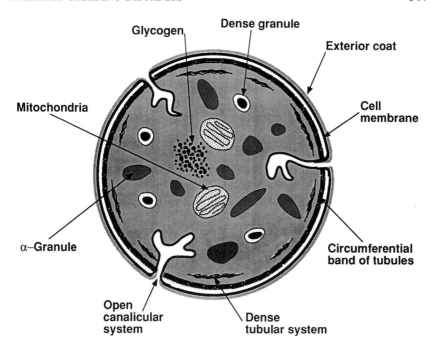

Figure 6. Ultrastructure of a normal platelet as viewed under electron microscopy. Adapted from White (1987).

a sol–gel zone and an organelle zone. The peripheral zone is made up of an exterior coat or glycocalyx, a lipoprotein membrane and a submembrane region that contains a regular system of filamentous elements. The platelet membrane glycoproteins (Ia, Ib, Ic, IIa, IIb, III, IV, V and IX) are located in the exterior coat. The sol–gel zone or cytoskeleton contains submembrane filaments, the circumferential band of microtubules located just beneath the cell membrane and microfilaments. The organelle zone contains mitochondria, perioxisomes, lysosomes, dense bodies and α-granules. Dense bodies are the storage sites for the non-metabolic pool of adenine nucleotides, adenosine diphosphate (ADP) and adenosine triphosphate (ATP), serotonin and calcium (Ca^{2+}). Alpha-granules contain platelet factor IV (PF4), β-thromboglobulin (β-TG), von Willebrand factor (vWf), thrombospondin, fibronectin, factor V, high molecular weight kininogen (HMWK) and platelet-derived growth factor (PDGF). In addition to the structures described, the platelet contains a complex membrane system. The dense tubular system (DTS) is smooth endoplasmic reticulum and is the site of calcium sequestration and prostaglandin synthesis. The surface-connected open canalicular system (OCS) provides access to the interior of the platelet for plasma constituents and is an egress route for the products of the platelet release reaction (for example ADP and thromboxane A_2).

Physiology of platelet thrombus formation

Following blood vessel injury, platelets rapidly adhere to adhesive glyco-proteins in the exposed subendothelium. In rapidly flowing blood this critical first step in platelet thrombus formation is mediated by interaction of the platelet surface membrane receptor complex GpIb/IX with von Willebrand factor (Weiss et al, 1978; Stel et al, 1985); binding of platelets to fibronectin may also be important under conditions of flow (Houdijk et al, 1985). Following initial interaction of platelets with vWf other adhesive events probably occur; the most important of these appears to be interaction of exposed collagen in the subendothelium with collagen receptors on platelet membrane glycoproteins Ia/IIa and IV (Santoro, 1986; Kunicki et al, 1988; Tandon et al, 1989). Adherence of platelets to exposed subendothelium (platelet adhesion) is associated with platelet activation, and a change in platelet shape from discs to spheres. Activated platelets spread on damaged subendothelium and release the contents of their storage granules to the exterior, a process that results in the activation of additional platelets. Following platelet activation, further growth of the platelet thrombus occurs

Table 5. Classification of the congenital platelet disorders. Modified from Rao (1990).

1. Defects in platelet–agonist interaction (receptor defects)
   1.1   Selective adrenaline defect
   1.2   Selective collagen defect
   1.3   Selective thromboxane A_2 defect

2. Defects in platelet–vessel wall interaction (disorders of adhesion)
   2.1   von Willebrand's disease
   2.2   Bernard–Soulier syndrome

3. Defects in platelet–platelet interaction (disorders of aggregation)
   3.1   Congenital afibrinogenaemia
   3.2   Glanzmann's thrombasthenia

4. Disorders of platelet secretion
   4.1   Storage pool deficiency
       4.1.1   δ-storage pool deficiency
       4.1.2   α-storage pool deficiency (gray platelet syndrome)
       4.1.3   αδ-storage pool deficiency
   4.2   Abnormalities in arachidonic acid pathway
       4.2.1   Impaired liberation of arachidonic acid
       4.2.2   Cyclo-oxygenase deficiency
       4.2.3   Thromboxane synthetase deficiency
   4.3   Primary secretion defect with normal granule stores and normal thromboxane
             synthesis
       4.3.1   Defects in calcium mobilization
       4.3.2   Defects in phosphatidylinositol metabolism
       4.3.3   Defects in myosin phosphorylation

5. Disorders of platelet–coagulant protein interaction
   Defect in factor Va–Xa interaction on platelets

6. Miscellaneous congenital disorders
   May–Hegglin anomaly
   Hermansky–Pudlak syndrome
   Chediak–Higashi syndrome

by cell-to-cell contact, a process known as aggregation. The essential requirement for platelet aggregation is an activation-dependent change in the glycoprotein GPIIb/IIIa complex that allows binding of adhesive proteins, in particular fibrinogen, to platelets.

Platelet activation plays a critical first step in the development of a platelet thrombus. During activation platelets contract and discharge the contents of their storage granules into the exterior; these chemical messengers (for example ADP) activate additional platelets which aggregate to form a platelet thrombus. The biochemistry of platelet activation involves first the interaction of a stimulating molecule (agonist) with a specific cell-surface receptor. The receptor then interacts with one of several coupling proteins in the platelet membrane to activate the enzyme phospholipase C; phospholipase C cleaves phosphatidylinositol or its phosphorylated derivatives to produce diacylglycerol (DGL) and inositol 1,4,5-triphosphate (IP3).

These messengers initiate further intracellular events that result in platelet contraction, shape change and secretion. The release of intracellular Ca^{2+} by IP3 is thought to play an important regulatory role in these events through an effect on a number of important Ca^{2+}-binding proteins including the regulator of myosin light chain kinase, calmodulin, phospholipase A_2 and Ca^{2+}-dependent proteins called calpains; these proteins may be involved in the polymerization of actin and other platelet cytoskeletal proteins.

Current knowledge of the structure and function of platelets can be used to classify the congenital platelet disorders (Table 5).

CONGENITAL PLATELET DISORDERS

Quantitative disorders: Congenital thrombocytopenias

Fanconi's syndrome

Fanconi's syndrome is an autosomal recessive disorder characterized by skeletal abnormalities (absent or hypoplastic thumbs, radial aplasia) renal anomalies, hyperpigmentation, short stature, microcephaly, deafness, strabismus and mental retardation. In chromosome studies peripheral blood lymphocytes show increased breaks. Haematological abnormalities reflect marrow hypoplasia and develop at age 5 to 10 years. A history of thrombocytopenia may preceed the appearance of pancytopenia due to marrow aplasia. Transformation to leukaemia occurs in some cases.

Thrombocytopenia–absent-radius (TAR) syndrome

Characteristic features of the TAR syndrome include bilateral absence of radii associated with thrombocytopenia. The disorder manifests early in infancy and may be fatal in as many as two thirds of cases. After the first year of life, gradual improvement can be expected, and patients with the TAR syndrome do not develop aplastic anaemia or leukaemia. The inheritance of the TAR syndrome is apparently autosomal recessive.

Wiskott–Aldrich syndrome

The Wiskott–Aldrich syndrome is an X-linked recessive disorder character-ized by thrombocytopenia, eczema and increased susceptibility to infection. A characteristic laboratory finding is the presence of small platelets. Bleeding commonly occurs in the first 6 months of life, and the clinical course of patients with Wiskott–Aldrich syndrome is often fatal with death due to infection, haemorrhage or lymphoreticular malignancy. Variants of the Wiskott–Aldrich syndrome include X-linked thrombocytopenia with failure to respond to microbial antigens (Cohn et al, 1975), and X-linked thrombocytopenia with no associated abnormalities.

Familial thrombocytopenias

A heterogeneous group of familial thrombocytopenias has been described with either X-linked or autosomal modes of inheritance. In some cases the disorder is associated with nephritis, deafness, large platelets and abnormal platelet forms (Epstein et al, 1972; Najean and Lecompte, 1990).

Qualitative disorders: Congenital disorders of platelet function

Current knowledge of platelet ultrastructure and physiology can be used to classify the congenital disorders of platelet function (Table 5).

Defects in platelet receptor–agonist interaction

Selective impairment in platelet responsiveness to adrenaline. Interaction of platelets with adrenaline is mediated by α_2-adrenergic receptors and results in several responses including exposure of fibrinogen receptors, an increase in intracellular ionized calcium, inhibition of adenylate cyclase activity, and platelet aggregation. Rao et al (1988) have described a family whose members had impaired aggregation and secretion responses only to adrenaline, associated with a decrease in the number of platelet α_2-adrenergic receptors. Three of the family members had a history of easy bruising with minimally prolonged bleeding times. A similar familial adrenaline defect has also been reported by Stormorken et al (1987) and Tamponi et al (1987). Despite these reports, the variability in aggregation response to adrenaline, even in otherwise normal individuals (O'Brien, 1964) indicates that the relationship of the selective adrenaline defect to bleeding manifestations still needs to be defined (Figures, 1986).

Selective impairment in platelet responsiveness to collagen. In 1986 Nieuwen-huis et al reported a patient with a bleeding disorder whose platelets were selectively unresponsive to collagen. The platelets from the patient were deficient in GPIa and the authors concluded that this platelet membrane glycoprotein contained the collagen receptor. Kehrel et al (1988) have reported a similar case in whom platelets responded to collagen only at high concentrations; the platelets of this patient were deficient in GPIa and thrombospondin.

Selective impairment in platelet responsiveness to thromboxane A_2. Although patients have been reported with selective impairment in responses to thromboxane A_2 (Lages et al, 1981; Samama et al, 1981; Wu et al, 1981) the highly unstable nature of this compound and the test systems employed to establish the selective deficiency cast doubt on the diagnosis.

Defects in platelet vessel-wall interaction

von Willebrand's disease. von Willebrand's disease (vWD) is an inherited bleeding disorder that is characterized by an autosomal dominant mode of inheritance, a prolonged bleeding time and mucocutaneous bleeding (reviewed in Berkowitz et al, 1989). The disorder was described by Erik von Willebrand in 1926 following studies in a family from the Finnish island of Foglo in the Åland archipelago (von Willebrand, 1926). vWD is the commonest inherited coagulation disorder with an estimated incidence of 125 per million persons (Holmberg and Nilsson, 1985). This figure may be an underestimate in some population groups; in a study of 1218 children in Northern Italy, Rodeghiero et al (1987) reported an incidence of 0.82%.

The primary defect in von Willebrand's disease is a quantitative or qualitative abnormality in von Willebrand factor (vWf), a large adhesive glycoprotein. Factor VIIIC circulates in plasma non-covalently bound to vWf. In its complexed form factor VIIIC is protected from rapid destruction. vWf plays a critical role in haemostasis by mediating adhesion of platelets to exposed subendothelium at sites of vessel injury. This key function of vWf involves the binding of this adhesive glycoprotein to a specific receptor on platelet membrane GPIb/IX (DeGroot and Sixma, 1987).

vWf is synthesized in endothelial cells where it is stored in Weibel–Palade bodies and in megakaryocytes. Synthesis of mature high-molecular weight vWf multimers, essential for haemostasis, involves first dimerization and subsequently multimerization of the basic 225 kD vWf subunit. Normal plasma contains an extremely wide range of vWf multimers ranging in molecular weight from 400 000 to more than 20 million D. The multimeric structure of vWf has been used to classify vWD into three basic types: I, II and III (Table 6).

Type I vWD accounts for approximately 80% of all cases (Table 7) and is characterized by a reduction in the amount of vWf; however, the full range of vWf multimers is present including the high molecular weight forms. Most type I cases present with reduced plasma levels of vWf, usually between 5 and 30%, and correspondingly low levels of ristocetin cofactor activity (functional vWf is required to promote the agglutination of platelets in the presence of the negatively charged antibiotic ristocetin). Factor VIIIC levels are characteristically decreased in proportion to the decrease in vWf. When factor VIIIC levels are low, bleeding is due to insufficient amounts of both circulating vWf and factor VIIIC. Bleeding manifestations in type I patients are more severe in those individuals who have reduced levels of platelet vWf (Gralnick et al, 1986).

Type II variants account for approximately 15% of cases and are characterized by a decrease or absence of large vWf multimers. A number of

Table 6. Classification of von Willebrand's disease. Modified from Berkowitz (1989).

Subtype	Features	Comments	Reference
Type I			
Platelet normal	Normal platelet vWf and ristocetin cofactor	Good haemostatic response to DDAVP	Mannucci et al (1985)
Platelet low	Decreased platelet vWf and ristocetin cofactor	Poor haemostatic response to DDAVP	Mannucci et al (1985)
Platelet discordant	Normal platelet vWf and decreased ristocetin cofactor	Poor haemostatic response to DDAVP	Mannucci et al (1985)
I, New York	Enhanced responsiveness to low concentrations of ristocetin; all vWf multimers present in plasma		Weiss (1986)
Type II			
IIA	Large and intermediate multimers absent in plasma and platelets	Increased proteolysis of vWf; variable response to DDAVP	Ruggeri & Zimmerman (1980)
IIB	Enhanced responsiveness to low concentrations of ristocetin; large vWf multimers absent in plasma present in platelets	Increased proteolysis of vWf; thrombocytopenia following DDAVP; few cases show recessive inheritance	Ruggeri et al (1980)
IIC	Large vWf multimers are absent; unique structural abnormality of multimers	Decreased proteolysis of vWf; recessive inheritance	Ruggeri et al (1982); Mannucci et al (1983)
IID	Large vWf multimers are absent; unique structural abnormality of individual multimers	Decreased proteolysis of vWf	Kinoshita et al (1984) Hill et al (1985)
IIE	Large vWf multimers are markedly decreased; unique structural abnormality of individual multimers	Decreased proteolysis of vWf	Zimmerman TS et al (1986)
IIF	Large vWf multimers are absent in plasma but present in platelets. Unique structural abnormality of individual multimers		Mannucci (1986a)
IIG	Unique structural abnormality of individual vWf multimers	Possible dominant inheritance	Gralnick et al (1987)
IIH	Unique structural abnormality of individual vWf multimers	Recessive inheritance	Mannucci (1986b)
Type III	Very low or undetectable levels of vWf, VIIIC and ristocetin cofactor Platelet vWf markedly decreased	Recessive inheritance	Zimmerman TS et al (1979)

Table 7. von Willebrand's disease (vWD) subtypes in a paediatric cohort.*

	Number of cases	%
Type I	42	75.0
Type II	11	19.6
Type III	3	5.4
	56	100.0

* Children ≤18 years of age followed by the haematology service, The Hospital for Sick Children, Toronto.

variants have been reported (Table 6). Subunit analysis of type II vWD patients has shown that proteolysis may be increased (types IIA and IIB) decreased (types IIE, IIF and IIH) or undetectable (types IIC and IID). Alteration in proteolysis of vWf multimers in type II vWD patients is a reflection of intrinsic abnormalities of the vWf molecule. The pathogenesis of bleeding in all type II variants is thought to be related to the reduction in concentration or absence of large vWf multimers (Figure 7). Bleeding may be more severe in patients who have decreased concentrations of both factor VIIIC and vWf.

Type III von Willebrand's disease is the least common of the three vWD types, but is the most severe. In some populations a relatively high frequency of type III vWD has been reported (Berlinger et al, 1986). Affected individuals are likely to present with major bleeding episodes early in life. Characteristic laboratory features included marked reduction in the level of vWf, ristocetin cofactor activity and factor VIIIC. Platelet vWf is markedly diminished, and the bleeding time is usually greater than 30 minutes. The inheritance pattern is typically recessive and affected individuals may be either homozygous or doubly heterozygous for the vWf defect (Figure 8).

Laboratory abnormalities in patients with type I vWD may be minimal and may vary both in affected individuals over time and between family members of an affected kindred (Abildgaard et al, 1980). Documentation of a reduction in the level of circulating vWf plus one other laboratory abnormality (a reduced ristocetin cofactor activity, a decrease in the level of factor VIIIC or a prolonged bleeding time) can be taken as evidence for a diagnosis of vWD. Repeat testing may be required to confidently diagnose vWD. The diagnosis of type II and III vWD variants is generally not difficult since these variants have characteristic laboratory features: reduction or absence of high molecular weight multimers in type II variants (Figure 7) and marked reduction in vWf, ristocetin cofactor activity and factor VIIIC in type III cases (Figure 8). Enhanced platelet aggregation at low levels of ristocetin is typical of type IIB von Willebrand's disease. This pattern of response also occurs in a rare type I variant—type I New York (Weiss and Sussman, 1986a). This disorder must be differentiated from pseudo-von Willebrand's disease in which a heightened affinity of platelets for normal vWf, and not a heightened vWf-platelet interaction due to an abnormal vWf, results in absence of the largest vWf multimers (Miller and Castella, 1982). In both conditions thrombocytopenia may be present.

The severity of bleeding in patients with vWD also varies considerably from affected individual to affected individual but is most severe in those patients with the most severe quantitative defect (type III cases). In such cases symptoms similar to those seen in haemophilic patients, including haemarthroses and muscular haematoma may develop. Individuals who make functionally abnormal vWf (type II variants) may have significant bleeding symptoms in spite of normal quantities of plasma vWf and may manifest symptoms comparable to the severity of bleeding seen in cases with type III (severe) vWD. In the majority of patients with vWD, however the abnormality is a mild or moderate quantitative defect of normal vWf (type I vWD) and bleeding manifestations are minimal or absent. The most common symptoms in such cases are easy bruising and bleeding from mucous membranes (epistaxis and menorrhagia). Excessive blood loss following dental extraction or other surgical procedures may occur, but is neither inevitable nor reproducible in any given patient with type I vWD.

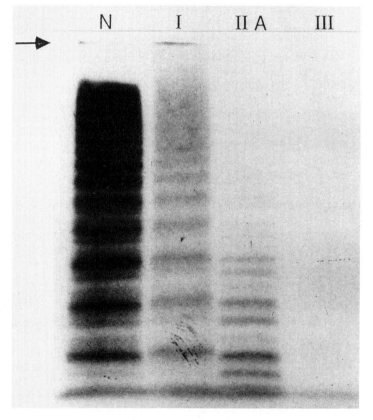

Figure 7. High resolution gel multimer pattern of plasma vWf from a normal subject (N), and patients with types I, IIA and III vWD. Note the repeating triplet patterns in normal plasma.

Finally, gastrointestinal bleeding has been reported in a subset of patients with vWD. These patients bleed profusely from the intestinal mucosa without an obvious source. In some cases the coexistence of vWD and hereditary haemorrhagic telangiectasia or angiodysplastic lesions have been reported (Quick, 1967; Conlon et al, 1973; Ramsay et al, 1976; Ahr et al, 1977). Episodes of gastrointestinal bleeding are often recurrent and in some patients are difficult to treat.

Bernard–Soulier syndrome. In 1948 Bernard and Soulier described a 5-month old infant who suffered recurrent episodes of spontaneous bleeding. The patient had a prolonged bleeding time and his platelets appeared large on a peripheral blood smear. A number of similar patients were subsequently described (Howard et al, 1973; Evensen et al, 1974; Caen et al, 1976; George et al, 1981). The disorder, now known as Bernard–Soulier syndrome, is transmitted in an autosomal recessive manner. Affected patients experience mucocutaneous bleeding, purpura, epistaxis, gingival bleeding, menorrhagia, gastrointestinal haemorrhage and haematuria. Bleeding into joints or muscles does not occur. The primary defect in patients with the Bernard–Soulier syndrome is a deficiency in the platelet membrane glycoprotein, GPIb

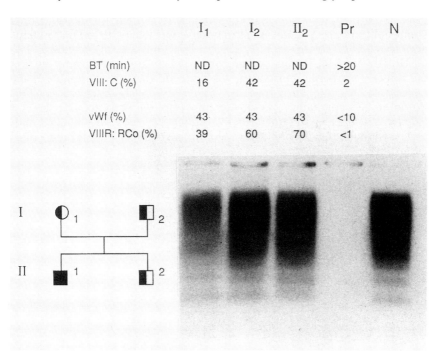

	I_1	I_2	II_2	Pr	N
BT (min)	ND	ND	ND	>20	
VIII: C (%)	16	42	42	2	
vWf (%)	43	43	43	<10	
VIIIR: RCo (%)	39	60	70	<1	

Figure 8. Low resolution gel analysis of a family with Type III vWD. Plasma from the propositus (Pr, II_1) shows a total absence of multimers. All multimeric forms were present in plasma samples from the parents and a brother of the propositus (I_1, I_2 and II_2). A normal plasma control (N) is shown on the extreme right of the gel. BT, bleeding time; VIII: C, coagulation factor VIII; vWf, von Willebrand factor; VIIIR: RCo, ristocetin cofactor.

(Nurden and Caen, 1975); GPIX and GPV have also been found to be deficient in affected patients (Berndt et al, 1983; Clemetson et al, 1982). The haemorrhagic disorder in patients with the Bernard–Soulier syndrome is explained by the fact that the α-chain of GPIb contains a specific receptor for vWf; platelets deficient in this glycoprotein fail to bind to vWf in the subendothelial matrix and as a result do not adhere to damaged blood vessels under conditions of flow. Platelets from patients with Bernard–Soulier disease aggregate normally in the presence of ADP, collagen and adrenalin, exhibit reduced aggregation responses to low concentrations of thrombin and fail to agglutinate in the presence of autologous plasma and the negatively charged antibiotic ristocetin.

Defects in platelet–platelet interaction

Glanzmann's thrombasthenia. Glanzmann's thrombasthenia was first reported in 1918 (Glanzmann, 1918) and is a hereditary bleeding disorder characterized by a normal platelet count and morphology, a prolonged bleeding time, absent or diminished clot retraction, defective platelet aggregation and an autosomal pattern of inheritance (Hardisty et al, 1964; Weiss and Kochwa, 1968; Coller et al, 1986). The biochemical defect in patients with Glanzmann's thrombasthenia is a reduction or functional abnormality in the platelet membrane glycoprotein, GPIIb/IIIa (Phillips and Agin, 1977; Nurden et al, 1985, 1987; Ginsberg et al, 1986). The GPIIb/IIIa complex mediates aggregation of activated platelets by binding the adhesive proteins fibrinogen, vWf and fibronectin. Thrombasthenic platelets fail to aggregate in response to physiological agonists such as ADP, thrombin and adrenalin; they do agglutinate in the presence of ristocetin (Figure 9). Thrombasthenic platelets attach normally to damaged sub-endothelium but fail to spread normally and do not form platelet aggregates (Weiss et al, 1986).

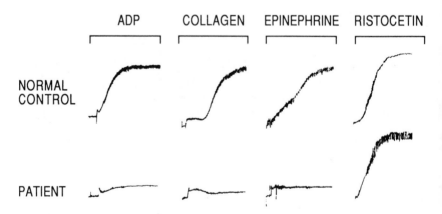

Figure 9. Platelet aggregation studies in a patient with Glanzmann's thrombasthenia showing absent responses to ADP, collagen and adrenalin (epinephrine) and a normal response to ristocetin.

Disorders of platelet secretion

δ-*Storage pool deficiency.* Storage pool disease (SPD) includes patients with deficiencies of dense granules (δ-SDP), α-granules (α-SDP) or both types of granules (αδ-SDP). δ-storage pool deficiency was first reported by Weiss et al (1969). Subsequent reports indicated that the total ATP and ADP platelet granule content in patients with δ-SDP was decreased (Holmsen and Weiss, 1972) as were other dense granule contents: calcium, pyrophosphates and serotonin (Lages et al, 1975). Patients with δ-STP have a mild to moderate bleeding disorder. In platelet aggregation studies of affected patients the second wave of aggregation with ADP and adrenalin is absent and the aggregation response to collagen is either markedly impaired or absent. The response to arachidonic acid is variable. Platelet storage pool deficiency has been reported in patients with prolonged bleeding times and normal platelet aggregation tests (Nieuwenhuis et al, 1977; Israels et al, 1990). The disorder has also been reported in association with α-granule deficiency (Weiss et al, 1979b) and with other inherited disorders such as the Hermansky–Pudlak syndrome, the Chediak–Higashi syndrome, the Wiskott–Aldrich syndrome and the thrombocytopenia–absent-radius (TAR) syndrome.

α-*Granule storage pool deficiency.* The term 'gray platelet' describes the morphological appearance of platelets in Romanovsky-stained peripheral blood smears prepared from patients with deficiency of α-granules. Platelets from these patients contain absent or markedly reduced α-granule proteins: PF4, βTG, vWf, thrombospondin, fibronectin, factor V, high molecular weight kininogen and platelet-derived growth factor. Affected patients have

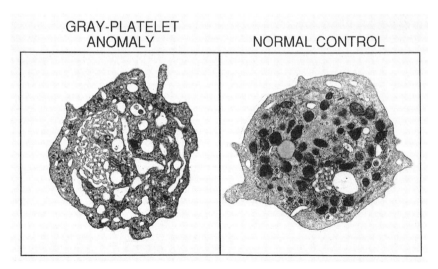

GRAY-PLATELET
ANOMALY   NORMAL CONTROL

Figure 10. Electron micrograph appearance of platelets from a patient with the gray platelet syndrome showing a virtual absence of α-granules. A normal platelet is shown for comparison.

mild thrombocytopenia, prolonged bleeding times and a life-long bleeding diathesis (Raccuglia, 1971; White, 1979; Gerrard et al, 1980; Levy-Toladano et al, 1981). The most consistent laboratory abnormality has been impairment in thrombin-mediated aggregation and secretion; aggregation responses to collagen and ADP are variable. Electron microscopy studies reveal virtual absence of alpha granules (Figure 10).

Abnormalities in platelet arachidonic acid pathways

Impaired liberation of arachidonic acid. A major response of platelets during activation is the release of arachidonic acid from membrane-bound phospholipids and its subsequent oxygenation to thromboxane A_2. Thromboxane A_2 forms an important positive feedback that enhances platelet activation. Rao et al (1984) have described four patients with platelet secretion defects associated with impaired liberation of arachidonic acid. They postulated that the impaired arachidonic acid liberation was secondary to a defect in Ca^{2+} mobilization that resulted in diminished activity of the Ca^{2+}-dependent enzyme phospholipase A_2, an enzyme that is involved in the release of arachidonic acid following thrombin stimulation of platelets.

Cyclo-oxygenase and thromboxane synthetase deficiency. Defects in thromboxane A_2 due to deficiencies of cyclo-oxygenase and thromboxane synthetase have been reported (Lagarde et al, 1978; Mestel et al, 1980; Pareti et al, 1980; Rak and Boda, 1980; Defreyn et al, 1981; Roth and Machuga, 1982; Horellou et al, 1983).

Platelet secretion defects with normal granule stores and normal thromboxane synthesis

Several studies have identified patients with a mild bleeding diathesis whose platelets have normal granule stores and normal thromboxane A_2 synthesis during stimulation (Rao et al, 1982; Lages and Weiss, 1988). This category also includes patients with the behavioural attention defect disorder (ADD) or minimal brain damage syndrome and easy bruising (Koike et al, 1984). Many affected patients have abnormalities in the aggregation and secretion responses to weak agonists (ADP, adrenalin) but not to relatively stronger agonists such as arachidonic acid or higher concentrations of collagen. The mechanism underlying the platelet dysfunction in these cases is unknown although defects in Ca^{2+} mobilization have been suggested. Platelet secretion defects with normal granule stores and normal thromboxane synthesis constitute the largest fraction of individuals diagnosed to have congenital platelet secretion defects and outnumber those with storage pool disease or defects in thromboxane A_2 synthetase.

Defects in Ca^{2+} mobilization. A number of key platelet processes are Ca^{2+}-dependent (for example the liberation of arachidonic acid and phosphorylation of myosin light chain). Patients with deficient Ca^{2+} mobilization have been reported (Hardisty et al, 1983; Rao et al, 1989).

Deficiency of platelet procoagulant activity

Platelets contain several coagulation factors in their granules and provide negatively charged lipid surfaces on which a number of key coagulation enzymatic reactions proceed (Walsh, 1985). Platelet factor 3 reflects the contribution of platelets to the interaction of factors Xa, V and Ca^{2+} in prothrombin activation. Isolated deficiency of platelet factor 3 has been reported (Girolami, 1973; Sultan et al, 1976; Weiss, 1979a). Detailed studies in one of these patients revealed a decreased binding of factor Xa by platelets due to a deficiency of factor Va binding sites on the platelet surface (Miletich et al, 1979).

Miscellaneous congenital platelet disorders

Hermansky–Pudlak syndrome

The Hermansky–Pudlak syndrome is a recessively inherited autosomal disorder characterized by oculocutaneous albinism, accumulation of ceroid-like material in reticuloendothelial cells of bone marrow and other tissues, and a haemorrhagic diathesis due to defective platelets (Hermansky and Pudlak, 1959). Dense bodies are reduced or virtually absent. Platelets from patients with Hermansky–Pudlak syndrome contain very low levels of serotonin, adenine nucleotides and Ca^{2+} (Weiss et al, 1974). As a result, platelets of affected patients do not secrete adequate amounts of these messengers and fail to develop secondary waves of aggregation when exposed to concentrations of ADP, adrenalin and thrombin that cause irreversible clumping of normal cells.

Chediak–Higashi syndrome

The Chediak–Higashi syndrome is a rare, autosomally-inherited disorder characterized by photophobia, nystagmus, pseudoalbinism, marked suscep-tibility to infection, hepatosplenomegaly, lymphadenopathy and early death. Platelets from patients with the Chediak–Higashi syndrome may be deficient in dense bodies and may contain the giant granule anomaly (White, 1976). Thrombocytopenia is common and is the chief cause of bleeding.

May–Hegglin anomaly

The May–Hegglin anomaly is characterized by the presence of giant platelets, thrombocytopenia (present in approximately one-third of cases) and basophilic granulocyte inclusions (Döhle bodies) in leukocytes. Platelets from affected individuals may contain giant granules (White, 1976; Hamilton et al, 1980). Some patients with this disorder have platelet function abnormalities (Lusher et al, 1968). The disorder is inherited in an autosomal dominant fashion and the majority of affected individuals do not have a significant bleeding disorder.

Miscellaneous

Platelet function abnormalities have also been reported in a number of miscellaneous congenital disorders including the Wiskott–Aldrich syndrome; the thrombocytopenia–absent-radius (TAR) syndrome; Epstein's syndrome (characterized by hereditary nephritis, thrombocytopenia and nerve deafness); hexokinase deficiency; glucose-6-phosphatase deficiency (type I glycogen storage disease); and a number of connective tissue disorders including osteogenesis imperfecta, Ehlers–Danlos syndrome and Marfan's syndrome.

LABORATORY EVALUATION OF PATIENTS WITH SUSPECTED CONGENITAL PLATELET DISORDERS

An abnormality of platelets, either quantitative or qualitative, should be suspected in patients with significant mucocutaneous bleeding: excessive bruising, epistaxis and menorrhagia. Muscle haematoma and haemarthroses are not characteristic of 'platelet bleeding' and suggest a defect in the coagulation system. Initial laboratory studies should include determination of the circulating platelet count and a careful examination of a well-stained blood smear to assess platelet size and presence of inclusion bodies. Studies to confirm or exclude a diagnosis of von Willebrand's disease should be performed and include a skin bleeding time, measurement of factors VIIIC, von Willebrand factor, ristocetin cofactor and an assessment of the multi-meric structure of plasma von Willebrand factor. In some cases these coagulation studies may need to be repeated several times before a diagnosis of vWD can be confidently excluded (Abildgaard et al, 1980). If these tests are not diagnostic or suggestive of a specific abnormality, platelet aggregation studies using standard agonists should be performed and platelet ultra-structure evaluated by electron microscopy. The results of these tests often define a subset of patients in whom further specialized testing is appropriate. Such testing may involve a biochemical study of the platelet-membrane glycoproteins and assessment of the complex sequence of intracellular events that lead to platelet activation, shape change and aggregation (for example assessment of calcium mobilization). These tests are generally available only in specialized reference laboratories. As in all congenital disorders a detailed family history plus a study of family members may be useful.

MANAGEMENT OF PATIENTS WITH CONGENITAL PLATELET DISORDERS

Management of patients with congenital platelet disorders depends on the nature of the abnormality and the clinical circumstance for which treatment is required. In patients with significant thrombocytopenia (platelet count $\leq 20 \times 10^9$ litre^{-1}), transfusion therapy using donor platelets is often indicated to either prevent or stop bleeding. In the patient who is not actively bleeding, and in whom an invasive procedure is not planned, life-threatening haemorrhage is unlikely if the circulating platelet count is $\geq 20 \times 10^9$ litre^{-1}. In most centres, prophylactic platelet transfusions are not given to such patients. This practice reflects the real risk of alloimmunization following repeated transfusion of pooled random donor platelets and the development of clinical refractoriness to such products. Prevention of allo-immunization may be possible through use of platelets that have been significantly depleted of contaminating leukocytes, or products that have been treated with ultraviolet-B irradiation to inactivate the antigen-presenting cells that are critical to the development of platelet allo-immunization. Once immunized, effective platelet support requires the infusion of compatible platelets selected by HLA typing and/or platelet cross-matching.

Many patients with platelet function disorders have a mild bleeding diethesis and require no therapy. If therapy is required, consideration should be given to use of DDAVP (Kobrinsky et al, 1984; Nieuwenhuis and Sixma, 1988). If platelet transfusion therapy is required to prevent or stop severe or life-threatening bleeding (for example in patients with the homozygous forms of Bernard–Soulier syndrome or Glanzmann's thrombasthenia), use of leukocyte-depleted single donor plateletpheresis concentrates should be considered to minimize the risk of platelet allo-immunization and the development of a platelet refractory state.

Management of patients with von Willebrand's disease requires knowledge of the patient's vWD subtype plus consideration of the clinical circumstance for which treatment is required. Most patients with type I vWD have a mild bleeding diethesis and require no treatment for control or prevention of bleeding; if therapy is required, DDAVP should be considered (Warrier and Lusher, 1983; de la Fuente de al, 1985; Mannucci, 1986). DDAVP is contraindicated in patients with type IIB vWD (because of the risk of thrombocytopenia) and is of no value in patients with severe type III vWD. In such cases effective treatment requires infusion of cryoprecipitate or a factor concentrate known to be effective in management of patients with vWD (Fukui et al, 1988; Berntorp and Nilsson, 1989; Cumming et al, 1990; Pasi et al, 1990).

DISORDERS OF BLOOD VESSELS

Hereditary haemorrhagic telangiectasia (Osler–Weber–Rendu disease)

Hereditary haemorrhagic telangiectasia is the most common of the inherited vascular disorders (Osler, 1901). The disease is inherited as an autosomal dominant trait and bleeding occurs from vascular lesions on the skin or mucous membranes. Lesions consist of dilated arterioles and capillaries lined by a thin endothelial layer. They are typical in appearance: 1–3 mm in diameter, flat, round, red or violet in colour, and they blanche on pressure. Histology of the abnormal vessels shows deficiency of supporting elastic fibres. Typical lesions occur most often on the nasal mucosa; lesions may also be present on the lips, oral mucosa, tongue, face, hands, oesophagus, stomach, rectum and, rarely, in the respiratory, gynaecological and urinary tracts. Epistaxis is the most common symptom and hypochromic anaemia secondary to occult bleeding from the gastrointestinal tract occasionally occurs.

Hereditary connective tissue disorders

Ehlers–Danlos syndrome

The Ehlers–Danlos syndrome is an uncommon disorder of connective tissues characterized by hyperextensible skin, hypermobile joints, fragile tissues and a bleeding tendency, mainly subcutaneous haematoma. There is a tendency for the skin to be easily broken and then to heal in paper-thin connective tissue scars. The bleeding disorder may be severe, and affected individuals may present with easy bruising, bleeding from gums after dental extraction, gastrointestinal bleeding and haemarthroses. Rupture of major arteries may occur in type IV (ecchymotic) Ehlers–Danlos syndrome. This disorder is associated with decreased levels of type III collagen which predominates in blood vessels and the gastrointestinal tract.

Pseudoxanthoma elasticum

This is a rare disorder of elastic tissues that is inherited as an autosomal trait. A characteristic feature of severely affected individuals is the presence of redundant folds of skin in the neck, face and axilla and inguinal regions. Spontaneous haemorrhage resulting from defective vessels may occur into the skin, eyes, kidney, joints, uterus and gastrointestinal tract. The common causes of death are subarachnoid and gastrointestinal haemorrhage.

Marfan's syndrome

Marfan's syndrome is characterized by skeletal abnormalities (arachnodactyly), long limbs, cardiovascular abnormalities (aortic wall defects) and dislocation of the lens (Pyeritz and McKusick, 1979). The syndrome is transmitted as an autosomal dominant trait. Affected individuals experience easy bruising and may bleed excessively at surgery.

Osteogenesis imperfecta

The defect is transmitted as an autosomal dominant trait and presents with brittleness of bones. Occasionally patients have a bleeding disorder which presents with bruising, epistaxis, haemoptysis and intracranial haemorrhage. The basic abnormality seems to be a defect in the amino acid composition of collagen fibres.

SUMMARY

Congenital bleeding disorders comprise a heterogeneous group of diseases that reflect abnormalities of blood vessels, coagulation proteins and platelets. Studies of these diseases, many of which are rare and several of which result in a mild bleeding diathesis only, have significantly increased our understanding of normal haemostasis. Two lessons have been learned. First, quantitative abnormalities of coagulation proteins and platelets are an important, but not the only, cause of significant haemorrhage; some cases of inherited bleeding disorders reflect synthesis of a dysfunctional coagulation protein or production of abnormal platelets. Diagnostic tests that reflect qualitative abnormalities are therefore important in the evaluation of selected patients with inherited bleeding disorders. Second, in occasional patients the inherited disorder is complex and reflects combined abnormalities of coagulation proteins alone or in association with platelet disorders.

In clinical practice it is useful to distinguish disorders that cause significant clinical bleeding from those that cause few or no symptoms. Examples of the former include severe deficiencies of factors VIII and IX, and the homozygous forms of factor II, V, VII, X, XI, XIII, fibrinogen and von Willebrand factor. Comparable platelet disorders include the inherited thrombocytopenias with platelet counts $< 20 \times 10^9$ litre^{-1} and the homozygous forms of Bernard–Soulier syndrome and Glanzmann's thrombasthenia. The most frequently encountered mild haemostatic abnormalities include type I von Willebrand's disease, the platelet storage pool deficiency syndromes and the mild and moderate forms of haemophilia A and B; occasionally heterozygous or homozygous forms of the rarer coagulation disorders, e.g. factor XI deficiency, may present with a mild bleeding diathesis. Finally, some disorders are entirely asymptomatic, e.g. factor XII deficiency and deficiencies of other contact coagulation factors.

Management of patients with inherited bleeding disorders should reflect knowledge of the specific disorder to be treated plus careful consideration of the clinical circumstance for which therapy is proposed. In all cases, once a decision to treat has been made, the safest efficacious therapy should be given (for example DDAVP in the treatment of patients with mild haemophilia A or type I von Willebrand's disease). Although blood products are now much safer and the risk of blood transmitted viral infections is low, there still remains a risk that transfusion of any blood product may be associated with serious side-effects. As a result, therapy should be given only after careful consideration of the risk: benefit ratio and not merely to treat an abnormal laboratory result. Finally, medications that are known to affect platelet function (George and Shattil, 1991) should be avoided, wherever possible, in individuals with known bleeding disorders.

Acknowledgement

The author is indebted to Nancy Fair for her patience and excellent secretarial assistance during preparation of this manuscript.

REFERENCES

Abildgaard CF & Harrison J (1974) Fletcher factor deficiency: family study and detection. *Blood* 43: 641–644.

Abildgaard CF, Suzuki Z, Harrison J et al (1980) Serial studies in von Willebrand's disease: variability versus 'variants'. *Blood* 56: 712–715.

Aggeler PM, White SG, Glendening MB et al (1952) Plasma thromboplastin component (PTC) deficiency: a new disease resembling hemophilia. *Proceedings of the Society for Experimental Biology and Medicine* 79: 692–694.

Ahr DJ, Rickles FR, Hoyer LW et al (1977) von Willebrand's disease and hemorrhagic telangiectasia. Association of two complex disorders of hemostasis resulting in life-threatening hemorrhage. *American Journal of Medicine* 62: 452–458.

Alexander B, Goldstein R, Landwehr G & Cook CD (1951) Congenital SPCA deficiency: a hitherto unrecognised coagulation defect with hemorrhage rectified by serum and serum fractions. *Journal of Clinical Investigation* 30: 596–608.

Aoki N, Saito H, Kamiya T et al (1979) Congenital deficiency of α_2-plasmin inhibitor associated with severe hemorrhagic tendency. *Journal of Clinical Investigation* 63: 877–884.

Berkowitz SD, Ruggeri ZM & Zimmerman TS (1989) von Willebrand's disease. In Zimmerman TS & Ruggeri ZM (eds) *Coagulation and Bleeding Disorders. The Role of Factor VIII and von Willebrand factor*, pp 215–259. New York: Marcel Dekker.

Berlinger SA, Seligsohn U, Zivelin A et al (1986) A relatively high frequency of severe (type III) von Willebrand's disease in Israel. *British Journal of Haematology* 62: 535–543.

Bernard J & Soulier JP (1948) Sur une nouvelle variété de dystrophie thrombocytaire hemorragipare congenitale. *Semaine des Hopitaux Paris* 24: 3217–3223.

Berndt MC, Gregory C, Chong BH et al (1983) Additional glycoprotein defects in Bernard–Soulier's Syndrome: confirmation of genetic basis by parental analysis. *Blood* 62: 800–807.

Berntorp E & Nilsson IM (1989) Use of a high-purity factor VIII concentrate (Hemate P) in von Willebrand's Disease. *Vox Sanguinis* 56: 212–217.

Bertina RM (1987) Factor IX variants. In Bloom AL & Thomas DP (eds) *Haemostasis and Thrombosis*, pp 437–441. London: Churchill Livingstone.

Bezeaud A, Guillin MC, Olmeda F, Quintana M & Gomez N (1979) Prothrombin Madrid: a new familial abnormality of prothrombin. *Thrombosis Research* 16: 47–58.

Bezeaud A, Drouet I, Soria C & Guillin MC (1984) Prothrombin Salakta: an abnormal prothrombin characterised by a defect in the active site of thrombin. *Thrombosis Research* 34: 507–518.

Biggs R, Douglas AS, MacFarlane RG et al (1952) Christmas disease: a condition previously mistaken for haemophilia. *British Medical Journal* 2: 1378–1382.

Blanchette V, Doyle J & Andrew M (1990) Haematological investigation in neonates. In Advancing Haematological Techniques. I. Cavill (ed.) *Baillière's Clinical Haematology* 2: 1019–1054.

Bloom AL (1987) Inherited disorders of blood coagulation. In Bloom AL & Thomas DP (eds) *Haemostasis and Thrombosis*, pp 393–436. London: Churchill Livingstone.

Board PG & Shaw DC (1983) Determination of the aminoacid substitution in human prothrombin type 3 (157 Glu→Lys) and the localisation of a third thrombin cleavage site. *British Journal of Haematology* 54: 245–254.

Board PG, Coggan M & Pidcock ME (1982) Genetic heterogeneity of human prothrombin (FII). *Annals of Human Genetics* 46: 1–9.

Bolton-Maggs PHB, Wan-Yin BY, McCraw AH et al (1988) Inheritance of bleeding in factor XI deficiency. *British Journal of Haematology* 69: 521–528.

Bray GL (1990) Recent advances in the preparation of plasma-derived and recombinant coagulation factor VIII. *Journal of Pediatrics* 117: 503–507.

Brettler DB & Levine PH (1989) Factor concentrates for the treatment of hemophilia: which one to choose? *Blood* 73: 2067–2073.

Briët E, Loeliger EA, van Tilburg NH & Veltkamp JJ (1976) Molecular variant of factor VII. *Thrombosis and Haemostasis* 35: 289–294.

Britten AFH (1967) Congenital deficiency of factor XIII (fibrin-stabilising factor): report of a case and review of the literature. *American Journal of Medicine* 43: 751–761.

Caen JP, Nurden AT, Jeannaeu C et al (1976) Bernard–Soulier syndrome: a new platelet glycoprotein abnormality. Its relationship with platelet adhesion to subendothelium and with the Factor VIII von Willebrand protein. *Journal of Laboratory and Clinical Medicine* **87:** 586–596.

Cash JD (1987) Blood replacement therapy. In Bloom AL & Thomas DP (eds) *Haemostasis and Thrombosis*, pp 585–606. London: Churchill Livingstone.

Clemetson KJ, McGregor JL, James E et al (1982) Characterization of the platelet membrane glycoprotein abnormalities in Bernard–Soulier syndrome and comparison with normal by surface-labeling techniques and high-resolution two-dimensional gel electrophoresis. *Journal of Clinical Investigation* **70:** 304–311.

Cohn J, Hauge M, Andersen V et al (1975) Sex-linked hereditary thrombocytopenia with immunological defects. *Human Heredity* **25:** 309–317.

Coller BS, Seligsohn U, Zivelin A et al (1986) Immunologic and biochemical characterization of homozygous and heterozygous Glanzmann thrombasthenia in the Iraqi-Jewish and Arab populations of Israel: comparison of techniques for carrier detection. *British Journal of Haematology* **62:** 723–735.

Colman LW, Bagdasarian A, Talamo RC et al (1975) Williams trait: human kininogen deficiency with diminished levels of plasminogen proactivator and prekallikrein associated with abnormalities of the Hageman factor-dependent pathways. *Journal of Clinical Investigation* **56:** 1650–1662.

Conlon CL, Weinger RS, Cimo PL et al (1973) Telangiectasia and von Willebrand's disease in two families. *Annals of Internal Medicine* **89:** 921–924.

Cumming AM, Fildes S, Cumming IR et al (1990) Clinical and laboratory evaluation of National Health Service factor VIII concentrate (8Y) for the treatment of von Willebrand's disease. *British Journal of Haematology* **75:** 234–239.

Daly HM & Haddon ME (1988) Clinical experience with a pasteurised human plasma concentrate in factor XIII deficiency. *Thrombosis and Haemostasis* **59:** 171–174.

Defreyn G, Machin SJ, Carreras LO et al (1981) Familial bleeding tendency with partial platelet thromboxane synthetase deficiency: reorientation of cyclic endoperoxide metabolism. *British Journal of Haematology* **49:** 29–41.

DeGroot PG & Sixma JJ (1987) Role of von Willebrand factor in the vessel wall. *Seminars in Thrombosis and Haemostasis* **13:** 416–424.

de la Fuente B, Kasper CK, Rickles FR & Hoyer LW (1985) Response of patients with mild and moderate hemophilia A and von Willebrand's disease to treatment with Desmopressin. *Annals of Internal Medicine* **103:** 6–14.

Denson KWE, Lurie A, De Cataldo F & Mannucci PM (1970) The factor-X defect: recognition of abnormal forms of factor X. *British Journal of Haematology* **18:** 317–327.

Denson KWE, Conrad J & Samama M (1972) Genetic variants of factor VII. *Lancet* **i:** 1234.

Donner M, Holmberg L & Nilsson IM (1987) Type IIB von Willebrand's disease with probable autosomal recessive inheritance and presenting as thrombocytopenia in infancy. *British Journal of Haematology* **66:** 349–354.

Duckert F, Jung E & Schmerling DH (1960) A hitherto undescribed congenital haemorrhagic diathesis probably due to fibrin-stabilizing factor deficiency. *Thrombosis et Diathesis Haemorrhagica* **5:** 179–186.

Dyerberg J & Stoffersen E (1980) Recurrent thrombosis in a patient with factor XIII deficiency. *Acta Haematologica* **63:** 278–282.

Eastman JR, Triplett DA & Nowakowski AR (1983) Inherited factor X deficiency. Presentation of a case with etiologic and treatment considerations. *Oral Surgery* **56:** 461–466.

Endo Y (1981) Congenital factor X deficiency and incomplete transverse paralysis. *Journal of the American Medical Association* **246:** 1708.

Epstein CJ, Shud MA, Piel CF et al (1972) Hereditary macrothrombocytopathia nephritis and deafness. *American Journal of Medicine* **52:** 299–310.

Evensen SA, Solum NO, Grothium KA et al (1974) Familial bleeding disorder with a moderate thrombocytopenia and giant blood platelets. *Scandinavian Journal of Haematology* **13:** 203–214.

Fair DS, Plow EF & Edgington TS (1979) Combined functional and immunochemical analysis of normal and abnormal human factor X. *Journal of Clinical Investigation* **64:** 884–894.

Figures WR, Scearce LM, Wachtfogel Y et al (1986) Platelet ADP receptor and $alpha_2$-adrenoreceptor interaction: Evidence for an ADP requirement for epinephrine-induced platelet activation and an influence of epinephrine on ADP binding. *Journal of Biological Chemistry* **261:** 5981–5986.

Forbes CD, Barr RD, Reid G et al (1972) Tranexamic acid in control of haemorrhage after dental extraction in haemophilia and Christmas disease. *British Medical Journal* **2:** 311–313.

Fried K & Kaufman (1980) Congenital afibrinogenaemia in 10 offspring of uncle–nice marriages. *Clinical Genetics* **17:** 223–227.

Fukui H, Nishino M, Terada S et al (1988) Hemostatic effect of a heat-treated factor VIII concentrate (Haemate P) in von Willebrand's disease. *Blut* **56:** 171–178.

George JN & Shattil SJ (1991) Medical Progress: The clinical importance of acquired abnormalities of platelet function. *New England Journal of Medicine* **324:** 27–39.

George JN, Reimann TA, Moake JL et al (1981) Bernard–Soulier disease: a study of four patients and their parents. *British Journal of Haematology* **48:** 459–467.

Gerrard JM, Phillips DR, Rao CHR et al (1980) Biochemical studies of two patients with the gray platelet syndrome. Selective deficiency of platelet alpha granules. *Journal of Clinical Investigation* **66:** 102–109.

Gershwin ME & Gude JK (1973) Deep vein thrombosis and pulmonary embolism in congenital factor VII deficiency. *New England Journal of Medicine* **288:** 141–142.

Gerwitz AM & Hoffman R (1990) Human megakaryocyte production. Cell biology and clinical considerations. *Hematology/Oncology Clinics of North America* **4:** 43–64.

Gill FM, Shapiro SS & Schwartz E (1978) Severe congenital hypoprothrombinemia. *Journal of Pediatrics* **93:** 264–266.

Ginsberg MH, Lightsey A, Kunicki TJ et al (1986) Divalent cation regulation of the surface orientation of platelet membrane glycoprotein IIb. Correlation with fibrinogen binding function and definition of a novel variant of Glanzmann's thrombasthenia. *Journal of Clinical Investigation* **78:** 1103–1111.

Girolami A, Molaro G, Calligaris A & deLuca G (1970a) Severe congenital factor X deficiency in a 5-month-old child. *Thrombosis et Diathesis Haemorrhagica* **24:** 175–184.

Girolami A, Molaro G, Lazzarin M et al (1970b) A 'new' congenital haemorrhagic condition due to the presence of an abnormal factor X (factor X Friuli): Study of a large kindred. *British Journal of Haematology* **19:** 179–192.

Girolami A, Brunetti A, Fioretti D et al (1973) Congenital thrombocytopathy (platelet factor 3 defect) with prolonged bleeding but normal platelet adhesiveness and aggregation. *Acta Haematologica* **50:** 116–123.

Girolami A, Bareggi G, Brunetti A & Sticchi A (1974) Prothrombin Padua: a 'new' congenital dysprothrombinemia. *Journal of Laboratory and Clinical Medicine* **84:** 654–666.

Girolami A, Falezza G, Patrassi G et al (1977) Factor VII Verona coagulation disorder: double heterozygosis with an abnormal factor VII and heterozygous factor VII deficiency. *Blood* **50:** 603–610.

Girolami A, Coccheri S, Palareti G et al (1978a) Prothrombin Molise: a 'new' congenital dysprothrombinemia, double heterozygosis with an abnormal prothrombin and 'true' prothrombin deficiency. *Blood* **52:** 115–125.

Girolami A, Fabris F, Zanon RDB et al (1978b) Factor VII Padua: A congenital coagulation disorder due to an abnormal factor VII with a peculiar activation pattern. *Journal of Laboratory and Clinical Medicine* **91:** 387–395.

Girolami A, Cattarozzi G, Dal Bo Zanon R et al (1979) Factor VII Padua$_2$: Another factor VII abnormality with defective Ox brain thromboplastin activation and a complex hereditary pattern. *Blood* **54:** 46–53.

Girolami A, Luzzatto G, Scattolo N & Zanolli FA (1983) A new family with classical factor X deficiency as demonstrated by electroimmunoassay. *Blut* **47:** 53–57.

Glanzmann E (1918) Hereditare hamorrhagische thrombasthenie: Ein Beitrag zur Pathologie der Blut plattchen. *Jährbuch der Kinderheilkunde* **88:** 1–41.

Godal HC, Madsen K & Nissen-Meyer R (1962) Thromboembolism in patients with total proconvertion (factor VII) deficiency. A report on two cases. *Acta Medica Scandinavia* **171:** 325–327.

Graham JB, Barrow EM & Hougie C (1957) Stuart clotting defect II. Genetic aspects of a new hemorrhagic state. *Journal of Clinical Investigation* **36:** 497–503.

Gralnick HR, Rick ME, McKeown LP et al (1986) Platelet von Willebrand factor: An important determinant of the bleeding time in type I von Willebrand's disease. *Blood* **68:** 58–61.

Gralnick HR, Williams SB, McKeown LP et al (1987) A variety of type II von Willebrand's disease with an abnormal type structure and discordant effects of protease inhibitors on plasma and platelet von Willebrand factor structure. *American Journal of Hematology* **24:** 259–266.

Greene WB & McMillan CW (1982) Surgery for scoliosis in congenital factor VII deficiency. *American Journal of Diseases of Children* **136:** 411–413.

Hamilton RW, Shaikh BS, Ottie JN et al (1980) Platelet function, ultrastructure, and survival in May–Hegglin anomaly. *American Journal of Clinical Pathology* **74:** 663–668.

Hardisty RM, Dormandy KM & Hutton RA (1964) Thrombasthenia. Studies on three cases. *British Journal of Haematology* **10:** 371–387.

Hardisty RM, Machin SJ, Nokes TJC et al (1983) A new congenital defect of platelet secretion: impaired responsiveness of the platelets to cytoplasmic free calcium. *British Journal of Haematology* **53:** 543–557.

Hathaway WE, Belhasen LP & Hathaway HS (1965) Evidence for a new plasma thromboplastin factor I. Case report, coagulation studies and physicochemical properties. *Blood* **26:** 521–532.

Hathaway WE, Christian MJ, Clark SL & Hasiba U (1984) Comparison of continuous and intermittent factor VIII concentrate therapy in hemophilia A. *American Journal of Haematology* **17:** 85–88.

Hellstern P, Kohler M, Schmengler K et al (1983) Arterial and venous thrombosis and normal response to streptokinase treatment in a young patient with severe Hageman factor deficiency. *Acta Haematologica* **69:** 123–126.

Hermansky F & Pudlak P (1959) Albinism associated with hemorrhagic diathesis and unusual pigmented reticular cells in the bone marrow: Report of two cases with histochemical studies. *Blood* **14:** 162–169.

Hilgartner MW (1989) Factor replacement therapy. In Hilgartner MW & Pchedly C (eds) *Haemophilia in the Child and Adult*, pp 1–26. New York: Raven Press.

Hill FG, Enayat MS & George AJ (1985) Investigation of a kindred with a new autosomal dominantly inherited variant type of von Willebrand's disease (possible type IID). *Journal of Clinical Pathology* **38:** 665–670.

Holmberg L & Nilsson IM (1985) Von Willebrand's disease. *Clinics in Haematology* **14:** 461–488.

Holmsen H & Weiss HJ (1972) Further evidence for a deficient storage pool of adenine nucleotides in platelets from some patients with thrombocytopathia 'storage pool disease'. *Blood* **39:** 197–209.

Horellou MH, Lecompte T, Lecrubier C et al (1983) Familial and constitutional bleeding disorder due to platelet cyclo-oxygenase deficiency. *American Journal of Haematology* **14:** 1–9.

Houdijk WMP, Sakariassen KS, Nievelstein PFEM & Sixma JJ (1985) Role of factor VIII–von Willebrand factor and fibronectin in the intraction of platelets in flowing blood with monomeric and fibrillar collagen types I and III. *Journal of Clinical Investigation* **75:** 531–540.

Hougie C, Barrow EM & Graham JB (1957) Stuart clotting defect. I. Segregation of an hereditary hemorrhagic state from the heterogenous group heretofore called 'stable factor' (SPA, proconvertin, factor VII) deficiency. *Journal of Clinical Investigation* **36:** 485–496.

Howard MA, Hutton RA & Hardisty RM (1973) Hereditary giant platelet syndrome. A disorder of a new aspect of platelet function. *British Medical Journal* **2:** 586–588.

Hynes HE, Owen CA Jr, Bowie EJW & Thompson JR Jr (1969) Development of the present concept of haemophilia. *Mayo Clinic Proceedings* **44:** 193–206.

Israels SJ, McNicol A, Robertson C & Gerrard JM (1990) Platelet storage pool deficiency: diagnosis in patients with prolonged bleeding times and normal platelet aggregation. *British Journal of Haematology* **75:** 118–121.

Kinoshita S, Harrison J, Lazerson J & Abildgaard CF (1984) A new variant of dominant type II von Willebrand's disease with aberrant multimeric pattern of factor VIII-related antigen (type IID). *Blood* **63:** 1369–1371.

Josso F, Monasterio de Sanchez J, Lavergne JM et al (1971) Congenital abnormality of the prothrombin molecule (factor II) in four siblings: prothrombin Barcelona. *Blood* **38:** 9–16.

Josso F, Rio Y & Beguin S (1982) A new variant of human prothrombin: prothrombin Metz, demonstration in a family showing double heterozygosity for congenital hypoprothrombinemia and dysprothrombinemia. *Haemostasis* **12:** 309–316.

Kahn MJP & Govaerts A (1974) Prothrombin Brussels, a new congenital defective protein. *Thrombosis Research* **5:** 145–146.

Kehrel B, Balleisen L, Kokott R et al (1988) Deficiency of intact thrombospondin and membrane glycoprotein Ia in platelets with defective collagen-induced aggregation and spontaneous loss of disorder. *Blood* **71:** 1074–1078.

Kelleher JF Jr, Gomperts E, Davis W et al (1986) Selection of replacement therapy for patients with severe factor VII deficiency. *American Journal of Pediatric Hematology/Oncology* **8:** 318–323.

Kitchens CS & Newcomb TF (1979) Factor XIII. *Medicine* **58:** 413–429.

Kluft C, Vellenga E, Brommer EJP & Wijngaards G (1982) A familial haemorrhagic diathesis in a Dutch family: an inherited deficiency of α_2-antiplasmin. *Blood* **59:** 1169.

Kobrinsky NL, Gerrard JM, Watson CM et al (1984) Shortening of bleeding time by 1-Deamino-8-D-Arginine vasopressin in various bleeding disorders. *Lancet* **i:** 1145–1148.

Koie K, Kamiya T, Ogata K et al (1978) α_2-plasmin-inhibitor deficiency (Miyasato disease). *Lancet* **ii:** 1334–1336.

Koike K, Rao AK, Holmsen H et al (1984) Platelet secretion defect in patients with the attention deficit disorder and easy bruising. *Blood* **63:** 427–433.

Kovalainen S, Myllyla VV, Tolonen U & Kokkanen E (1979) Recurrent subarachroid haemorrhages in patient with Hageman factor deficiency. *Lancet* **i:** 1035–1036.

Kunicki TJ, Nugent DJ, Staats SJ et al (1988) The human fibroblast class II extracellular matrix receptor mediates platelet adhesion to collagen and is identical to the platelet glycoprotein Ia-IIa complex. *Journal of Biological Chemistry* **263:** 4516–4519.

Lacombe M-J, Varet B & Levy J-P (1975) A hitherto undescribed plasma factor acting at the contact phase of blood coagulation (Flaujeac factor): case report and coagulation studies. *Blood* **46:** 761–768.

Lagarde M, Byron PA, Vargaftig BB & Dechavanne M (1978) Impairment of platelet thromboxane A_2 generation and of the platelet release reaction in two patients with congenital deficiency of platelet cyclo-oxygenase. *British Journal of Haematology* **38:** 251–266.

Lages B & Weiss HJ (1988) Heterogenous defects of platelet secretion and responses to weak agonists in patients with bleeding disorders. *British Journal of Haematology* **68:** 53–62.

Lages B, Scrutton MC, Holmsen H et al (1975) Metal ion contents of gel-filtered platelets from patients with storage pool disease. *Blood* **46:** 119–130.

Lages B, Malmsten C, Weiss HJ & Samuelsson B (1981) Impaired platelet response to thromboxane A_2 and defective calcium mobilization in a patient with a bleeding disorder. *Blood* **57:** 545–552.

Lane DA & Southan C (1987) Inherited abnormalities of fibrinogen synthesis and structure. In Bloom AL & Thomas DB (eds) *Haemostasis and Thrombosis*, pp 442–451. London: Churchill Livingston.

Lechner K, Mahr G, Margariteller P & Deutsch E (1979) Factor X Vorarlberg, a new variant of hereditary factor X deficiency. *Thrombosis and Haemostasis* **42:** 58 (abstract).

Levy-Toledano S, Caen JP, Breton-Gorius J et al (1981) Gray platelet syndrome: α-granule deficiency. Its influence on platelet function. *Journal of Laboratory and Clinical Medicine* **98:** 831–848.

Lorand L, Losowsky MS & Miloszewski KJM (1980) Human factor XIII: Fibrin stabilizing factor. *Progress in Haemostasis and Thrombosis* **5:** 245–290.

Lusher JM (1987) Diseases of Coagulation: The fluid phase. In Nathan DG & Oski FA (eds) *Haematology of Infancy and Childhood*, pp 1239–1342. London: WB Saunders.

Lusher JM, Schneider J, Mizukami I & Evans RK (1968) The May–Hegglin anomaly: platelet function, ultrastructure and chromosome studies. *Blood* **32:** 950–961.

Lutcher CL (1976) A new expression of high molecular weight kininogen (HMW-kininogen) deficiency. *Clinical Research* **24:** 440 (abstract).

Machin SJ, Winter MR, Davies SC & Mackie IJ (1980) Factor X deficiency in the neonatal period. *Archives of Diseases of Childhood* **55:** 406–408.

Mammen EF (1974) Congenital abnormalities of fibrinogen molecule. *Seminars in Thrombosis and Haemostasis* **1:** 184–201.

Mannucci PM (1986) Desmopressin (DDAVP) for treatment of disorders of hemostasis. *Progress in Hemostasis and Thrombosis* pp 19–45.

Mannucci PM, Lombardi R, Pareti FI et al (1983) A variant of von Willebrand's disease characterized by recessive inheritance and missing triplet structure of von Willebrand factor multimers. *Blood* **62:** 1000–1005.

Mannucci PM, Lombardi R, Bader R et al (1985) Heterogeneity of Type I von Willebrand's disease: evidence for a subgroup with an abnormal von Willebrand factor. *Blood* **66:** 796–802.

Mannucci PM, Lombardi R, Federici AB et al (1986a) A new variant of type II von Willebrand's disease with aberrant multimeric structure of plasma but not platelet von Willebrand factor (Type IIF). *Blood* **68:** 269–274.

Mannucci PM, Lombardi R, Leltreade A (1986b) High-resolution multimeric analysis identifies a new variant of type II von Willebrand's disease (type IIH) in an autosomal recessive manner. *R.C. Clin Lab* **16:** 237a.

Marder VJ & Shulman NR (1964) Clinical aspects of congenital factor VII deficiency. *American Journal of Medicine* **37:** 182–194.

Mariani G & Mazzucconi MG (1983) Factor VII congenital deficiency. Clinical picture and classification of the variants. *Haemostasis* **13:** 169–177.

Mariani G, Mannucci PM, Mazzucconi MG & Capitanio A (1978) Treatment of congenital factor VII deficiency with a new concentrate. *Thrombosis and Haemostasis* **39:** 675–682.

Matthay KH, Koerper MA & Ablin AR (1979) Intracranial haemorrhage in congenital factor VII deficiency. *Journal of Pediatrics* **94:** 413–415.

Mazzucconi MG, Mandelli F, Mariani G et al (1977) A CRM-positive variant of factor-VII deficiency and the detection of heterozygotes with the assay of factor-like antigen. *British Journal of Haematology* **36:** 127–135.

Mestel F, Oetliker O, Beck E et al (1980) Severe bleeding associated with defective thromboxane synthetase (letter) *Lancet* **i:** 157.

Michalski C, Bal F, Burnouf T & Goudemand M (1988) Large scale production and properties of solvent-detergent treatment factor IX concentrate from human plasma. *Vox Sanguinis* **55:** 202–210.

Miles LA, Plowe F, Donnelly KJ et al (1982) A bleeding disorder due to a deficiency of α_2-antiplasmin. *Blood* **59:** 1236–1251.

Miletich JP, Kane WH, Hofman SL et al (1979) Deficiency of factor Xa-factor Va binding sites on the platelets of a patient with a bleeding disorder. *Blood* **54:** 1015–1022.

Miller JL & Castella A (1982) Platelet-type von Willebrand's disease. Characterization of a new bleeding disorder. *Blood* **60:** 790–794.

Najean Y & Lecompte T (1990) Genetic thrombocytopenia with autosomal dominant transmission: a review of 54 cases. *British Journal of Haematology* **74:** 203–208.

Nieuwenhuis HK & Sixma J (1988) 1-Desamino-8-D-arginine vasopressin (Desmopressin) shortens the bleeding time in storage pool deficiency. *Annals of Internal Medicine* **108:** 65–67.

Nieuwenhuis HK, Ackerman JW & Sixma JJ (1977) Patients with a prolonged bleeding time and normal aggregation tests may have storage pool deficiency: studies on one hundred and six patients. *Blood* **70:** 620–623.

Nieuwenhuis HK, Sakariassen KS, Houdijk WPM et al (1986) Deficiency of platelet membrane glycoprotein Ia is associated with a decreased platelet adhesion to subendothelium: a defect in platelet spreading. *Blood* **68:** 692–695.

Nurden AT & Caen JP (1975) Specific roles for platelet surface glycoproteins in platelet function. *Nature* **255:** 720–722.

Nurden AT, Didry D, Kieffer N & McEver RP (1985) Residual amounts of glycoproteins IIb and IIIa may be present in the platelets of most patients with Glanzmann's thrombasthenia. *Blood* **65:** 1021–1024.

Nurden AT, Rosa J-P, Fournier D et al (1987) A variant of Glanzmann's thrombasthenia with abnormal glycoprotein IIb-IIIa complexes in the platelet membrane. *Journal of Clinical Investigation* **79:** 962–969.

O'Brien JR (1964) Variability in the aggregation of human platelets by adrenaline. *Nature* **202:** 1188–1190.

Oh-Ishi S, Keno A, Uchida Y et al (1981) Abnormalities in the contact activation through factor XII in Fujiwara trait. A deficiency in both high and low molecular weight kininogens with low level of prekallikrein. *Tohoku Journal of Experimental Medicine* **133:** 67–80.

Osler W (1901) On a family form of recurrent epistaxis associated with telangiectasia of the skin and mucous membranes. *Bulletin of the Johns Hopkins Hospital* **12:** 333–337.

Owen CA, Henriksen RA, McDuffie FC & Mann KG (1978) Prothrombin Quick: a newly identified dysprothrombinemia. *Mayo Clinic Proceedings* **53:** 29–33.

Owren PA (1947) Parahaemophilia. Haemorrhagic diathesis due to absence of a previously unknown clotting factor. *Lancet* **i:** 446–448.

Pareti F, Mannucci PM, D'Angelo A et al (1980) Congenital deficiency of thromboxane and prostacyclin. *Lancet* **i:** 898–900.

Pasi KJ, Williams MD, Enayat MS & Hill FGH (1990) Clinical and laboratory evaluation of the treatment of von Willebrand's disease patients with heat-treated factor VIII concentrate (BPL 8Y). *British Journal of Haematology* **75:** 220–233.

Phillips DR & Agin PP (1977) Platelet plasma membrane glycoproteins. Evidence for the presence of nonequivalent disulfide bonds using nonreduced–reduced two dimensional gel electrophoresis. *Journal of Biological Chemistry* **252:** 2121–2126.

Pyeritz RE & McKusick VA (1979) The Marfan syndrome: Diagnosis and management. *New England Journal of Medicine* **300:** 772–777.

Quick AJ (1967) Telangiectasia: its relation to the Minot–von Willebrand syndrome. *American Journal of Medical Science* **254:** 585–601.

Rabiet MJ, Jandrot-Perrus M, Boissel JP et al (1984) Thrombin Metz: characterization of the dysfunctional thrombin derived from a variant of human prothrombin. *Blood* **63:** 927–934.

Raccuglia G (1971) Gray platelet syndrome. A variety of qualitative platelet disorder. *American Journal of Medicine* **51:** 818–828.

Ragni MV, Lewis JH, Spero JA & Hasiba U (1981) Factor VII deficiency. *American Journal of Haematology* **10:** 79–88.

Rak K & Boda Z (1980) Hemostatic balance in congenital deficiency of platelet cyclo-oxygenase. *Lancet* **ii:** 44.

Ramsay DM, MacLeod DAD, Buist TAS & Heading RC (1976) Persistent gastrointestinal bleeding due to angiodysplasia of the gut in von Willebrand's disease. *Lancet* **ii:** 275–278.

Rao AK (1990) Congenital disorders of platelet function. *Haematology/Oncology Clinics of North America* **4:** 65–86.

Rao AK, Willis J, Hassel B et al (1982) Congenital platelet secretion defect with normal storage pools and arachidonic metabolism. *Circulation* **66(II):** 299.

Rao AK, Koike K, Willis J et al (1984) Platelet secretion defect associated with impaired liberation of arachidonic acid and normal myosin light chain phosphorylation. *Blood* **64:** 914–921.

Rao AK, Willis J, Kowalska MA et al (1988) Differential requirements for platelet aggregation and inhibition of adenylate cyclase by epinephrine. Studies of a familial alpha 2-adrenergic receptor defect. *Blood* **71:** 494–501.

Rao AK, Kowalska MA & Disa J (1989) Impaired cytoplasmic ionized calcium mobilization in inherited platelet secretion defects. *Blood* **74:** 664–672.

Ratnoff OD & Colopy JE (1955) A familial hemorrhagic trait associated with a deficiency of clot-promoting fraction of plasma. *Journal of Clinical Investigation* **34:** 601–613.

Ratnoff OD, Busse RJ & Sheon RP (1968) The demise of John Hageman. *New England Journal of Medicine* **279:** 760–761.

Rimon A, Schiffman S, Feinstein DI & Rapaport SI (1976) Factor XI activity and factor XI antigen in homozygous and heterozygous factor XI deficiency. *Blood* **48:** 165–174.

Rizza CR & Matthews JM (1984) The management of patients with coagulation factor deficiencies. In Biggs R & Rizza CR (eds) *Human Blood Coagulation, Haemostasis and Thrombosis*, pp 273–318. Oxford: Blackwell Scientific.

Rodeghiero F, Castaman G & Dini E (1987) Epidemiological investigation of the prevalence of von Willebrand's disease. *Blood* **69:** 454–459.

Rosenthal RL, Dreskin OH & Rosenthal M (1953) New hemophilia-like disease caused by deficiency of a third plasma thromboplastin factor. *Proceedings of the Society for Experimental Biology and Medicine* **82:** 171–174.

Roth GJ & Machuga ET (1982) Radioimmune assay of human platelet prostaglandin synthetase. *Journal of Laboratory and Clinical Medicine* **99:** 187–196.

Rubio R, Almagro D, Cruz A & Corral JF (1983) Prothrombin Habana: a new dysfunctional molecule of human prothrombin associated with a true prothrombin deficiency. *British Journal of Haematology* **54:** 553–560.

Ruggeri ZM & Zimmerman TS (1980) Variant von Willebrand's disease: characterization of two subtypes by analysis of multimeric composition of factor VIII/von Willebrand factor in plasma and platelets. *Journal of Clinical Investigation* **65:** 1318–1325.

Ruggeri ZM, Pareti FI, Mannucci PM et al (1980) Heightened interaction between platelets and factor VIII/von Willebrand factor in a new subtype of von Willebrand's disease. *New England Journal of Medicine* **302:** 1047–1051.

Ruggeri ZM, Nilsson IM, Lombardi R et al (1982) Aberrant multimeric structure of von Willebrand factor in a new variant of von Willebrand's disease (type IIC). *Journal of Clinical Investigation* **70:** 1124–1127.

Samama M, Lecrubier C, Conard J et al (1981) Constitutional thrombocytopathy with subnormal response to thromboxane A_2. *British Journal of Haematology* **48:** 293–303.

Santoro SA (1986) Identification of a 160,000 dalton platelet membrane protein that mediates the initial divalent-cation dependent adhesion of platelets to collagen. *Cell* **46:** 913–920.

Schwartz RS, Abildgaard CF, Aledort LM et al (1990) Human recombinant DNA-derived antihemophilic factor (factor VIII) in the treatment of hemophilia A. *New England Journal of Medicine* **323:** 1800–1805.

Seeler RA (1972) Parahemophilia Factor V deficiency. *Medical Clinics of North America* **56:** 119–125.

Seligsohn U (1978) High gene frequency of factor XI (PTA) deficiency in Ashkenazi Jews. *Blood* **51:** 1223–1228.

Shapiro SS (1975) Prothrombin San Juan: a new complex dysprothrombinemia. In Hemker HC & Veltkamp JJ (eds) *Prothrombin and related coagulation factors*, pp 205–212. Leiden: Leiden University Press.

Shapiro SS, Martinez J & Holburn RR (1969) Congenital dysprothrombinemia: an inherited structural disorder of human prothrombin. *Journal of Clinical Investigation* **48:** 2251–2259.

Shapiro SS, Maldonado M, Fradera J & McCord S (1974) Prothrombin San Juan: a complex new dysprothrombinemia. *Journal of Clinical Investigation* **53:** 73 (abstract).

Shifter T, Machtey I & Creter D (1984) Thromboembolism in congenital factor VII deficiency. *Acta Haematologica* **71:** 60–62.

Stel HV, Sakariassen KS, de Groot PG et al (1985) von Willebrand factor in the vessel wall mediates platelet adherence. *Blood* **65:** 85–90.

Stormorken H, Lyperg T, Hakvaag L et al (1987) Dissociation of the aggregating effect and the inhibitory effect upon cyclic adenosine diphosphate in human platelets. *Thrombosis Research* **45:** 363.

Sultan Y, Brouet JC & Devergie A (1976) Isolated platelet factor 3 deficiency. *New England Journal of Medicine* **294:** 1121.

Tamponi G, Pannocchia A, Ardruino C et al (1987) Congenital deficiency of alpha-2-adrenoceptors on human platelets: Description of two cases. *Thrombosis and Haemostasis* **58:** 1012–1016.

Tandon NN, Kralisz U & Jamieson GA (1989) Identification of glycoprotein IV (CD36) as a primary receptor for platelet-collagen adhesion. *Journal of Biological Chemistry* **264:** 7576–7583.

Telfer TP, Denson KW & Wright DR (1956) A 'new' coagulation defect. *British Journal of Haematology* **2:** 308–316.

Triplett DA, Brandt JT, Batard MAM et al (1985) Hereditary factor VII deficiency: heterogeneity defined by combined functional and immunochemical analysis. *Blood* **66:** 1284–1287.

von Willebrand EA (1926) Hereditar pseudohemofili. *Finska Lakaresalestkapets Handlingar* **67:** 7–112.

Waldman R, Abraham JP, Rebuck JW et al (1975) Fitzgerald factor: a hitherto unrecognised coagulation factor. *Lancet* **i:** 949–950.

Walsh PN (1985) Platelet-mediated platelet coagulant protein interactions in hemostasis. *Seminars in Hematology* **22:** 178–186.

Walsh PN, Rizza CR, Matthews JM et al (1971) Epsilon-aminocaproic acid therapy for dental extractions in haemophilia and Christmas disease: a double-blind controlled trial. *British Journal of Haematology* **20:** 463–475.

Warrier AI & Lusher JM (1983) DDAVP: A useful alternative to blood components in moderate hemophilia A and von Willebrand disease. *Journal of Pediatrics* **102:** 228–233.

Weigner RS, Rudy C, Moake JL, Olson JD & Cimo PL (1980) Prothrombin Houston: a dysprothrombin identifiable by crossed immunoelectrofocusing and abnormal echis carinatus venom activation. *Blood* **55:** 811–816.

Weiss HJ & Kockwa S (1968) Studies of platelet function and proteins in 3 patients with Glanzmann's thrombasthenia. *Journal of Laboratory and Clinical Medicine* **71**: 153–165.

Weiss HJ & Sussman II (1986) A new von Willebrand variant (type I, New York): increased ristocetin—induced platelet aggregation and plasma von Willebrand factor containing the full range of multimers. *Blood* **68**: 149–156.

Weiss HJ, Chervenick PA, Zalusky R & Factor A (1969) A familial defect in platelet function associated with impaired release of adenosine diphosphate. *New England Journal of Medicine* **281**: 1264–1270.

Weiss HJ, Tschopp TB, Rogers J & Brand H (1974) Studies of platelet 5-hydroxytryptamine (Serotonin) in storage pool disease and albinism. *Journal of Clinical Investigation* **54**: 421–432.

Weiss HJ, Turitto VT & Baumgartner HR (1978) Effect of shear rate on platelet interaction with subendothelium in citrated and native blood. I Shear rate dependent decrease of adhesion in von Willebrand's disease and Bernard–Soulier syndrome. *Journal of Laboratory and Clinical Medicine* **92**: 750–764.

Weiss HJ, Vicic WJ, Lages BA & Rogers J (1979a) Isolated deficiency of platelet procoagulant activity. *American Journal of Medicine* **67**: 206–213.

Weiss HJ, Witte LD, Kaplan KL et al (1979b) Heterogeneity in storage pool deficiency: studies on granule-bound substances in 18 patients including variants deficient in α-granules, platelet factor 4, β-thromboglobulin and platelet-derived growth factor. *Blood* **54**: 1296–1319.

Weiss HJ, Turitto VT & Baumgartner HR (1986) Platelet adhesion and thrombus formation on subendothelium in platelets deficient in glycoproteins IIb–IIIa, Ib and storage granules. *Blood* **67**: 332–330.

White JG (1979) Ultrastructural studies of the gray platelet syndrome. *American Journal of Pathology* **95**: 445–462.

White JG (1987) Platelet ultrastructure. In Bloom AL & Thomas DP (eds) *Haemostasis and Thrombosis*, pp 20–46. London: Churchill Livingstone.

White JG & Gerrard JM (1976) Ultrastructural features of abnormal blood platelets. *American Journal of Pathology* **83**: 590–632.

Winkelman L, Sims GE, Haddon ME et al (1986) A pasteurised concentrate of human plasma factor XIII for therapeutic use. *Thrombosis and Haemostasis* **55**: 402–405.

Wu KK, LeBreton GC, Tai H-H & Chen Y-C (1981) Abnormal platelet response to thromboxane A_2. *Journal of Clinical Investigation* **67**: 1801–1804.

Wuepper KD (1973) Prekallikrein deficiency in man. *Journal of Experimental Medicine* **138**: 1345–1355.

Zimmerman R, Ehlers W, von Voss H et al (1979) Congenital factor VII deficiency: A report of four new cases. *Blut* **38**: 119–125.

Zimmerman TS, Abildgaard CF & Meyer D (1979) The factor VIII abnormality in severe von Willebrand's disease. *New England Journal of Medicine* **301**: 1307–1310.

Zimmerman TS, Dent JA, Ruggeri ZM & Nannini LH (1986) Subunit composition of plasma von Willebrand factor. Cleavage is present in normal individuals, increased in IIA and IIB von Willebrand's disease, but minimal in variants with aberrant structure of individual oligomers (types IIC, IID and IIE). *Journal of Clinical Investigation* **77**: 947–951.

3

Paediatric HIV infection

ELAINE J. ABRAMS
MARTHA F. ROGERS

As the first decade of the acquired immunodeficiency syndrome (AIDS) epidemic draws to a close, the depth of our understanding about infection with human immunodeficiency virus (HIV) has grown dramatically. Since the first case report of this disease in a child in 1982, the aetiological agent, HIV, has been identified and analysed, the modes of transmission have been clarified, and the pathophysiology of the infection has been described (Centers for Disease Control, 1982; Amman et al, 1983; Barre-Sinoussi et al, 1983; Oleske et al, 1983; Rubinstein et al, 1983; Gallo et al, 1984; Scott et al, 1984; Fauci, 1988). The spectrum of disease in children is better understood, and is slowly being recognized as a chronic, multisystem disease. Antiretroviral medications are becoming the standard of care for the HIV-infected child, and a large battery of medications are available for treatment of opportunistic infections and secondary complications of the disease. Finally, the importance of social, economic, and psychological factors is increasingly appreciated as HIV infection has become more prevalent in the paediatric age group.

This chapter provides an overview of HIV infection in children. The epidemiology of the disease, modes of transmission, early diagnosis, the spectrum of disease, and treatments will be summarized with an emphasis on clinical issues.

EPIDEMIOLOGY AND TRANSMISSION

The World Health Organization (WHO) estimates that approximately 500 000 cases of AIDS in women and children, largely unreported, occurred during the first 10 years of the HIV pandemic (Chin, 1990). During the 1990s an additional 3 million women and children are expected to die from this infection. In the United States, as of 30 September 1990, more than 2500 children with AIDS, less than 13 years of age, have been reported to the Centers for Disease Control (CDC). An additional 585 cases for adolescents aged 13–19, have also been reported.

Perinatal transmission of the virus from an infected woman to her child is the primary route of exposure for the paediatric population (Table 1)

Table 1. Risk factors associated with AIDS in children (less than 13 years of age). Reported to the CDC (United States) as of 31 December 1989 and the World Health Organization (European Region) as of 31 December 1989.

Risk factor	Number and (%) of children	
	United States	Europe
Perinatally acquired	1614 (81)	513 (70)
Mother i.v. drug user	826 (51)	242 (33)
Heterosexual contact	627 (39)	168 (23)
Mother transfusion-recipient	34 (2)	12 (2)
Mother's risk unknown	127 (8)	91 (12)
Transfusion-acquired	212 (11)	101 (14)
Haemophilia	106 (5)	71 (10)
Other unknown	63 (3)	46 (6)
TOTAL	1995 (100)	731 (100)

(Oxtoby, 1990). Eighty-one percent of children with AIDS reported to the CDC in the United States and 70% in Europe were perinatally infected. Similar percentages are estimated for children in countries in sub-Saharan Africa and the Caribbean. Because of the introduction of HIV screening of the blood supply and the adoption of viral-inactivation measures for factor concentrates in many countries, the perinatal route of infection will account for an increasingly large proportion of new cases in children. Though no cases of AIDS have yet been reported, a number of children with HIV disease are thought to have become infected after being sexually abused by an HIV-infected adult.

Parental intravenous drug use is the primary risk factor for perinatal transmission in the United States and Europe. Fifty percent of perinatally acquired AIDS cases reported to the CDC in the United States identify maternal intravenous drug use as the risk factor for infection. An additional 21% report sexual contact with an intravenous drug-using partner. In comparison, heterosexual contact is the primary mode of transmission to women in high prevalence areas of Africa and the Caribbean.

Among adolescents (age 13–19) reported to CDC in the United States, 27% reported a history of homosexuality, 11% used i.v. drugs, 4% reported both homosexuality and i.v. drug use, 13% reported heterosexual contact, 39% had acquired HIV from blood/blood products and 6% remain undetermined. Younger adolescents are more likely to have become infected by transfusion of contaminated blood products. With increasing age, risk factors begin to parallel the adult population with sexual contact and intravenous drug use accounting for infection in the majority of cases.

Cases in women and children have increased at similar rates in the United States: in 1989, 3098 new cases in women aged 15 to 44 years and 585 new cases in children due to perinatally acquired infection were reported. For children this represents a 38% increase over cases diagnosed in 1988 (Centers for Disease Control, 1990). These two groups, women with AIDS and children with perinatally acquired AIDS are presently the fastest growing groups in the United States.

The majority of children with AIDS have been infants or toddlers; however, older children are now being diagnosed with increasing frequency. Among children reported to the CDC as of December 1989, the median age at time of diagnosis of AIDS was 1.1 years (range 1 month to 10 years) for perinatally acquired cases, 4.5 years (range 4 months to 12 years) for transfusion-associated cases, and 9.7 years (range 9 months to 12 years) for haemophilia-associated cases. These data reflect cumulative cases occurring since surveillance for AIDS began at CDC in 1981. Currently reported cases, however, differ somewhat in age at diagnosis. Since transmission of AIDS through transfusions virtually stopped in 1985, children developing AIDS in 1990 via this route received their transfusion at least 5 years ago. Thus all these children currently being diagnosed are at least 5 years of age. Likewise, among children with haemophilia-associated infection, virtually all received contaminated factor products at least 5 years ago. Since perinatal transmission continues to occur, infants, toddlers and older children are currently being diagnosed.

The demographic characteristics of children with HIV infection may differ depending on the route of transmission. The demographic characteristics of children with perinatally acquired HIV infection reflect the characteristics of their mothers, most of whom are intravenous drug users or partners of men who abuse drugs. In the United States, infection rates among intravenous drug users have been highest in the north east and other east coast cities, and among poor, inner city, largely minority populations. Thus children with perinatally acquired HIV infection in the United States have largely been of Black or Hispanic ethnicity living in impoverished urban areas along the east coast. In Europe, the largest number of paediatric AIDS cases have been reported from France, Spain, Italy, Romania, Germany and the United Kingdom.

Children with transfusion-acquired HIV infection reflect the population of children receiving transfusions. Thus newborns with perinatal conditions requiring transfusions, children with chronic anaemias, and others receiving multiple transfusions have been at greatest risk.

PERINATAL TRANSMISSION

Perinatally-acquired infection refers to the transmission of HIV from an infected mother to her child during pregnancy, at the time of delivery, or during the postpartum period via breast-feeding. The timing of transmission from mothers to infants is unknown, but can occur at all three times. Intrauterine transmission has been substantiated by identification of the virus in 15–20 week fetuses (Jovaisas et al, 1985; Sprecher et al, 1986). HIV has also been cultured from cord blood samples (Ryder et al, 1989). In addition, an HIV-related dysmorphism with craniofacial abnormalities has been described, though not substantiated (Marian et al, 1986; Qazi et al, 1988). This would imply, however, early antenatal infection.

Transmission may occur during labour and delivery when the infant is exposed to infected maternal blood and secretions, similar to hepatitis B.

However, the mode of delivery (vaginally vs. caesarean) appears to have little impact on the infection status of the child (Lapointe, 1985; Minkoff et al, 1987).

Several cases of transmission of HIV during breast-feeding have been reported in women who were infected when they were transfused with contaminated blood in the postpartum period (Oxtoby, 1988). However, the likelihood of transmission with breast-feeding, particularly in women already infected during pregnancy, and the potential protective role of breast milk remain to be elucidated. Presently, breast-feeding is not recommended for HIV-infected women in the United States and most European countries. In developing countries, where alternatives for infant nutrition are limited, breast-feeding is still encouraged. In these situations, the risk of morbidity and mortality in non breast-fed infants is substantial due to the limited availability of infant formula and clean water for reconstitution.

Estimates of the rate of perinatal transmission from an infected mother to her child range from 20–40%. Several large longitudinal studies in Europe, Africa and the United States which attempt to determine the rate of transmission as well as the factors associated with infection have been underway for several years (European Collaborative Study, 1988; Italian Multicentre Study, 1988; Blanche, et al, 1989; Hira et al, 1989; Thomas et al, 1989; Halsey et al, 1990). The majority of studies in Europe and the United States estimate transmission rates at approximately 20–30%. Studies from less developed areas are complicated by high infant mortality rates and the difficulties in establishing the diagnosis of HIV infection (Lallemant et al, 1989; Ryder et al, 1989).

A number of associated risk factors for transmission are presently under evaluation. One study suggested that women with symptomatic infection or decreased T4 (CD4) cell counts are more likely to transmit infection (Ryder et al, 1989). Women with a history of an infected child may also be more likely to transmit during a subsequent pregnancy (Scott et al, 1988). Recent investigations have focused attention on antibodies to epitopes of gp120. These antibodies were more likely to be found in mothers who did not transmit HIV to their children when compared to transmitting mothers (Goedert et al, 1989a; Rossi et al, 1989). The implications for such a marker are great, but these initial studies include only a small number of women and children, and have not been confirmed by larger studies in other laboratories. Additional studies are necessary before conclusions can be drawn. Finally, a host of other factors which may influence transmission including cofactor viral infections, maternal drug use, and socio-economic issues need to be evaluated. Antiviral medication during pregnancy may also impact on viral transmission, but clinical studies will be necessary to elucidate this question.

Thus, despite slowly accumulating information about risk and rate of transmission, the outcome of any specific pregnancy to an infected woman cannot be predicted. Appropriate counselling should be provided to high-risk women who are pregnant or considering pregnancy. Non-judgemental counselling, comprehensive medical and social services, and the full range of options including termination should be offered to the HIV-infected, pregnant woman. Since HIV screening is presently not incorporated as a routine part of prenatal care in most parts of the world, many women first learn of their HIV status when their child is identified as infected. In addition, a large subset of women at high risk for HIV receive erratic or no prenatal care, either because they have inadequate access to health services and/or they are active drug users.

DEFINITION OF INFECTION

The identification of the HIV-infected infant is complicated by passive maternal transmission of the HIV antibody during pregnancy. Virtually all infants born to HIV-positive women will test antibody-positive at birth regardless of whether the infant is actually infected. Hence the presence of the HIV antibody reflects maternal infection status and identifies the child at risk for HIV disease (Pyun et al, 1987a). As many as 80% of HIV antibody-positive infants will lose maternal antibody during the first 15 months of life and serorevert to HIV antibody-negative. The median age of seroreversion to HIV antibody-negative was 9.8 months with a range of 2.0 to 18.0 months in the New York City Collaborative Maternal Infant Transmission Study (Abrams et al, 1990).

Children who become seronegative and are clinically well and immuno-logically normal are very unlikely to be infected. Several investigators have reported the presence of virus in a small subset of clinically well children who lost maternal antibody (European Collaborative Study, 1988; Italian Multi-centre Study, 1988). In addition, antibody-negative, HIV-infected children with clinical evidence of disease have been identified (Borkowsky et al, 1987; Pyun et al, 1987b). However, the majority of seroreverters have no detectable evidence of infection (Abrams et al, 1990). At our Center, at Harlem Hospital, we continue to follow HIV seroreverters on a yearly basis, repeating HIV antibody and basic immunological studies.

The definition of HIV infection in children under 13 years of age presently used in the United States and Europe is delineated in Table 2 (Centers for Disease Control, 1987a). Identification of the virus or viral products (p24 antigen) and/or significant clinical and immunological abnormalities con-sistent with paediatric HIV infection are necessary before the perinatally infected child under 15 months of age can be classified as infected. The presence of the HIV antibody in a perinatally infected child greater than 15 months of age or one exposed to the virus via modes other than perinatal transmission is indicative of HIV infection (Table 2).

The majority of children with perinatal infection begin to manifest clinical symptoms between 4 and 6 months of age although the latency or incubation period (time between infection and onset of symptoms) can be quite long, up to 10 years or longer. For children who have received contaminated blood, the period of time between transfusion of contaminated blood to the diagnosis of AIDS (incubation period) is somewhat longer than with perinatally-acquired disease; the median incubation period is 3.5 years for transfusion vs. 1.7 years for perinatally-acquired cases (Jones et al, 1991). In general, the incubation period for children is much shorter compared with adults.

Table 2. Centers for Disease Control Classification System for human immunodeficiency virus (HIV) infection in children under 13 years of age.

Infants and children under 15 months of age with perinatal infection
1. Virus in blood or tissues
       or
2. HIV antibody
       and
   evidence of both cellular and humoral immune deficiency
       and
   one or more categories in Class P–2
       or
3. Symptoms meeting CDC case definition for AIDS

Older children with perinatal infection and children with HIV infection acquired through other modes of transmission
1. Virus in blood or tissues
       or
2. HIV antibody
       or
3. Symptoms meeting CDC case definition for AIDS

For perinatally-acquired infection, early elevation of immunoglobulins, particularly IgG, may be the first evidence of immune dysfunction. Hypogammaglobulinaemia can also be found, but is less common. The presence of persistent anaemia and an elevated erythrocyte sedimentation rate have also been helpful as early indicators of infection in our clinical practice.

Lymphocyte subset abnormalities have proven less useful as early diagnostic criteria during infancy. Normal absolute values for CD4 cells are generally higher in healthy children when compared with the adult population: 3000 cells mm^{-3} in year one with a gradual decrease to 1500–2000 cells mm^{-3} by year two, compared with 1000 cells mm^{-3} in a healthy adult (Yanase et al, 1986; Nirven et al, 1990). Significant depression of CD4 cell number as well as reversal of the CD4/8 ratio occur commonly during HIV infection in children, but are often late manifestations.

EARLY DIAGNOSIS

Early diagnosis of HIV infection in the infant optimizes medical management and offers the potential for initiation of antiviral treatment. Unlike adults, the presence of HIV antibody in young infants does not define HIV infection (see p. 336). Several techniques are available, generally on an experimental basis, to identify the young infected child including virus culture, p24 antigen assays, polymerase chain reaction (PCR), in vitro antibody production, and HIV-specific IgA/IgM (Husson et al, 1990). For example, HIV has been successfully cultured from newborn samples, but the high cost, the need for large blood volumes and the time-consuming nature of the technique have precluded its wide use in the clinical setting. Viral activity has been widely monitored by the presence of p24 antigen, a viral structural protein, in clinical and treatment studies of HIV-infected adults and children (Borkowsky et al, 1989). Since p24 antigen is usually not detected when excess serum antibody is present, as in infants with maternal antibody, this technique has rarely proven valuable for early diagnosis. The polymerase chain reaction (PCR) is a molecular genetic technique of gene amplification, and holds great promise for early detection of infection in the perinatal period. HIV proviral DNA is enzymatically amplified several fold via a series of denaturing and annealing processes. Amplified HIV genetic material is then detected by a labelled probe. Positive results reflect the presence of proviral DNA in the host genome. In our study of infants prospectively followed from birth, PCR detected approximately 65% of infants who developed AIDS in the first 18 months of life and 10% of infants with a less severe course of disease when these infants were tested in the neonatal period. Over 90% of infected infants test PCR positive by 6 months of age (Rogers et al, 1989). Several other studies have also shown a high rate of concordance between viral culture and PCR (Edwards et al, 1989; Krivine et al, 1990), but further standardization is necessary before this technique can be used widely.

In vitro HIV antibody production is another laboratory technique which holds promise for the early identification of the infected infant (Slade et al, 1989). Production of anti-HIV IgG by the infant, as differentiated from passively transmitted antibody, would substantiate infant infection. A B-cell enriched population of lymphocytes from the infant is thoroughly washed to eliminate any maternal IgG. These cells are cultured and the supernatant is tested for HIV-specific IgG. While preliminary data are promising prospective studies are necessary before this technique can be applied to the clinical setting.

Unlike IgG, IgM and IgA do not cross the placenta. The presence of HIV-specific IgM or IgA would reflect the immune response of the infant to HIV. Earlier tests for HIV-specific IgM did not prove useful in the diagnosis of infants (Ryder and Hassig, 1988). However, Weiblen et al (1990) recently described an improved method for detection of both IgA and IgM and successfully identified IgA in 42 of 64 samples from 38 infected infants less than 12 months of age. Further studies must be conducted to clarify the role of this technique in the early identification of the infected infant.

In the absence of reliable laboratory diagnostic techniques for the diagnosis of HIV infection in infants, the diagnosis of HIV infection remains in the hands of the clinician. Most commonly, the antibody–positive child is identified as infected by the presence of persistent clinical and immunological abnormalities consistent with HIV disease. In the absence of virological confirmation, the diagnosis should be made cautiously and thoughtfully over time.

CLINICAL SPECTRUM OF DISEASE

The spectrum of clinical disease for the HIV-infected child continues to be clarified. Originally described primarily as a series of immunological abnormalities with consequent infectious complications, time and experience has furthered our understanding. Manifestations and severity of disease vary from child to child, often leading to a pattern of chronic disease with multisystem involvement.

HIV infection in childhood differs significantly from the adult disease. Children present early in the infection, often exhibiting symptoms by the sixth month of life. Immunological abnormalities and clinical manifestations differ as well. Children are more likely to have recurrent bacterial infections, and a chronic pneumonitis known as lymphoid interstitial pneumonitis (LIP); Kaposi's Sarcoma is rarely seen in the paediatric age group, and with the exception of *Pneumocystis carinii* pneumonia (PCP), opportunistic infections are less common in children than in adults. HIV-infected children with haemophilia appear to have characteristics similar to both the adult and paediatric populations; PCP is less common than in adults with haemophilia-associated AIDS and LIP is seen infrequently when compared with the perinatal population (Jason et al, 1988; Goedert et al, 1989b). The overall course of the disease for all children with HIV infection closely resembles the course of adults—there is a progressive deterioration of immune status, chronic clinical abnormalities, and ultimate demise. A review of the CDC classification provides a format to describe the multiple manifestations of this infection seen in children less than 13 years of age (Table 3).

Table 3. Summary of the classification of HIV infection in children under 13 years of age.

Class P–0 Indeterminate infection

Class P–1 Asymptomatic infection
    Subclass A   Normal immune function
    Subclass B   Abnormal immune function
    Subclass C   Immune function not tested

Class P–2 Symptomatic infection
    Subclass A   Non-specific findings
    Subclass B   Progressive neurological disease
    Subclass C   Lymphoid interstitial pneumonitis
    Subclass D   Secondary infectious disease
       Category D–1   Specified secondary infectious disease listed in the CDC surveillance
                        definition for AIDS
       Category D–2   Recurrent bacterial infection
       Category D–3   Other specified secondary infectious diseases
    Subclass E   Secondary cancers
       Category E–1   Specified cancers listed in the CDC surveillance definition for AIDS
       Category E–2   Other cancers possibly secondary to HIV
    Subclass F   Other diseases possibly due to HIV infection

---

   Perinatally-exposed infants and children described above whose infection status is indeterminate are classified as P–0. A child determined to be HIV-infected (Table 2) will fall into one of two mutually exclusive categories based on the presence or absence of clinical symptoms. Asymptomatic children are classified as P–1 and are further subclassified by the immune status. Overall, this group is relatively small. At our institution, only 1 child in 25 with infection will fall into the P–1 classification.

   Symptomatic children are classified as P–2 and are further subdivided by manifestation of disease.

Non-specific manifestations

Most children with symptomatic disease fall into this category, exhibiting any of a constellation of non-specific, HIV-related symptoms. Children must have two or more persistent, unexplained findings including at least two months of fever, failure-to-thrive or weight loss of greater than 10% of baseline, hepatomegaly, splenomegaly, generalized lymphadenopathy, parotitis, and persistent or recurrent diarrhoea.

Lymphadenopathy is often the first physical finding; axillary nodes in an infant or young child may be the initial clue of infection. Hepatospleno-megaly and poor growth are also frequently noted early in the course of the disease. Children may begin to fall off their predicted growth curve as early as 4 weeks of age. Older children may deviate from expected growth patterns during the course of an intercurrent illness or may experience a progressive weight loss secondary to the advancement of the primary disease.

Poor growth has been reported in asymptomatic HIV-infected children with haemophilia. A recent study by Brettler et al (1990) examined growth rates in a cohort of 36 asymptomatic, HIV-positive children with haemo-philia (Brettler et al, 1990). The data suggest that a decrease of >15 percentile points in height or weight for age on two repeated measurements may be a predictive marker for the development of other HIV-related symptoms.

Progressive neurological disease

Early in the description of the infection it became clear that HIV had a predilection for the nervous system. Manifestations of HIV brain disease in childhood reflect direct disruption of neurological function as manifested by loss of developmental milestones or intellectual ability, impaired brain growth, and/or progressive symmetrical motor deficits including paresis, abnormal tone, pathological reflexes, ataxia or gait disturbances (Ultman et al, 1985; Epstein et al, 1986; Belman et al, 1988; European Collaborative Study, 1990). Computer tomography scans classically reveal cerebral atrophy with concomitant ventricular enlargement. Calcifications of the basal ganglia and frontal lobes may be noted as well. Clinical abnormalities often precede radiographic findings. Electroencephalograms reveal non-specific abnormalities and cerebral spinal fluid may be notable for a mild pleocytosis or elevated protein for age. HIV antigen and virus have been demonstrated in the cerebrospinal fluid and brain in children with peri-natally acquired infection.

Neurological disease may be the presenting and/or only manifestation of HIV infection, but is most frequently seen in children with significant clinical and immunological abnormalities. The course may be static, or slowly, intermittently, or rapidly progressive.

Several distinct, age-related patterns of neurological involvement in children with HIV infection have been noted in our population. A subset of children display evidence of significant brain involvement early in the course of disease: absence of head growth, development of abnormal reflexes or persistence of neonatal reflexes, and stagnation in the development of motor and social skills form a cluster of abnormalities in the very young child. Often associated with absolute growth failure, these children remain infantile in development with advancing age and many die within the first 12 to 18 months.

Another subset of children have developed a spastic tetraparesis associated with decreased velocity of head growth during the first year of life. A number of toddlers who appeared neurologically intact have shown evidence of acute brain involvement with loss of developmental milestones, hypertonicity, abnormal reflexes and acquired microcephaly. For instance, these children can lose the ability to walk, talk and control basic functions including swallowing and bowel control.

Many of the children we follow, older than 5 years, also have a range of neurological developmental abnormalities including learning disabilities, poor attention span, speech delay, abnormal reflexes and gait disturbances.

Finally, many children with HIV infection have been found to be developmentally delayed. Developmental delay may be the result of a series of intrauterine and environmental factors contributing to the child's deviation from the normal expectations of social and psychological growth. HIV may contribute to these abnormalities: several prospective studies of children at risk for HIV disease are presently working to clarify this issue.

Lymphoid interstitial pneumonitis

Chronic pulmonary disease is a major source of morbidity and mortality in the paediatric age group. Lymphoid interstitial pneumonitis (LIP) is a chronic, interstitial pneumonitis seen primarily in children with HIV disease (Grieco and Chinoy-Acharya, 1985; Joshi et al, 1985; Rubinstein et al, 1986). Histologically, the disease is characterized by diffuse interstitial and peribronchiolar infiltration by lymphocytes and plasma cells (Kornstein et al, 1986). EBV DNA and HIV RNA have been identified in the lung tissue of children with this diagnosis, but the aetiology is unknown (Andiman et al, 1985).

In the absence of a histological diagnosis, the presence of a chronic pneumonitis on X-ray, at least 2 months in duration, characterized by bilateral reticulonodular interstitial infiltrates often associated with hilar and mediastinal adenopathy can lead to the diagnosis of LIP. However, other causes of interstitial pneumonitis including PCP, tuberculosis and cytomegalovirus must be excluded.

Debate exists about the reliability of diagnosing LIP on X-ray (Bradford et al, 1988; Zimmerman et al, 1987). Several institutions have reported a high rate of reliability when correlating radiographic and pathologic diagnoses. In most cases, classic radiological and clinical findings and a negative bronchoscopic evaluation for other pathogens, are satisfactory to confirm the diagnosis of LIP. Open lung biopsy is still performed at some institutions, providing reliable confirmation of this disease.

A distinct pattern of disease often identifies children with LIP. This subset of children tend to have lymphoproliferative disease—they often sustain excellent growth, appearing chubby and round secondary to good weight gain, but minimal change in height growth velocity. Large, prominent adenopathy and parotid enlargement also contribute to a 'healthy' appearance. Digital clubbing may be seen as well. Immunologically, these children are often hypergammaglobulinaemic with concomitant high levels of CD4 and CD8 cells. However, CD4/CD8 ratio may be diminished or reversed. The median survival time for children with this diagnosis is 91 months (Scott et al, 1989).

LIP has a variable course of progression ranging from rapidly to slowly, or intermittently progressive. Over the course of several years, some children may become progressively hypoxic, developing oxygen dependency, limitation of activity, secondary cardiac dysfunction and ultimate respiratory failure. Other children stabilize with a mild chronic hypoxia, intermittent acute respiratory exacerbations and a moderate state of pulmonary debilitation. These children appear to be at higher risk for recurrent respiratory infections. Intermittent episodes of bronchospasm have also been noted in children with LIP. For older children, the clinical prominence of LIP may decrease or resolve over time. Three children in our cohort with biopsy proven LIP, ages 7 through 11, have resolution of X-ray findings. Evidence of chronic lung disease remains with clubbing, mild hypoxia and abnormal pulmonary function tests consistent with restrictive disease. Theoretically, progression of HIV disease, with lymphocyte depletion, may result in the resolution of pulmonary lymphocytic infiltrates, leaving only chronic, fibrotic changes.

Treatment of LIP includes good pulmonary toilet, the use of bronchodilators and β-adrenergic agents, and the use of corticosteroids. The prescription of steroids remains controversial, but some investigators report a clinical improvement or levelling off of the rate of progression with the addition of corticosteroid therapy. This medication should only be used with biopsy-proven disease in the absence of other infectious agents. Frequent evaluation of changes in respiratory status are essential. Finally, supplemental oxygen may be necessary to sustain optimal respiratory performance.

Secondary infectious diseases

Opportunistic infections

Children with HIV disease are at risk for the opportunistic infections included in Table 4.

In 1988 and 1989 39% of children with AIDS in the United States reported to CDC States had *Pneumocystis carinii* pneumonia (PCP). PCP frequently presents during the first year of life, and can be the first indication of HIV disease (Leibovitz et al, 1990). Clinical presentation often includes the report of non-specific upper respiratory symptoms followed by tachypnea and hypoxia. On chest X-ray the findings can be minimal initially with rapid progression to fluffy infiltrates which evolve to a diffuse interstitial pneumonitis. Clinically, the disease progression is often fulminant with progressive hypoxia and respiratory failure. Older children with end-stage disease and CD4 cell depletion are also at high risk for PCP. The development of PCP is an ominous sign—many children die within days; the mean survival for children with PCP is 1 month following diagnosis (Bernstein et al, 1989; Scott et al, 1989).

Table 4. AIDS-related diagnoses in children less than 13 years of age reported to CDC in the United States, 1981 to September 1990.

AIDS-indicator disease	Paediatric cases Number	(%)*
Bacterial infections, multiple or recurrent	569	(22)
Candidiasis of bronchi, trachea, or lungs	107	(4)
Candidiasis of oesophagus		
definitive diagnosis	245	(9)
presumptive diagnosis	140	(5)
Coccidiodomycosis, disseminated or extrapulmonary	0	(0)
Cryptococcosis, extrapulmonary	30	(1)
Cryptosporidiosis, causing chronic diarrhoea	84	(3)
Cytomegalovirus disease other than retinitis	226	(9)
Cytomegalovirus retinitis		
definitive diagnosis	14	(1)
presumptive diagnosis	15	(1)
HIV encephalopathy (dementia)	261	(10)
Herpes simplex, with oesophagitis, pneumonia, or chronic mucocutaneous ulcers	87	(3)
Histoplasmosis, disseminated or extrapulmonary	11	(0)
Isosporiasis, causing chronic diarrhoea	1	(0)
Kaposi's sarcoma		
definitive diagnosis	18	(1)
presumptive diagnosis	0	(0)
Lymphoid interstitial pneumonia/pneumonitis		
definitive diagnosis	402	(15)
presumptive diagnosis	261	(10)
Lymphoma, Burkitt's or equivalent term	22	(1)
Lymphoma, immunoblastic, large cell, or equivalent term	14	(1)
Lymphoma, primary in brain	12	(0)
Mycobacterium avium or *M. kansasii*, disseminated		
definitive diagnosis	125	(5)
presumptive diagnosis	4	(0)
M. tuberculosis, extrapulmonary		
definitive diagnosis	5	(0)
presumptive diagnosis	0	(0)
Mycobacterial disease, other, disseminated		
definitive diagnosis	15	(1)
presumptive diagnosis	12	(0)
Pneumocystis carinii pneumonia		
definitive diagnosis	819	(31)
presumptive diagnosis	208	(8)
Progressive multifocal leukoencephalopathy	11	(0)
Toxoplasmosis of brain		
definitive diagnosis	14	(8)
presumptive diagnosis	8	(0)
HIV wasting syndrome	346	(13)

* The sum of percentages is greater than 100%, because some patients have more than one disease.

A high index for suspicion of PCP in the at-risk child facilitates early diagnosis and the initiation of appropriate treatment. The diagnosis can be made on deep tracheal aspirate or bronchoalveolar lavage of secretions which are stained with Gomori's methenamine silver nitrate stain or modified toluidine blue O technique (Leigh, 1985; Ognibene et al, 1989). Treatment should be initiated early with trimethoprim–sulfamethoxazole (co-trimoxazole) for a 14 to 21 day course. Pentamidine may be substituted in the course of co-trimoxazole allergy or poor response to treatment.

Guidelines for PCP prophylaxis are under development, but the following suggestions may be helpful. Co-trimoxazole $10\,\mathrm{mg\,kg^{-1}}$, should be given three times a week in two divided doses to all children who survive an episode of PCP. At Harlem Hospital, all HIV-infected children less than 15 months of age, receive PCP prophylaxis. Older children with an absolute CD4 count less than 500 are also placed on prophylaxis. Monthly intravenous pentamidine ($4\,\mathrm{mg\,kg^{-1}}$ monthly) is an alternative for children with co-trimoxazole sensitivity. Studies evaluating the efficacy of inhaled pentamidine in the paediatric population are presently underway.

Other opportunistic infections seen in the paediatric age group include candidiasis (primarily oesophageal), disseminated cytomegalovirus, *Mycobacterium avium intracellulare*, toxoplasmosis and chronic or disseminated herpes simplex virus. The management of these infections, at times found in combination, make the care of these children exceedingly complex.

Recurrent bacterial infections

Unlike adults, children with HIV disease appear to be at high risk for serious bacterial infections such as meningitis, bacteraemia, pneumonia, sepsis, osteomyelitis and abscesses (Bernstein et al, 1985; Krasinski et al, 1988). Common pathogens include *Streptococcus pneumoniae*, *Haemophilus influenzae*, *Staphylococcus aureus*, and Salmonella species. *Staphylococcus epidermidis*, and Gram-negative organisms including *Pseudomonas* and *Enterobacteriacae* are important to consider in the child receiving multiple or long-term antibiotics, children with central venous catheters, and children with long hospital stays. As with any immunocompromised child, the presence of fever in an HIV-infected child may herald the presence of a bacterial infection. Thus an appropriate evaluation and antibiotic therapy should be initiated promptly. The recognition of the role of bacterial disease and the liberalization of the use of antibiotics has probably lead to a decrease in the morbidity and mortality in this population.

Monthly intravenous immunoglobulin (IVIg) has been identified as potentially effective for the reduction of the rate of bacterial infections in this population (Gupta et al, 1986; Shaad et al, 1988). The efficacy of this drug is presently being evaluated in a large, placebo-controlled trial in the United States. Individual clinicians may opt to use IVIg for a subset of children with recurrent bacterial disease. The role of prophylactic antibiotics as well as early immunization with *H. influenzae B* vaccine and Pneumovax (pneumococcal vaccine) have not been evaluated.

Other bacterial infections often seen in the HIV-infected child include recurrent and chronic otitis media, sinusitis, and skin and soft tissue infections. Though not considered major infections, these diseases can contribute to significant morbidity and often require aggressive and chronic treatment. Hearing loss and language delay may result from chronic ear disease.

Other infections

Oral candidiasis may be one of the first indications of HIV disease in the infant. Particularly severe candidiasis and/or poor response to an appropriate course of treatment may provide the earliest information about a young child's disease status. Oral thrush often interferes with feeding and may progress to oesophageal disease. Treatment with oral nystatin may not be sufficient and the use of clotrimazole troches or ketoconazole suspension may be indicated. Prophylactic nystatin for the child on antibiotics may diminish or prevent recurrent infection.

Complications of viral infections, including primary varicella, recurrent herpes zoster, and measles, have been reported in this population (Pawha et al, 1988).

Secondary cancers

Kaposi sarcoma has been reported in 1% of children with AIDS (Table 4). A number of children with lymphomas have been reported as well as rhabdomyosarcoma of the gall bladder and Burkitt's lymphoma, but in general malignancies are rarely seen in the paediatric population.

Other diseases

Whether the result of direct organ involvement, immune deregulation, or secondary infection, HIV disease can manifest with multisystem involvement.

Hepatitis with elevation of transaminases can be attributed to HIV infection. Cardiac abnormalities including abnormal rhythms, abnormal function, pericardial effusions and cardiomyopathy have been reported as well (Steinherz et al, 1986; Stewart et al, 1989; Lipshultz et al, 1989). Renal involvement can manifest as nephrotic syndrome with focal and segmental glomerular sclerosis, proteinuria, azotaemia and progressive renal failure (Connor et al, 1988; Strauss et al, 1989). Pancreatitis and primary eye disease have also been reported.

Haematological abnormalities

Haematological manifestations of HIV infection have been well described in the adult literature (Zon et al, 1987; Costello, 1988; Zon and Groopman, 1988). Unfortunately, similar descriptions are unavailable for children. Though systematic haematologic data are being collected in multiple prospective studies of paediatric disease and by the treatment trials, little information about the haematological complications of the disease in children has been published.

Thrombocytopenia is a common haematological abnormality in the paediatric population; it is estimated that 10–15% of infected children will have thrombocytopenia at some point during the course of the disease. Saulsbury et al (1986) described immune-mediated thrombocytopenia as the initial presentation of HIV disease in three infants. Bone marrow evaluation in HIV-related thrombocytopenia usually reveals a normal or increased megakaryocyte population. Antiplatelet-associated IgG and serum antibody to platelets have been found in the majority of these children. In the adult population, hypothesized mechanisms for thrombocytopenia include complement and immune complex deposition, autoantibodies directed against a specific target protein of the platelet membrane, and extracorpuscular hyperdestruction, usually within the spleen (Walsh et al, 1983; Stricker et al, 1985; Karpatkin, 1988; Rossi et al, 1990).

While increased peripheral destruction may account for most instances of thrombocytopenia, one case report of a 3-month-old child with thrombocytopenia revealed an absence of megakaryocytes in the presence of normal erythroid and granulocyte precursors (Weinblatt et al, 1987). In our clinic, a 2-month-old child presented with severe anaemia and thrombocytopenia. Bone marrow examination showed the absence of erythroid and megakaryocyte precursors. In this child a spontaneous increase in haematocrit and platelet count occurred without treatment.

The natural course of thrombocytopenia appears to vary. Some children have a spontaneous resolution, while others present with a waxing and waning or an intermittent picture. Fluctuations in platelet count may occur with acute changes in the overall disease status of the child, perhaps reflecting a response to secondary infections.

Bone marrow evaluation is generally indicated for a persistent platelet count less than $50 \times 10^9/mm^3$. Normal megakaryocyte population is consistent with immune-mediated destruction and the use of intravenous immunoglobulin is the recommended therapy. Response to this treatment also appears to vary (Bussel and Haimi, 1988). A substantial and permanent increase in platelet count has been documented for a number of children. Some children may require monthly infusions to sustain adequate platelet numbers. A number of children appear to lose sensitivity to the medication and require increasingly frequent infusions. Ellaurie et al (1988) have reported that of 15 children with immune-mediated idiopathic thrombocytopenia purpura treated with IVIg, 40% (6) responded with an increase in platelet count. Five of the six responders relapsed within 3 weeks to 3 months. Prednisone, danazol, AZT, and anti-Rh globulin have been reported as useful treatments in the adult population, but no data is available in children (Oksenhendler et al, 1988; Pottage et al, 1988; Swiss Group for Clinical Studies, 1988; Weinblatt et al, 1988). In light of the increased susceptibility to bacterial infections in the HIV-infected child, splenectomy is not recommended.

Anaemia, a common finding in symptomatic HIV infection in children, is often an early indicator of HIV infection. Most children develop a normocytic, normochromic anaemia with an inappropriately low reticulocytosis. A number of children in our population have developed a macrocytic anaemia with normal B12 and folate levels. In our clinical experience, falling haemoglobin levels correlate with a general progression of the disease. Some children have become transfusion-dependent, particularly in light of chronic cardiopulmonary abnormalities and oxygen dependence. Children with LIP and chronic hypoxia may have normal haemoglobin levels for age, but because of poor oxygenation remain relatively anaemic.

In adults as well as children, the haemoglobin level appears to be inversely related to severity of disease. The anaemia, generally characterized as normochromic, normocytic in type, is thought to be caused by ineffective erythropoiesis. An inappropriately low production of erythropoietin in response to anaemia may also play an important aetiological role (Spivak et al, 1989; Fischl et al, 1990). Despite a high incidence of direct antiglobulin tests, haemolysis occurs infrequently. Parvovirus infection of the bone marrow has been described in one case of aplastic anaemia in an HIV-infected adult (Mitchell et al, 1990).

Anaemia in children also probably results primarily from ineffective erythropoiesis, but acute and chronic haemolysis can occur as well. Nutritional deficiencies must be evaluated, particularly in the chronically ill child with failure-to-thrive. A standard evaluation for anaemia including indices, reticulocyte count, iron studies, electrophoresis and Coombs test should be conducted when anaemia is diagnosed or when significant changes in haemoglobin are noted. Bone marrow aspiration is only necessary for profound anaemia, usually when haemoglobin drops below $6 \, g \, dl^{-1}$.

Leukopenia is also seen in the HIV-infected child, but the incidence is not well documented. Neutropenia may be the result of drug toxicity or coincident viral or bacterial infection. One case report describes the presence of neutropenia associated with an antibody directed against neutrophils in a 12-month-old male with symptomatic HIV infection (McCance-Katz et al, 1987). Neutropenia and/or pancytopenia may be seen in end-stage disease. Obviously, neutropenia may further compromise immune status and increase susceptibility to secondary infectious agents.

Lymphopenia is seen less frequently in the paediatric population than the adult. Lymphocytosis with neutropenia has also been seen, particularly in children with LIP pneumonia. Depletion of lymphocytes appears to correlate with increasing severity of disease, and is most frequently seen as a late manifestation.

Abnormalities of coagulation are not commonly seen in the HIV-infected child. Coagulopathy may result from deficient factor production secondary to hepatic disease and disseminated intravascular coagulation with bacterial sepsis can occur. Burns et al (1988) reported an acquired anticoagulant-circulating inhibitor of coagulation in three children with asymptomatic elevation of activated partial thromboplastin time. Lupus anticoagulant and anticardiolipin antibody have also been reported in the adult population (Bloom et al, 1986; Cohen et al, 1986). Finally, one case of autoimmune haemolytic anaemia and two cases of thrombotic thrombocytopenic purpura have been described in adults (Nair et al, 1988; Rapoport et al, 1988).

While information about the status of the bone marrow is limited in the childhood population, a wide range of abnormalities have been described in HIV-infected adults including plasmacytosis, myelodysplastic features, increased reticulin, fat necrosis and lymphocytic aggregation (Namiki et al, 1987; Treacy et al, 1987; Mir et al, 1989). Sandaus and Scudder (1989) described bone marrow findings in eight paediatric patients with HIV infection: in general they appeared normocellular. Lymphoid aggregates were found in three of five patients biopsied, but other abnormalities observed in the adult population were not noted in this small series. Ryan et al (1987) reported on seven patients with bone marrow aspirations: six were normocellular, one hypocellular. Other abnormalities included an increase in myeloid precursors, and increase of plasma cells. Bone marrow evaluation is generally performed for evaluation of cytopenia and/or the identification of potential secondary infectious agents.

CRITERIA FOR THE DIAGNOSIS OF AIDS

The definition of AIDS was developed for surveillance purposes to track the HIV epidemic. The diagnosis of AIDS must be differentiated from the classifications presented in Table 3 and described in the previous pages (Centers for Disease Control, 1987b). In general, children in class P–2, subclasses B, C, D–1, D–2, and E–1 meet the CDC definition of AIDS.

CARE OF THE HIV-INFECTED CHILD

General management issues

Many centres providing care for HIV-infected children recognize the need to provide comprehensive services including preventive, well-child care. The multiple, complex medical and social problems of these families often require centralized care for the entire family, providing medical, social and psychological services (Abrams and Nicholas, 1990). The traditional fragmentation of care with subspeciality involvement may appear burdensome for many infected families. Centralization and co-ordination of services facilitate the provision of quality care.

Vaccinations

The immunization of the HIV-infected child remains somewhat controversial. The efficacy and immune response of the infected child to primary immunizations has not been well documented; there are concerns that the vaccine may trigger increased HIV activity; the use of live viruses, generally contraindicated in the immunocompromised child, may possibly lead to disseminated infection although very few cases have been described (Peter and Zaia, 1990). These issues should be weighed against the risks of acquiring the infection in a given community and the potential morbidity and

Table 5. Recommendation for routine immunization of HIV-infected children: WHO and ACIP (Special Program on AIDS and Expanded Immunization, 1987; Immunization Practices Advisory Committee, 1988).

	ACIP		WHO	
	Asymptomatic	Symptomatic	Asymptomatic	Symptomatic
OPV	No	No	Yes	Yes
IPV	Yes	Yes		
DPT	Yes	Yes	Yes	Yes
Measles*	Yes	Yes†	Yes	Yes
HbCV	Yes	Yes		
Pneumococcal	Yes	Yes		
Influenza	No	Yes		

* Administered as MMR, live measles, mumps, and rubella viruses in a combined vaccine in the United States and United Kingdom.
† Administration of MMR vaccine should be considered for all HIV-infected children, regardless of symptoms.
OPV, oral polio vaccine; IPV, inactivated polio virus; DPT, diptheria pertussis tetanus; HbCV, Haemophilus b conjugate vaccine.

mortality associated with the primary infection. Table 5 outlines WHO and the Immunization Practices Advisory Committee (ACIP) immunization recommendations (Immunization Practices Advisory Committee, 1986, 1988; Special Program on AIDS, 1987).

Oral polio vaccine (OPV) is recommended by WHO for all children in developing nations. To date, no vaccine-associated cases of paralytic polio have been reported in an HIV-infected child. Inactivated polio vaccine (IPV) is available in the United States and is recommended for HIV-positive children. Because polio virus is excreted in the stool of the immunized infant, IPV is also suggested for all children residing with HIV-infected individuals.

WHO recommends measles vaccination for all HIV-positive children. ACIP recommends live measles vaccine immunization of asymptomatic HIV-infected children and consideration of immunization for symptomatic children. In the United States and United Kingdom it is given with mumps and rubella as MMR. During a measles outbreak, infants 6–11 months of age should receive monovalent measles vaccine and should be revaccinated with MMR at 12 months of age or older. In addition, children with symptomatic HIV infection exposed to measles should receive intramuscular immuno-globulin (IG) prophylaxis ($0.5\,\mathrm{ml\,kg^{-1}}$) regardless of vaccination status.

Haemophilus b conjugate vaccine (HbCV), pneumococcal vaccine and influenza vaccine should be administered to the HIV-infected child, where available. Varicella-zoster immune globulin is also recommended after exposure to this virus.

NUTRITION, GROWTH AND DEVELOPMENT

Many factors may interfere with the normal attainment of growth in the HIV-infected child. Intrauterine exposure to alcohol and/or drugs as well as poor prenatal care may have an impact on growth expectations. Environmental factors including financial resources, availability of appropriate, nutritional alimentation, and dietary patterns within families may also be important. Finally, manifestations of the infection including persistent oral or mucosal disease secondary to candida and/or herpes, respiratory compromise, neurological compromise, chronic diarrhoea and gastrointestinal infections may significantly limit caloric intake (McCloughlin et al, 1989).

Aggressive nutritional therapy is frequently required for the HIV-infected child (Leung, 1989). Active involvement of a nutritionist and gastroenterologist in the treatment programme may prove essential. Feeding regimens should be implemented in a stepwise fashion. The use of elemental and concentrated formulas has proven invaluable for growth enhancement in our population. Intermittent and continuous nasogastric tube feedings may be necessary to sustain adequate calorific intake (Fennoy and Leung, 1990). Some centres have relied upon the placement of gastric tubes, citing easier management in the household. Hyperalimentation has also proven useful to maintain caloric intake for the hospitalized child during an acute intercurrent illness, when other modes of feeding cannot be accomplished. However, parental nutrition is frequently not a long-term option for the HIV-infected child at home.

The same intrauterine and environmental factors affecting the physical growth of the HIV-infected child may also affect his/her intellectual and psychological development. The role of a psychologist in the care programme cannot be underestimated. Sequential psychometric testing should be included in the general assessment and care of the HIV-infected child. Many young children appear to be developmentally delayed, while older infected children may have speech and language abnormalities, and learning disabilities. Again, aggressive assessment and the development of a treatment regimen is imperative. Children may require special services including infant stimulation, early intervention programmes and special educational settings. Those with neurological manifestations of the infection often require physical and occupational therapy, and special equipment or appliances in the household.

The psychological needs of the HIV-infected child are too often forgotten. The tendency of the medical community to focus on treatment of the disease, rather than on the child; the fact that many of the children are preverbal allowing us to relate primarily to the caretaker; and the secrecy and discrimination around this particular infection have worked to the disadvantage of the child. Working individually and independently with the child is essential to reduce psychological stress. Openly discussing the nature of the disease, allowing the child to express fantasies and fears, answering questions simply and honestly, and involving the child in plans for care allow the child to exert some control over their disease. For the older child, the need to maintain as normal a lifestyle as possible cannot be overemphasized. Excellent models for this approach have already been established in other fields where children must deal with chronic and/or fatal diseases.

Pain management is becoming an increasingly important issue in the care of the HIV-infected child. Frequent, often painful procedures are common in the management of this disease. Intercurrent infections of the oropharynx, oesophagus and gastrointestinal tract, as well as neurological complications may be quite painful. The use of standard relaxation techniques, anticipatory guidance, and a growing battery of pain medications for children should be incorporated into the care plan.

AN APPROACH TO HIV INFECTION IN PAEDIATRICS

The diagnosis and treatment of specific disease entities and opportunistic infections in the HIV-infected child is beyond the scope of this chapter (Pawha, 1988; Falloon et al, 1989; Wiznia and Nicholas, 1990). Several issues have been addressed above, but more detailed descriptions are outlined in a series of review papers. A general approach to the disease, however, deserves emphasis. Despite a relatively high rate of mortality, HIV is becoming a chronic disease of childhood. The introduction of anti-viral therapy, and improved treatment of opportunistic and intercurrent infections will prolong the lives of these children. Children with the infection must learn to cope with the limitations set by their disease.

HIV disease was initially viewed as a series of immunological abnormalities. With time, our understanding of the nature of this disease has broadened: Despite a predilection for the immune system, HIV can cause multisystem disease. Multisystem involvement becomes more likely with increasing duration of illness. Medical care should also include routine surveillance for the onset of new organ system involvement. Early detection may facilitate successful treatment and new abnormalities can often be diagnosed with a thorough physical examination and basic screening tests, including complete blood count, urinanalysis, chest X-ray, and electro-cardiogram.

Prophylactic treatment is another essential component in the care of the HIV-infected child. Prophylaxis for PCP and the use of intravenous immunoglobulin have been previously discussed. Prophylaxis for recurrent otitis media, other bacterial infection and recurrent herpes simplex, may be necessary for some children.

ANTIRETROVIRAL TREATMENT

The introduction of antiretroviral treatment for HIV infection has significantly altered our approach to the disease. While care initially focused on the treatment of the manifestations of the disease and secondary complications of immune system deterioration, we are now able to treat the infection directly. The use of AZT for children with symptomatic HIV infection is quickly becoming the standard of care in the developed world (Pizzo, 1990; Pizzo and Wilfert, 1990; Warrier and Lusher, 1990). Unfortunately, high cost and unavailability have limited access to this medication in developing countries.

Azidothymidine is a nucleoside analogue which interferes with normal viral replication (Yarchoan et al, 1989). An oral suspension with good bioavailability is available and the drug penetrates the central nervous system. Efficacy studies in adults have revealed a significant decrease in mortality and morbidity in individuals with severe symptomatic disease (Fischl et al, 1987). Further studies have also revealed improved immune status for patients with less severe, asymptomatic infection (Volberding et al, 1990).

In a phase one trial of AZT in children, 21 children who received intravenous medication showed significant subjective and objective improvement (Pizzo et al, 1988). Improvement in neurological status, neurodevelopmental scores, physical findings, weight gain, and immune status were reported. An initial trial of intermittent oral medication revealed findings of improved weight gain, decreased hepatosplenomegaly and lowering of IgG and IgM levels (McKinney et al, 1990). Additional trials of AZT in the infected child are presently under way.

In the United States, AZT is approved for infected children greater than 3 months of age. The recommended starting dose in children is $180\,mg\,m^{-2}$ q6 hours. A dosing regimen of $120\,mg\,m^{-2}$ q6 hours may be effective and less toxic for children with mild to moderate symptoms, and is presently under evaluation. Individual clinicians may opt to begin treatment at reduced doses ($90–120\,mg\,m^{-2}$) in children with severe bone marrow and liver function abnormalities, but efficacy at these doses remains to be determined.

Side-effects of AZT include bone marrow toxicity, liver function abnormalities, clinical myositis and non-specific findings including nausea, headache and vomiting (Richman et al, 1987). Dose reduction to $120\,mg\,m^{-2}$ (or two thirds the starting dose) or temporary discontinuation of treatment are indicated for anaemia and neutropenia. Medication can be continued, and/or the initial dose reinstituted with normalization of laboratory values. Severe anaemia may require transfusion. AZT will also cause a macrocytosis of the erythroid cell line, often a useful guide to monitor patient compliance. Recombinant erythropoietin shows some promise for treatment of AZT-related anaemia in the adult population (Fischl et al, 1990). No studies have been conducted in children.

Elevations of transaminases may also be dose-limiting. Systemic findings are not commonly reported in children. In our experience, AZT is relatively well tolerated in children with mild to moderate symptoms of infection. As the disease progresses, however, the rate of side-effects appears to increase and often limits use of the medication.

Other medications presently under evaluation for treatment of HIV infection include dideoxyinosine (ddI), dideoxycytidine (ddc) and soluble recombinant CD4 (CD4). The introduction of antiviral agents, alone or in combination are heralding a pattern of treatment parallel to chemotherapy for paediatric oncology patients. Future therapeutic regimens may include long-term, intermittent, intravenous therapy in combination with oral agents to treat the primary infection, along with a myriad of medications for prophylaxis and treatment of secondary diseases.

SOCIAL ISSUES

The bulk of the children with HIV infection come from disorganized, often poor families. Absence of community resources, limited access to health-care and social services, suspicion of the medical care community, and active parental drug use, may compromise the care of the HIV-infected child. Many of these social issues must be addressed before appropriate treatment can be successfully initiated.

Unlike other chronic diseases of childhood, HIV is also a family disease. Often, the identification of the HIV-infected child heralds the identification of infected parents and siblings. Uninfected siblings may suffer the psycho-logical consequences of witnessing the deterioration or death of other family members. Extended family members may be called upon to provide direct and supportive care. Twenty-seven percent of the children followed at our Center live with an extended family member; 25% reside in traditional foster care homes. For those with blood product-related disease, family members are generally intimately involved in daily care and management of the infected child. A therapeutic approach incorporating the needs of the entire family unit may significantly enhance the care of the index child.

Care of the children at risk for, or infected with, HIV requires a multi-disciplinary team approach. The family should be provided with on-site, general and subspecialty paediatric, social and psychological services. This will create the appropriate environment for the care and treatment of this complex, chronic disease. Community and clerical support, when available should be accessed as well. Creative mechanisms for addressing the needs of these families may need to be developed to successfully engage them in care.

Increasing numbers of children with HIV disease and progress in treatment and management of the infection will continue to provide a challenge for the health-care professional into the twenty-first century.

REFERENCES

Abrams EJ & Nicholas SW (1990) Pediatric HIV infection. *Pediatric Annals* 19: 482–487.
Abrams EA, Rogers MR, Ou C et al (1990) Lack of proviral sequences in children who have lost maternal antibody following birth to HIV (+) mothers. Fifth International Conference on AIDS: San Francisco Abstract Th.C.47.
Amman AG, Cowan MJ, Wara DW et al (1983) Acquired immune deficiency in an infant: possible transmission by means of blood products. *Lancet* i: 956–958.
Andiman W, Eastman R, Martin K et al (1985) Opportunistic lymphoproliferations associated with Epstein–Barr viral DNA in infants and children with AIDS. *Lancet* ii: 1390–1393.
Barre-Sinoussi F, Chermann JC, Rey F et al (1983) Isolation of a T-lymphotropic retrovirus from a patient at risk for acquired immune deficiency syndrome (AIDS). *Science* 220: 868–871.
Belman AL, Diamond G, Dickson D et al (1988) Pediatric acquired immunodeficiency syndrome: Neurologic syndromes. *American Journal of Disease of Children* 142: 29–35.
Bernstein LJ, Kreiger BZ, Novick B et al (1985) Bacterial infection in the acquired immuno-deficiency synderome of children. *Pediatric Infectious Disease Journal* 4: 472–475.
Bernstein LJ, Bye MR & Rubinstein A (1989) Prognostic factors and life expectancy in children with acquired immunodeficiency syndrome and pneumocystis carinii pneumonia. *American Journal of Diseases of Children* 143: 775–778.

Blanche S, Rouzioux C, Guihard Moscato ML et al (1989) A prospective study of infants born to women seropositive for human immunodeficiency virus type 1. *New England Journal of Medicine* 320: 1643–1648.

Bloom EJ, Abrams DI & Rodgers G (1986) Lupus anticoagulant in the acquired immunodeficiency syndrome. *Journal of the American Medical Association* 256: 491–493.

Borkowsky W, Krasinski K, Paul D et al (1987) Human-immunodeficiency-virus infections in infants negative for anti-HIV by enzyme-linked immunoassay. *Lancet* i: 1168–1171.

Borkowsky W, Krasinski K, Paul D et al (1989) Human immunodeficiency virus type 1 antigenemia in children. *Journal of Pediatrics* 14: 940–945.

Bradford BF, Abdenour GE, Frank JL et al (1988) Usual and unusual radiologic manifestations of acquired immunodeficiency syndrome (AIDS) and human immunodeficiency virus (HIV) infection in children. *Radiologic Clinics of North America* 26: 341–353.

Brettler DB, Forsberg A, Bolivar E et al (1990) Growth failure as a prognostic indicator for progression to acquired immunodeficiency syndrome with hemophilia. *Journal of Pediatrics* 117: 584–588.

Burns ER, Krieger BZ, Bernstein L & Rubinstein A (1988) Acquired circulating anticoagulants in children with acquired immunodeficiency syndrome. *Pediatrics* 82: 763–765.

Bussel JB & Haimi JS (1988) Isolated thrombocytopenia in patients infected with HIV: Treatment with intravenous gammaglobulin. *American Journal of Hematology* 28: 79–84.

Centers for Disease Control (1982) Unexplained immunodeficiency and opportunistic infections in infants—New York, New Jersey, California. *Morbidity and Mortality Weekly Report* 31: 665–667.

Centers for Disease Control (1987a) Classification system for human immunodeficiency virus (HIV) infection in children under 13 years of age. *Morbidity and Mortality Weekly Report* 36: No. 15: i–vi.

Centers for Disease Control (1987b) Revision of CDC surveillance case definition for acquired immunodeficiency syndrome. *Morbidity and Mortality Weekly Report* 36: 1S–15S.

Centers for Disease Control (1990) Update: Acquired Immunodeficiency Syndrome—United States, 1989. *Morbidity and Mortality Weekly Report* 39: 81–86.

Chin J (1990) Current and future dimensions of HIV/AIDS pandemic in women and children. *Lancet* 336: 221–224.

Cohen AJ, Philips TM & Kessler CM (1986) Circulating coagulation inhibitors in the acquired immunodeficiency syndrome. *Annals of Internal Medicine* 104: 175–180.

Connor E, Gupta S, Joshi V et al (1988) Acquired immunodeficiency syndrome-associated renal disease in children. *Journal of Pediatrics* 113: 39–44.

Costello C (1988) Haematological abnormalities in human immunodeficiency virus (HIV) disease. *Journal of Clinical Pathology* 41: 711–715.

Edwards JR, Ulrich PP, Weintrub PS et al (1989) Polymerase chain reaction compared with concurrent viral cultures for rapid identification of human immunodeficiency virus infection among high-risk infants and children. *Journal of Pediatrics* 115: 200–203.

Ellaurie M, Burns ER, Bernstein LJ et al (1988) Thrombocytopenia and human immunodeficiency virus in children. *Pediatrics* 82: 905–908.

Epstein LG, Sharer LR, Oleske JM et al (1986) Neurologic manifestations of human immunodeficiency virus infection in children. *Pediatrics* 78: 678–687.

European Collaborative Study (1988) Mother-to-child transmission of HIV infection. *Lancet* ii: 1039–1042.

European Collaborative Study (1990) Neurologic signs in young children with human immunodeficiency virus infection. *Pediatric Infectious Disease Journal* 9: 402–406.

Falloon J, Eddy J, Weiner L & Pizzo P (1989) Human immunodeficiency virus infection in children. *Journal of Pediatrics* 114: 1–30.

Fauci A (1988) The human immunodeficiency virus: Infectivity and mechanisms of pathogenesis. *Science* 239: 617–622.

Fennoy I & Leung J (1990) Refeeding and subsequent growth in the child with AIDS. *Nutrition in Clinical Practice* 5: 54–58.

Fischl MA, Richman DD, Grieco MH et al (1987) The efficacy of azidothymidine (AZT) in the treatment of patients with AIDS and AIDS-related complex: A double-blind, placebo-controlled trial. *New England Journal of Medicine* 317: 185–191.

Fischl M, Galpin JE, Levine JD et al (1990) Recombinant human erythropoietin for patients with AIDS treated with zidovudine. *New England Journal of Medicine* 322: 1488–1493.

Gallo RC, Salhuddin SZ, Popovic M et al (1984) Frequent detection and isolation of cytopathic retroviruses (HTLV-III) from patients with AIDS and at risk for AIDS. *Science* **224:** 500–503.

Goedert JJ, Kessler CM, Aledort LM et al (1989b) A prospective study of human immuno-deficiency virus type 1 infection and the development of AIDS in subjects with hemophilia. *New England Journal of Medicine* **321:** 1141–1148.

Goedert JJ, Mendez H, Drummond JE et al (1989a) Mother-to-infant transmission of human immunodeficiency virus type1L association with prematurity or low anti-gp120. *Lancet* **ii:** 1351–1354.

Grieco MH & Chinoy-Acharya (1985) Lymphocytic interstitial pneumonia associated with the acquired immune deficiency syndrome. *American Review of Respiratory Diseases* **131:** 952–955.

Gupta A, Novick BE & Rubinsteins A (1986) Restoration of suppressor T cell function in children with acquired immunodeficiency syndrome (AIDS) following intravenous immunoglobulin. *American Journal of Diseases in Children* **140**(2): 143–146.

Halsey NA, Boulos R, Holt E et al (1990) Transmission of HIV-1 infections from mothers to infants in Haiti. Impact on childhood mortality and malnutrition. *Journal of American Medical Association* **264:** 2088–2092.

Hira S, Kamanga J, Bhat GJ et al (1989) Perinatal transmission of HIV-1 in Lusaka, Zambia. *British Medical Journal* **299:** 1250–1252.

Husson RN, Comeau AM & Hoff R (1990) Diagnosis of human immunodeficiency virus infection in infants and children. *Pediatrics* **86:** 1–10.

Immunization Practices Advisory Committee (1986) Immunization of children infected with human T-lymphotropic virus type III/lymphadenopathy-associated virus. *Morbidity and Mortality Weekly Report* **25:** 595–598; 603–606.

Immunization Practices Advisory Committee (1988) Immunization of children infected with human immunodeficiency virus: supplementary statement. *Morbidity and Mortality Weekly Report* **37:** 181–183.

Italian Multicentre Study (1988) Epidemiology, clinical features, and prognostic factors of paediatric HIV infection. *Lancet* **ii:** 1043–1045.

Jason JM, Stehr-Green J, Holman RC et al (1988) Human immunodeficiency virus infection in hemophiliac children. *Pediatrics* **82:** 565–570.

Jones DC, Byers RH, Bush TJ et al (1991) The epidemiology of transfusion-associated AIDS in Children in the United States, 1981–1989. *Pediatrics* (in press).

Joshi VV, Oleske JM, Minnefore AB et al (1985) Pathologic pulmonary findings in children with the acquired immunodeficiency syndrome: a study of ten cases. *Human Pathology* **16:** 241–246.

Jovaisas E, Koch MA, Schafer A et al (1985) LAV/HTLV-III in a 20-week fetus. *Lancet* **ii:** 1129.

Karpatkin S (1988) Immunologic thrombocytopenic purpura in HIV-seropositive homo-sexuals, narcotic addicts and hemophiliacs. *Seminars in Hematology* **25:** 219–229.

Kornstein MJ, Pietra GG, Hoxie JA & Conley ME (1986) The pathology and treatment of interstitial pneumonitis in two infants with AIDS. *American Review of Respiratory Disease* **133:** 1196–1198.

Krasinski K, Borkowsky W, Bonk S et al (1988) Bacterial infections in human immuno-deficiency virus-infected children. *Pediatric Infectious Disease Journal* **7:** 323–328.

Krivine A, Yakudima A, Le May ML et al (1990) A comparative study of virus isolation, polymerase chain reaction, and antigen detection in children of mothers infected with human immunodeficiency virus. *Journal of Pediatrics* **116:** 372–376.

Lallemant M, Lallemant-Le-Coeur S, Cheynier D et al (1989) Mother–child transmission of HIV-1 and infant survival in Brazzaville, Congo. *AIDS* **3:** 643–646.

Lapointe N, Michaud J, Pekovic D et al (1985) Transplacental transmission of HTLV-III virus. *New England Journal of Medicine* **312:** 1325–1326.

Leibovitz E, Rigaud M, Pollack H et al (1990) Pneumocystis carinii pneumonia in infants infected with the human immunodeficiency virus with more than 450 CD4 T lymphocytes per cubic millimeter. *New England Journal of Medicine* **323:** 531–533.

Leigh M (1985) Diagnosis of PCP in pediatric patients using bronchoscopic bronchoalveolar lavage. *Pediatric Infectious Disease Journal* **4:** 408.

Leung J (1989) An approach to feeding HIV-infected infants and toddlers. *Topics in Clinical Nutrition* **4:** 27.

Lipschultz SE, Chanock S, Sanders SP et al (1989) Cardiovascular Manifestations of human Immunodeficiency Virus Infection in Infants and Children. *American Journal of Cardiology* **63:** 1489–1497.

Marion RW, Wisnia AA, Hutcheon RG, Rubinstein A (1986) Human T-cell lymphotropic virus type III (HTLV-III) embryopathy: a new dysmorphic syndrome associated with intrauterine HTLV-III infection. *American Journal of Diseases of Children* **140:** 638–640.

McCance-Katz EF, Hoecker JL & Vitale NB (1987) Severe neutropenia associated with antineutrophil antibody in a patient with acquired immunodeficiency syndrome-related complex. *Pediatric Infectious Disease Journal* **6:** 417–418.

McCloughlin LL, Nord KS, Joshi VV et al (1989) Severe gastrointestinal involvement in children with acquired immunodeficiency syndrome. *Journal of Pediatric Gastroenterology and Nutrition* **6:** 517–524.

McKinney RE, Pizzo PA, Scott GC et al (1990) Safety and tolerance of intermittent intravenous and oral zidovudine therapy in human immunodeficiency virus infected pediatric patients: a phase I study. *Journal of Pediatrics* **116:** 641–647.

Minkoff H, Nanda D, Menez R et al (1987) Pregnancies resulting in infants with acquired immunodeficiency syndrome or AIDS-related complexes. *Obstetrics and Gynecology* **69:** 285–287.

Mir N, Costello C, Luckit J & Lindley R (1989) HIV-disease and bone marrow changes: A study of 60 cases. *European Journal of Haematology* **42:** 339–343.

Mitchell SA, Welch JM, Weston-Smith S et al (1990) Parvovirus infection and anaemia in a patient with AIDS: case report. *Genitourinary Medicine* **66:** 95–96.

Nair JM, Bellevue R & Bertoni M (1988) Thrombotic thrombocytopenic purpura in patient with AIDS-related complexes: A report of two cases. *Annals of Internal Medicine* **109**(3): 209–212.

Namiki TS, Boone DC & Meyer PR (1987) A comparison of bone marrow findings in patients with acquired immunodeficiency syndrome (AIDS) and AIDS related conditions. *Hematological Oncology* **5:** 99–106.

Nirven P, Skuza C, Chadwick E et al (1990) Age related changes of lymphocyte phenotypes in healthy children. *Pediatric Research* **27:** 155A.

Ognibene G, Gill V, Pizzo PA et al (1989) Induced sputum to diagnose PCP in immunosuppressed pediatric patients. *Journal of Pediatrics* **115:** 430–433.

Oksenhendler E, Bierling P, Brossard Y et al (1988) Anti-RH immunoglobulin therapy for human immunodeficiency virus-related immune thrombocytopenic purpura. *Blood* **71:** 1499–1502.

Oleske J, Minnefore A, Cooper R et al (1983) Immune deficiency syndrome in children. *Journal of the American Medical Association* **249:** 2345–2349.

Oxtoby MJ (1988) Human immunodeficiency virus and other viruses in human milk: placing the issues in broader perspective. *Pediatric Infectious Disease Journal* **7:** 825–835.

Oxtoby MJ (1990) Perinatally acquired human immunodeficiency virus infection. *Pediatric Infectious Disease Journal* **9:** 609–619.

Pawha S (1988) Human immunodeficiency virus infection in children: nature of immunodeficiency, clinical spectrum and management. *Pediatric Infectious Disease Journal* **7:** S61–S71.

Pawha S, Biron K, Lim W et al (1988) Continuous varicella-zoster infection associated with acyclovir resistance in a child with AIDS. *Journal of the American Medical Association* **260:** 2879–2882.

Peter G & Zaia JA (1990) Vaccines for Infection and HIV-1. In Pizzo PA & Wilfert CM (eds) *Pediatric AIDS. The Challenge of HIV Infection in Infants, Children and Adolescents*, pp 651–668. Baltimore: Williams and Wilkins.

Pizzo PA (1990) Considerations for the evaluation of antiretroviral agents in infants and children infected with human immunodeficiency virus: a perspective from the National Cancer Institute. *Reviews of Infectious Diseases* **12:** S561–S569.

Pizzo PA & Wilfert CM (1990) Treatment considerations for children with human immunodeficiency virus infection. *Pediatric Infectious Disease Journal* **9:** 690–699.

Pizzo PA, Eddy J, Falloon J et al (1988) Effect of continuous intravenous infusion of zidovudine (AZT) in children with symptomatic HIV infection. *New England Journal of Medicine* **319:** 8989–8996.

Pottage JC, Benson CA, Spear JB et al (1988) Treatment of human immunodeficiency virus-related thrombocytopenia with zidovudine. *Journal of the American Medical Association* **260**: 3045–3048.

Pyun KH, Ochs HD & Dafford MT (1987a) Perinatal infection with human immunodeficiency virus: specific antibody response by the neonate. *New England Journal of Medicine* **317**: 611–614.

Pyun KH & Ochs HD et al (1987b) Seronegativity and paediatric AIDS. *Lancet* **i**: 1152–1153.

Qazi QH, Sheikh TM, Fikrig S, Menikoff H (1988) Lack of evidence for craniofacial dysmorphism in perinatal human immunodeficiency virus infection. *Journal of Pediatrics* **112**: 7–11.

Rapoport AP, Rowe JM & McMican A (1988) Life-threatening autoimmune hemolytic anemia in a patient with acquired immune deficiency syndrome. *Transfusion* **28**: 190–191.

Richman DD, Fischl MA, Grieco MH et al (1987) The toxicity of azidothymidine (AZT) in the treatment of patients with AIDS and AIDS-related complex: A double-blind, placebo-controlled trial. *New England Journal of Medicine* **317**: 192–197.

Rogers MF, Ou CY, Rayfield M et al (1989) Use of the polymerase chain reaction for early detection of the proviral sequences of human immunodeficiency virus in infants born to seropositive mothers. *New England Journal of Medicine* **320**: 1649–1654.

Rossi P, Moschese V, Broliden PA et al (1989) Presence of maternal antibodies to human immunodeficiency virus 1 envelope glycoprotein gp120 epitopes correlates with the uninfected status of children born to seropositive mothers. *Proceedings of the National Academy of Science, USA* **86**: 8055–8058.

Rossi G, Gorla R, Stellini R et al (1990) Prevalence, clinical and laboratory features of thrombocytopenia among HIV-infected individuals. *AIDS Research and Human Retroviruses* **6**: 261–269.

Rubinstein A, Sicklick M, Gupta A et al (1983) Acquired immunodeficiency with reversed T4/T8 ratios in infants born to promiscuous and drug-addicted mothers. *Journal of the American Medical Association* **249**: 2350–2356.

Rubinstein A, Morecki R, Silverman B et al (1986) Pulmonary disease in children with acquired immune deficiency syndrome and AIDS-related complex. *Journal of Pediatrics* **108**: 498–503.

Ryan B, Connor E, Minnefor A et al (1987) Human immunodeficiency virus (HIV) infection in children. *Hematology/Oncology Clinics of North America* **1**: 381–395.

Ryder RW & Hassig SE (1988) The epidemiology of perinatal transmission of HIV *AIDS* **2**(suppl. 1): S83–S89.

Ryder R, Nsa W, Hassig S et al (1989) Perinatal transmission of the human immunodeficiency virus type 1 to infants of seropositive women in Zaire. *New England Journal of Medicine* **320**: 1637–1642.

Sandhaus LM & Scudder R (1989) Hematologic and bone marrow abnormalities in pediatric patients with human immunodeficiency virus (HIV) infection. *Pediatric Pathology* **9**: 277–288.

Saulsbury FT, Boyle RJ, Wykoff RF & Howard TH (1986) Thrombocytopenia as the presenting manifestation of human T-lymphotropic virus type III infection in infants. *Journal of Pediatrics* **109**: 30–34.

Scott BG, Buck BE & Leterman JG (1984) Acquired immunodeficiency syndrome in infants. *New England Journal of Medicine* **310**: 76–81.

Scott GB, Hutto C, Matrucci T et al (1988) Probability of perinatal infections in infants of HIV-1 positive mothers. Fourth International Conference on AIDS: Stockholm Abstract #6583.

Scott GB, Hutto C, Makuch R et al (1989) Survival in children with perinatally acquired human immunodeficiency virus type I infection. *New England Journal of Medicine* **321**: 1791–1796.

Shaad VB, Granella-Berradoni A & Pawet B (1988) Intravenous immunoglobulin in symptomatic pediatric HIV infection. *European Journal of Pediatrics* **147**(3): 300–303.

Slade HB, Pica RV & Pahwaq SG (1989) Detection of HIV-specific antibodies in infancy by isoelectric focusing and affinity immunoblotting. *Journal of Infectious Diseases* **160**: 126–130.

Special Programme on AIDS and Expanded Programme on Immunization (1987) *Human immunodeficiency virus infection and routine childhood immunization* (WHO/EPI/GAG WP.8 Rev.1). Geneva: World Health Organization.

Spivak JL, Barnes DC, Fuchs E & Quinn TC (1989) Serum immunoreactive erythropoietin in HIV-infected patients. *Journal of the American Medical Association* **261**: 3104–3107.

Sprecher S, Sopumenkoff G, Puissant F et al (1986) Vertical transmission of HIV in a 15-week fetus. *Lancet* **ii**: 288–289.

Steinherz LJ, Brochstien JA & Robins J (1986) Cardiac involvement in congenital acquired immunodeficiency syndrome. *American Journal of Diseases in Children* **140**: 1241–1244.

Stewart JM, Kaul A, Gromish DS et al (1989) Symptomatic cardiac dysfunction in children with human immunodeficiency virus. *American Heart Journal* **117**: 140–144.

Strauss J, Abitbol C, Zilleruelo G et al (1989) Renal disease in children with the acquired immunodeficiency syndrome. *New England Journal of Medicine* **321**: 625–630.

Stricker RB, Abrams DI, Corash L & Shuman MA (1985) Target platelet antigen in homosexual men with immune thrombocytopenia. *New England Journal of Medicine* **313**: 1375–1380.

Swiss Group for Clinical Studies on the Acquired Immunodeficiency Syndrome (AIDS) (1988) Zidovudine for the treatment of thrombocytopenia associated with human immunodeficiency virus (HIV). *Annals of Internal Medicine* **109**: 718–721.

Thomas PA & New York City Perinatal HIV Transmission Collaborative Study Group (1989) Early predictors and rate of perinatal HIV Disease. Fifty International Conference on AIDS: Montreal, Abstract ThAO7.

Treacy M, Lai L, Costello C & Clark A (1987) Peripheral blood and bone marrow abnormalities in patients with HIV related disease. *British Journal of Haematology* **65**: 289–294.

Ultman MH, Belman AL, Ruff H et al (1985) Developmental abnormalities in infants and children with acquired immune deficiency syndrome (AIDS) and AIDS-related complex. *Developmental Medicine and Child Neurology* **27**: 563–571.

Volberding PA, Lagakos SW, Koch MA et al (1990) Zidovudine in asymptomatic human immunodeficiency virus infection: A controlled trial in persons with fewer than 500 CD4-Positive cells per cubic millimeter. *New England Journal of Medicine* **322**: 941–949.

Walsh CM, Nardi MA & Karpatkin S (1983) On the mechanism of thrombocytopenic purpura in sexually active homosexual men. *New England Journal of Medicine* **311**: 635–639.

Warrier I & Lusher J (1990) Retrovir therapy in hemophiliac children with symptomatic human immunodeficiency virus infection: efficacy and toxicity. *American Journal of Pediatric Hematology/Oncology* **12**: 160–163.

Weinblatt ME, Scimeca PG, James-Herry AG & Pahwa S (1987) Thrombocytopenia in an infants with AIDS. *American Journal of Diseases of Children* **141**: 15.

Weinblatt ME, Kochen J & Ortega J (1988) Danazol for children with immune thrombocytopenic purpura. *American Journal of Diseases of Children* **142**: 1317–1319.

Weiblen BJ, Lee FK, Cooper ER et al (1990) Early diagnosis of HIV infection in infants by detection of IgA HIV antibodies. *Lancet* **335**: 988–990.

Wiznia AA & Nicholas SW (1990) Organ system involvement in HIV-infected children. *Pediatric Annals* **19**: 475–481.

Yanase Y, Tango T, Okumura K, Tada T & Kawasaki T (1986) Lymphocyte subsets identified by monoclonal antibodies in healthy children. *Pediatric Research* **20**: 1147–1151.

Yarchoan R, Mitsya H, Myers C & Broder S (1989) Clinical pharmacology of 3'-azido-2',3'-dideoxythymidine (zidovudine) and related dideoxynucleosides. *New England Journal of Medicine* **321**: 726–738.

Zimmerman BL, Haller JO, Price AP et al (1987) Children with AIDS—is pathologic diagnosis possible based on chest radiographs. *Pediatric Radiology* **17**: 303–307.

Zon LI & Groopman JE (1988) Hematologic manifestations of the human immunodeficiency virus (HIV). *Seminars in Hematology* **25**: 208–213.

Zon LI, Arkin C & Groopman JE (1987) Haematologic manifestations of the human immune deficiency virus (HIV). *British Journal of Haematology* **66**: 251–256.

4

The management of haemoglobinopathies

SALLY C. DAVIES
BEATRIX WONKE

The haemoglobinopathies are disorders which result either from the synthesis of structurally abnormal haemoglobin (Hb) chains (the Hb variants), or from the defective synthesis of Hb chains (the thalassaemia syndromes). They are the most commonly inherited genetic disorders worldwide with some 240 000 infants born annually with major haemoglobinopathies and at least 190 million carriers worldwide. They are all inherited in a Mendelian recessive manner so that persons with the carrier, or trait, states are generally healthy. Patients manifesting clinically significant disease may be homozygous for any one condition or compound heterozygotes for two or more haemoglobinopathy genes which interact.

The haemoglobinopathies have arisen as a result of mutations and deletions in and around the globin genes on chromosomes 16 and 11. While these mutations occurred spontaneously they have persisted within particular ethnic groups because of the selective advantage against *Plasmodium falciparum* malaria offered by the carrier states. The haemoglobinopathies are therefore rarely found in the autochthonous Northern European populations but have come to Europe and North America with the population migrations (WHO, 1987). As a result the patients in Northern Europe are generally found domiciled in industrial conurbations, often associated in groups related to their countries of origin.

PATHOPHYSIOLOGY OF HOMOZYGOUS β THALASSAEMIA AND SICKLE CELL DISEASE

Homozygous β thalassaemia is an inherited disorder of Hb resulting from an unbalanced rate of β globin chain synthesis. As a direct result of the basic genetic defect the β thalassaemic red cells contain an excess amount of Hb subunits. Following oxidation, these subunits generate free oxygen radicals such as superoxide and hydroxy radicals. These oxygen radicals start a chain of oxidative events which leads to the formation of methaemoglobin and hemichromes. Hemichromes are known as Heinz bodies in β thalassaemia. Heinz bodies are monomeric unstable chains which bind to different membrane proteins altering the normal structure and function which leads to early death of the red blood cells before the erythroblasts are well haemo-globinized (Shinar and Rachmilewitz, 1990). This ineffective erythropoiesis leads to anaemia, increased production of erythropoietin and an expansion of the bone marrow of 15–30 times normal. This marrow expansion results in distortion and fragility of the bones and an increased blood volume. The reticuloendothelial cells become congested by these abnormal cells and consequently hepatosplenomegaly develops, which increases the anaemia and causes thrombocytopenia and neutropenia. The child's growth and maturation are retarded. The overactive marrow also enhances gastro-intestinal iron absorption resulting in haemosiderosis. In the absence of diagnosis and treatment most patients with β thalassaemia major die before the age of 5 years, Modell and Berdouskas (1984). With recommended treatment, which will be discussed in detail, all the above-mentioned compli-cations are avoidable or treatable and consequently the overall prognosis is now open-ended.

Sickle cell disease (SCD) is a generic term for a family of haemoglobin disorders having in common the inheritance of the sickle β globin gene (β^s). Sickle cell anaemia is the homozygous state (SS) when the β^s gene is inherited from both parents. The other commonly encountered SCDs result from the coinheritance of β^s with either a β thalassaemia gene (Sβ^o or Sβ$^+$) or with another β chain structural variant such as β^c which gives rise to haemoglobin SC.

The β^s gene has a point mutation in the DNA from adenine to thiamine resulting in amino acid substitution of valine for glutamic acid at the sixth position of the β globin chain so that the β^s protein chains gel on deoxy-genation. These liquid crystals distort the red blood cells into their pathog-nomonic rigid sickle shape. It is blockage by the sickled cells of the microvasculature that gives rise to the pathology associated with SCD.

INHERITANCE AND GENETIC LESIONS OF β THALASSAEMIA MAJOR AND SICKLE CELL DISEASE

When two carriers (trait) mate there is a one in four chance in each pregnancy that they will produce an affected child. This is so whether the parents carry the same trait, in which case the child is homozygous, or different haemo-globinopathy traits, when the child is a double heterozygote.

β Thalassaemia carriers may have a slightly reduced Hb and typically low red blood cell indices (Hb 11–13 g dl^{-1}, MCH <27 pg, and a red cell count >5.0 × 10^{12} L^{-1}). The diagnosis is confirmed with a raised HbA$_2$ (>3.6%). Hb F levels are variable.

Once 'at risk' couples are identified, a clear explanation about the significance of the condition is essential; the genetic risk being the most important information, followed by advice about the various prenatal diagnostic possibilities for the purpose of prevention. Safe and accurate prenatal diagnosis is possible in all cases of SCD and the majority of cases before 12 weeks of gestation by chorionic villus sampling (CVS). Diagnosis by CVS depends on gene mapping. By March 1990, 91 point mutations had been discovered in β thalassaemia major (Kazazian, 1990). Each major population group, Mediterranean, Indian, Chinese and Afro-Caribbean/ African has its own spectrum of β thalassaemia mutations. Prenatal diagnosis has led to a marked reduction in the incidence of β thalassaemia in Europe (Cao et al, 1984; Modell et al, 1984).

HOMOZYGOUS β THALASSAEMIA

The disease commonly presents during the first year of life, although occasionally a severe transfusion-dependent patient presents at 3 to 4 years of age—these cases are now called *late onset thalassaemia major*. Those patients with homozygous β thalassaemia who manifest a mild course and are therefore transfusion-independent are called *thalassaemia intermedia* (see below).

Affected infants can present with a variety of symptoms including: failure to thrive, poor weight gain, feeding problems and irritability. Fever, diarrhoea and vomiting with a distended abdomen and increasing pallor may alert parents that their child has a serious disease, while the clinical findings often only reveal anaemia and sometimes splenomegaly.

An accurate diagnosis can be made from a simple blood test which always shows a severe degree of anaemia with microcytosis and hypochromia. The red cells show strikingly abnormal morphological appearances with microcytosis, hypochromia, anisocytosis, poikilocytosis, distorted red cells and a variable number of erythroblasts relating to the degree of anaemia. Hb electrophoresis confirms the diagnosis with elevated fetal haemoglobin (HbF) levels, reduced or absent adult haemoglobin (HbA) and a variable haemoglobin A_2 (HbA_2).

DNA studies should be undertaken in order to define the precise genetic lesion. This gives both information about the possibility of CVS sampling for future pregnancies and also as to the probable disease severity (β thalassaemia major or intermedia).

Management of homozygous β thalassaemia

Blood transfusions

The recommended treatment for homozygous β thalassaemia involves regular (three-weekly or more frequent) blood transfusions, not allowing the Hb level to fall below $10 \, \text{g} \, \text{dl}^{-1}$. This ensures erythroid marrow suppression and preserves excellent health with normal growth and development. It is a clinical decision as to when to start regular blood transfusion. In the majority of cases the decision to transfuse is obvious. In the few others the decision should be based on clinical parameters rather than any set Hb level. All children should be followed and monitored carefully for signs of anaemia, heart failure, splenomegaly, variable Hb level, lassitude, poor weight gain and low growth velocity.

In practice, one aims to transfuse not more than $20 \, \text{ml} \, \text{kg}^{-1}$ body weight of packed filtered red cells over a period of 2–3 hours. The post-transfusion Hb should not rise above 15.0 g dl^{-1} as higher levels increase blood viscosity and the risk of thrombosis and result in unnecessarily high blood consumption. Patients with cardiac failure or very low initial Hb levels (≤ 5.0 g dl^{-1}) should receive 5 ml kg^{-1} body weight of packed filtered red cells in 3–4 hours.

The effectiveness of blood transfusion can be measured by the rate of Hb fall. In splenectomized patients this is in the order of 1 g of Hb a week, while in non-splenectomized patients it may be as high as 1.5 g of Hb a week. The frequency of blood transfusions can be calculated from the rate of Hb fall. When the Hb fall is greater than expected, as calculated above, then the following causes should be considered: alloimmunization of red cells, hypersplenism or even poor quality of blood used for transfusion.

Side-effects of transfusion

Chronic transfusions may be associated with serious side-effects. *Allosensitization* of clinically important blood group antigens occurs in up to 25% of the multiply-transfused thalassaemia patients. Therefore, patients' ABO, rhesus, Kell, Kidd and Duffy systems should be typed at diagnosis or before institution of transfusion therapy and patients' blood should always be matched with donor blood in ABO, rhesus and Kell systems.

Febrile, urticarial transfusion reactions, *cytomegalovirus* (CMV) infection and immunosuppression occur when transfused blood is not filtered. These complications can easily be avoided by simple filtration of the units of blood at the bedside of the patient. These filters have a 99.6% white cell removal efficiency in minimal time and easy handling. Not more than two units can be transfused through each of the available systems; Miramed (Italy), PALL (America), Sepacell (Japan) and Cellselect (Holland) which take one per filter.

The most common cause of death in homozygous β thalassaemia is heart failure secondary to *iron overload*. The second commonest cause is liver failure due to *transfusion-transmitted viruses* in thalassaemic patients. It is therefore essential that donor blood should be tested for *hepatitis B virus* (Moroni et al, 1984). Hepatitis B vaccination should be administered to all newly diagnosed thalassaemic patients and to those older patients who lack demonstrable antibodies to hepatitis B virus. Low-dose intradermal hepatitis B vaccination has been found to be protective against hepatitis B virus and considerably more cost-effective than the conventional dose recommended by the manufacturers of the vaccine (Mok et al, 1989).

Transfusion-associated non-A, non-B hepatitis (*hepatitis C*) remains the most important problem in multiply-transfused thalassaemia major patients. In a recent report, the incidence of positive antibodies to Hepatitis C virus was 23.2% in multiply-transfused thalassaemia major patients (Wonke et al, 1990). Over 60% of these infections progress to chronic active hepatitis and eventually to cirrhosis. All chronically-transfused thalassaemic patients should be tested for HCV antibodies and patients suffering from chronic active hepatitis should be considered for treatment with α interferon

(Donohue et al, 1990). Blood transfusions will become safer with the introduction of donor screening for anti-HCV.

Since the introduction of anti-HIV donor screening, the risk of acquisition of *human immunodeficiency virus* (HIV) by transfusion has been reduced to 1 in 150 000 units (Cumming et al, 1989). Thalassaemia patients infected with HIV should be informed, counselled and appropriately investigated. The European Mediterranean WHO Working Group on Haemoglobinopathies is currently studying the HIV seropositive thalassaemia patients. The aim of this study is to learn about factors (e.g. splenectomy and altered immunity) affecting the natural history of HIV and to give information and recommendations regarding treatment. Preliminary data were reported at the Cooley Care meeting in Athens in June 1990 (Girot, 1990). Over 100 thalassaemia patients of both sexes, collected from more than 12 countries, have been reported to be anti-HIV positive. The disease appears to have a slow evolution, 2 years or longer, and the rate of progression to symptomatic disease is 26% after 6 years of seropositivity. Recommendations of this group include the following; all HIV seropositive thalassaemia patients are to be monitored clinically and investigated every 6 months. Particular emphasis should be placed on the following clinical problems; lymphadenopathy, constitutional disorder, neurological problems, secondary infections and secondary cancers. Investigations should include the following; absolute $CD4^+$ (T-helper cells) lymphocyte count, presence of P^{24} antigen, loss of P^{24} antibody, serum IgG, IgA levels and erythrocyte sedimentation rate (ESR).

The treatment of symptomatic patients should be routine, while for those asymptomatic seropositive thalassaemia patients with a falling $CD4^+$ count it remains controversial. Low-dose zidovudine (AZT) should, we believe, be used when the absolute $CD4^+$ counts are $\leq 5 \times 10^9 L^{-1}$. The efficacy in preventing disease of the central nervous system and the development of resistance is unknown (Swart and Weller, 1990), but at such low doses prophylactic AZT has minimal marrow toxicity.

Chelation therapy

Maintenance transfusion preserves excellent health but, without treatment of iron overload, it leads to severe iron damage. Excess iron resulting from transfusions leads to endocrine disturbances, growth retardation, failure of puberty, and diabetes. Death in early life is generally the result of intractable heart failure.

At present the only way to avoid this outcome is by regular subcutaneous (s.c.) infusion of the iron-chelating agent desferrioxamine (DF) from a small portable syringe driver pump, over 8 to 12 hours, at least five to six nights a week. Iron overload is monitored by serum ferritin assay. Monitoring urinary iron excretion over 24 hours is the best way to appraise DF therapy, as serum ferritin levels may not reflect the true extent of iron overload.

Chelation therapy should commence by the time the serum ferritin has reached $1000 \mu g L^{-1}$; this, in practice, is around the twelfth to fourteenth transfusion. It is easiest to start early in order to habituate the child and family to the burdensome regimen.

It is important not to over-chelate these infants, when the iron burden is still low, in order to avoid DF-related toxicity. The initial recommended dose is $20 \, mg \, kg^{-1}$ 4 or 5 nights each week. $100 \, mg$ oral vitamin C supplements should be given on the days of infusion, as this increases urinary iron excretion. In the older, more iron-overloaded patients, DF should not exceed $50 \, mg \, kg^{-1}$ body weight, with $200 \, mg$ oral vitamin C.

In patients with cardiac complications continuous intravenous (i.v.) infusion of DF in doses of up to $200 \, mg \, kg^{-1}$ body weight for 24 hours has been used in an attempt to reverse cardiomyopathy (Marcus et al, 1984). In our centre, once early cardiomyopathy secondary to iron overload is diagnosed by MUGA scan (multiple gated imaging with Tc^{99}-labelled autologous red cells) the DF treatment is intensified. This usually entails the insertion of an intravenous delivery system (Port-a-Cath or Hickman line) which allows continuous i.v. DF infusions. We use low-dose DF (between 3–4 g in 24 hours) with low-dose vitamin C (200 mg) oral supplementation.

Combined regular transfusion and iron chelation therapy (optimal treatment) appears to ensure good health in the long term and, if DF chelation begins before the age of 10 years and is complied with then the patient can be expected to survive, free of cardiac disease for an indefinite duration.

Desferrioxamine toxicity

Desferrioxamine chelation treatment is burdensome, painful, expensive and lifelong. If DF is infused subcutaneously it tends to leave painful lumps at the site of injection because of the relatively slow absorption of the drug. This problem may be solved either by the addition of small doses of hydrocortisone added to the DF (1 to 2 mg per syringe) or by increasing the volume of the solution. Poor hygiene techniques can give rise to the development of infection and abscesses, even requiring surgical drainage as well as antibiotics. It is, therefore, essential that the parents are fully instructed in the correct techniques and provided with the proper equipment (swabs, butterfly needles, sterile water and syringes). Hypersensitivity occasionally develops to DF but most patients can be successfully desensitized by using small repeated injections of DF with gradually increasing doses.

Both ophthalmic and oto-toxicity have now been described in patients receiving high dose i.v. DF or inappropriately high doses of s.c. DF for their degree of iron overload (Olivieri et al, 1986). Tables 1 and 2 summarize the symptoms, signs and clinical investigation of the ophthalmic complications. While the cataracts, which are a rare complication, do not improve on reducing the DF dose, the retinal symptoms do.

The risk of oto-toxicity is also related to the dose of DF and is most commonly encountered in children with low serum ferritin levels ($\leq 2000 \, \mu g \, l^{-1}$) who have received DF treatment in doses $\geq 50 \, mg \, kg^{-1}$ daily dose. We therefore recommend that hearing tests are performed yearly and if hearing loss is demonstrated then the DF dose is adjusted. The more severely affected children, who may present with speech or school problems, may require hearing aids and a change of chelation agent. Calcium diethylene

Table 1. Ophthalmological changes in desferral toxicity seen by clinical examination.

Symptoms and signs	Method of assessment	Pathological changes
Retinal appearance	Fundoscopy	Pigmentary changes, oedema, vessels narrowed, later atrophic changes (N.B. anterior eye changes also occur.)
Blurred vision	Visual acuity	Variable decrease in VA*
Tunnel vision	Perimetry	Peripheral field loss, possible annular scotoma, RP-like; collapse of field with small and dim targets*
Night blindness	Adaptometry	Variable increase of rod and cone thresholds
Reduced light and colour sensation	Colour tests particularly blue/ yellow (tritan)	100-Hue test show tritan axis loss*, contrast sensitivity reduced for low spatial frequencies*

* Abnormalities may be detected before subjective disturbances begin: useful for monitoring retinal state.

Table 2. Ancillary ophthalmological tests.

Ancillary tests	Findings
Fluorescein angiography	Pigmentary changes lead to window defects; oedema
Electro-oculography (EOG)	May be reduced acutely, unreliable
Ganzfeld electroretinography (ERG)	Loss of scotopic sensitivity*, delayed responses*
Pattern electroretinography (PERG)	Reduced responses*
Visual evoked potentials (VER)	Delayed responses*

*Abnormalities may be detected before subjective disturbances begin: useful for monitoring retinal state.

triamine pantacetic acid (Ca-DTPA) with oral zinc supplementation may be used. The plasma zinc levels should be monitored. In the severe cases recovery is a rare occurrence. These children will require additional speech therapy and support (Wonke et al, 1989a).

The toxic effect of high doses of DF on skeletal growth is still unclear. It is known that DF inhibits DNA synthesis, fibroblast proliferation, collagen formation and may also cause zinc deficiency.

Patients who received inappropriately high doses of DF when their iron burden is minimal frequently complain of pain in the hips, lower back and have difficulty in walking, with growth arrest or a reduction of growth velocity. The body measurements of children and adults are dispropor-tionate: characteristically they have a short trunk with discrepancy between pubis–heel and crown–pubis and span measurements. Swelling of the wrists and knees and genu valgum of variable severity is often found. These patients have almost always a normal onset of puberty and pubertal development. Once the epiphyses have fused (puberty) alteration of the chelation regimen cannot improve growth. In pre-pubertal children reduction in the DF dose and oral zinc supplementation can achieve a partial improvement but they never regain their original centile. Growth hormone treatment is being piloted in these children but, as yet, the data is incomplete.

Infection with *Yersinia* spp. is a common complication in DF-treated patients (Porter and Huehns, 1989). The *Yersinia* family of bacteria has a low pathogenicity but an unusually high requirement for iron. They do not secrete a siderophore but have receptors for ferrioxamine and become pathogenic when more iron is available in the tissues, as in thalassaemic patients on DF. Thus *Yersinia* presents an important hazard to any patient receiving this drug.

Clinicians should be alert to the possibility of *Yersinia* infection in any child who presents with an abdominal complaint, including: acute abdomen, pain, diarrhoea, vomiting, fever and sore throat. DF treatment must be stopped immediately. Appropriate cultures of stool, in discussion with the microbiologist, should be taken. Empirical treatment must be commenced as a medical emergency with either an aminoglycoside or co-trimoxazole.

For the future, an effective cheap non-toxic oral iron chelator would clearly provide a better alternative. Many compounds are currently under investigation. Porter et al (1989) have reviewed this topic. Clinical trials are being undertaken in several centres with the oral chelator 1-2 dimethyl-3-hydroxy pyrid-4-one (L1). In the longest trial reported to date, (Bartlett et al, 1990) nine patients with β thalassaemia major, aged between 12 and 38 years, of both sexes were given daily L1 for up to 15 months. The drug was generally well tolerated with no significant side-effects in the thalassaemics. Three patients developed muscle and joint pains and one of these had an anti-rheumatoid factor that rose from $1:80$ to $1:640$ after six months on treatment. L1 therefore, appears to be a safe iron-chelation agent in thalassaemics.

Complications of β thalassaemia major

Most of the complications of thalassaemia major are attributable to iron overload. This may be the result of economic circumstances, late onset of chelation therapy or poor compliance with DF therapy.

In iron overload the excess iron which is deposited in the tissues causes damage. The mechanisms by which iron damages the organs have only recently been identified. Toxicity begins when the iron load in a particular tissue exceeds the tissue or blood binding capacity of iron, and free non-transferrin iron appears. This 'free iron' is a catalyst of the production of oxygen species that damage cells and peroxidize membrane lipids leading to cell destruction (Shinar and Rachmilewitz, 1990).

Liver has a large capacity to produce proteins which bind the iron and store it in the form of ferritin and haemosiderin. Heart cells generate only small amounts of storage proteins and are therefore sensitive to 'free iron'-induced oxygen radicals. Therefore, cardiomyopathy frequently occurs with relatively little iron in the myocardial cells (Gutteridge and Halliwell, 1989).

Cardiac complications

Normal myocardial function requires adequate tissue oxygen, as chronic anaemia increases cardiac output by increasing stroke volume. Iron deposition in the heart causes cardiac complications including; hypertrophy, dilatation, degeneration of myocardial fibres and myocardial fibrosis. The extent of damage is directly related to the transfusional iron load in the absence of, or with poor compliance to, chelation therapy (Wonke et al, 1989b).

In our experience, clinical assessment, chest X-ray, electrocardiogram, 24-hour ECG monitoring and even echocardiography are relatively insensitive techniques in detecting early myocardial damage before the onset of clinically apparent disease. Furthermore, age, serum ferritin levels, number of units transfused, liver disease and sexual maturation do not correlate with cardiac abnormality (Wonke et al, 1989b). MUGA scan is the most sensitive method to evaluate early damage and it also helps in monitoring cardiac function after intensification of DF chelation therapy (Aldouri et al, 1990; see i.v. chelation).

Reduced growth

Iron-overloaded thalassaemic children of both sexes show reduced growth around the age of 10 to 11 years. The cause of this is not fully understood, but several mechanisms have been reported: growth hormone deficiency secondary to pituitary damage by haemosiderosis (Pintor et al, 1986); defective hepatic synthesis of somatomedin (TGF-1) (Saenger et al, 1980); sex steroid deficiency. Serum ferritin levels are usually high and bone age is at least 2 years behind chronological age. Treatment for these patients consists of intensification of chelation therapy and in cases of growth hormone deficiency replacement therapy is indicated.

Hypothyroidism

Hypothyroidism is observed in >17% of iron-overloaded patients (Sabato et al, 1983). It affects both sexes equally and occurs after the age of 10 years. Three types of thyroid dysfunction have been recognized in thalassaemics; pre-clinical, mild and overt hypothyroidism. Classical symptoms of hypothyroidism in patients with pre-clinical or mild hypothyroidism are absent, whereas in overt hypothyroidism a whole spectrum of clinical features have been observed; growth retardation, decreased activity, dry skin, cardiac failure and pericardial effusion. The thyroid gland is not usually enlarged (see Table 3). Treatment depends on the severity of the organ failure. Replacement with L-thyroxine is recommended in symptomatic patients. In the remaining patients, intensification of iron chelation may improve thyroid dysfunction.

Table 3. Investigations for hypothyroidism.

Hypothyroidism	Serum T_4	Serum FT_4	Serum TSH	TSH response to TRH
Pre-clinical	Normal	Normal	Marginally increased	Increased
Mild	Marginally low	Marginally low	Elevated	Exaggerated
Overt	Low	Low	Elevated	Exaggerated

Hypoparathyroidism

The incidence of hypocalcaemia related to hypoparathyroidism, in iron-overloaded thalassaemic patients is 7% (Wonke and De Sanctis, 1991). The majority are older than 15 years of age; males are more commonly affected than females (3:1). It is almost always associated with bone complications; spontaneous fractures which are slow to heal, genu valgum of variable severity and short stature. Serum calcium is low, phosphate high and the PTH low or inappropriate for the serum calcium level. There is also a low excretion of 1,25 dihydroxycholecalciferol $(1,25(OH)_2D)$. There is a reduction of 24-hour urinary calcium and phosphate. Treatment is with oral vitamin D or one of its analogues. If high serum phosphate concentrations persist a phosphate binder is recommended.

Diabetes mellitus

The incidence of diabetes mellitus (DM) in iron-overloaded patients varies between 8 and 14.5% (Wonke and De Sanctis, in press). The onset of DM in the majority of patients is in the late teens and both sexes are affected equally. Frequently, impaired oral glucose tolerance precedes frank diabetes. This is asymptomatic while DM itself presents with the classical symptoms accompanied by ketosis or ketoacidosis. In asymptomatic patients treatments, including carbohydrate-reduced diet or an oral hypo-glycaemic agent, are controversial. In our experience carbohydrate-reduced diet, together with vigorous iron-chelation therapy, improves biochemical diabetes. In symptomatic patients insulin treatment is essential; metabolic control can be difficult to achieve.

Patients with insulin-dependent diabetes have a higher incidence of cardiac failure, liver cirrhosis and cerebral thromboembolism. Diabetic retinopathy is a rare complication; albuminuria may be present at the time of diagnosis or during the course of the disease.

Sexual complications

In a large study of 1240 thalassaemic patients 41% of males and 45% of females over the age of 15 years were pre-pubertal (De Sanctis, personal communication). Many of the affected patients began DF therapy well after the age of 10 years. In a smaller study data suggest that long-term DF therapy, begun before the age of 10, may ensure, in the majority of patients, normal sexual function (Bronspiegel et al, 1990). The clinical presentation is variable. Some patients have delayed puberty, defined, as a complete lack of pubertal development in girls by their 13th birthday and boys by their 14th birthday. A few patients have arrested puberty which is characterized by lack of progression of puberty for 12 months or longer with reduced or absent growth velocity.

In the majority of cases primary hypogonadism is present. In these patients there are no signs of puberty at the age of 18 years; they are also short and their weight corresponds to their height. Secondary hypogonadism occurs where hypogonadism develops after complete pubertal maturation. In males this is

Table 4. Pituitary and gonadal function tests in thalassaemic patients.

Sexual maturation	Basal plasma gonadotrophins	Gonadotrophins response to GnRH	Basal plasma sexual steroids	Sexual steroids response to HCG or HMG
Delayed puberty	Pre-pubertal range	Reduced response	Low	Normal response
Arrested puberty	Low	Reduced response	Low	Normal response
Primary hypogonadism	Low	Poor or absent response	Low	Normal or reduced response
Secondary hypogonadism	Low	Reduced or absent response	Low	Variable response (normal, low, absent)

manifested by impotence and in females with secondary amenorrhoea, weight gain, hot flushes and bone pain. Another characteristic clinical finding in male thalassaemic patients is the reduced beard appearance and the absence of facial acne during puberty. These aspects are not fully understood. Diagnostic findings are summarized in Table 4.

Treatment of delayed puberty depends on the following factors; age, severity of iron overload, chronic liver disease and presence of psychological problems resulting from delayed puberty. Teenagers with psychological problems need hormone treatment in order to minimize the risk of complete rejection of thalassaemia treatment (DF chelation and even transfusion). Treatment should be withheld in the well chelated age groups without psychological problems but regular follow up is necessary.

Patients with pubertal arrest are treated with oestrogen/progesterone or i.m. testosterone. In hypogonadism treatment consists of oral sexual steroids. In secondary hypogonadism replacement therapy is indicated. Induction of fertility in both sexes is a frequent request. This involves the co-operation of the haematologist and the reproductive endocrinologist. Experience in this field is limited but encouraging.

Bone change

The bone changes commonly found in the older thalassaemic patients are the result of inadequate transfusion in childhood. These changes are due to the expansion of the bone marrow mass secondary to the anaemia. The changes may be mild, moderate or severe. The characteristic facial appearance with bossing, flat nose, mongoloid slant of the eyes and prominent molar eminences (or protrusions) are permanent disfigurations. In extreme cases these can cause nasal airway obstruction, speech defect and difficulties with eating. Cosmetic surgery is required as improved treatment has no affect on bone changes. Cortical thinning of the long bones leads to spontaneous fractures which are slow to heal, often resulting in deformities. Premature fusion of the epiphyses of the humerus and femur results in shortening of the arms or legs and considerable restriction in movement. With time, osteo-arthritic changes develop in the affected joints. Treatment is palliative only. The most serious complication is spinal cord compression, either from collapsed vertebrae or extramedullary haematopoiesis in the spinal canal. Surgical intervention or radiotherapy is necessary to treat these cases. Bone changes are entirely preventable by optimal treatment.

Cholelithiasis is associated with all haemolytic anaemias. In patients with sickle cell anaemia the biliary calculi are reported to occur in 10–37% of cases (Bond et al, 1987; Webb et al, 1989). The incidence of gallstones in thalassaemia appears to be about the same as in sickle cell anaemia; it also occurs as early as 10 years of age. Prophylactic cholecystectomy to protect patients from future formation of gallstones has been proposed by Feretis et al (1985).

Hypersplenism

Optimal treatment usually prevents splenomegaly. Inadequate transfusion invariably leads to massive hypersplenism caused by extramedullary haematopoiesis. Hypersplenism is associated with worsening of anaemia (Hb fall is greater than $1.5\,g\,l^{-1}$ per week), neutropenia and even thrombocytopenia. Splenectomy should not be undertaken before the age of 5 years due to the risk of overwhelming pneumococcal sepsis in infants. Treatment with pneumococcal vaccine should precede elective surgery by 3 to 4 weeks and penicillin prophylaxis is recommended for life after splenectomy. In patients with β thalassaemia intermedia post-splenectomy high platelet counts may cause thromboembolic complications. Low dose soluble aspirin 75 mg daily or an antiplatelet aggregating agent is recommended.

Bone marrow transplantation

Bone marrow transplantation is the only cure available for thalassaemia at present. For transplantation a histocompatible bone marrow donor is required. A suitable bone marrow donor is a sibling or occasionally a parent, where parents are first cousins. In younger patients on optimal treatment the overall success rate is 94% whilst in patients of older age groups with liver fibrosis or liver enlargement the survival rate is 65–75% (Lucarelli et al, 1990). Mortality results from infections, heart problems and graft versus host disease. The world experience of bone marrow transplantation is shown in Figure 1. Bone marrow transplantation is far less expensive than the cumulative cost of conventional life-long treatment, so it is reasonable to set up transplant centres in countries with a high incidence of thalassaemia. It is also recommended in those children, both with thalassaemia and sickle cell disease (Vermylen et al, 1988), where conventional treatment is not readily available.

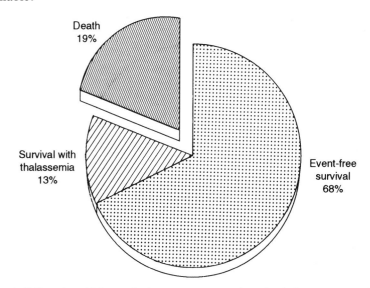

Figure 1. Collected world figures for bone marrow transplantation in homozygous β thalassaemia, to December 1989.

The improved survival in homozygous β thalassaemia means that we must recognize and manage the psychosocial problems associated with the disease. Patients and their families require support and psychosocial intervention at an early age in order to maximize their full integration into society (Politis et al, 1990).

β THALASSAEMIA INTERMEDIA

In β thalassaemia intermedia the clinical picture is milder than β thalassaemia major despite the same pattern of inheritance as homozygous β thalassaemia. It is a clinical definition based on the patient's rare requirements for blood transfusion. The Hb level is usually above $7.0\,\mathrm{g}\,\mathrm{dl}^{-1}$, red cell indices are as in β thalassaemia major and Hb electrophoresis shows variable levels of HbA,

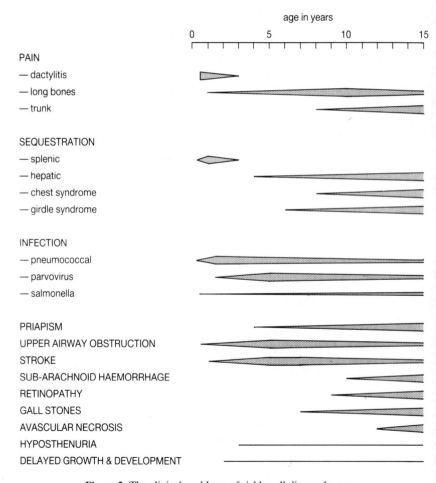

Figure 2. The clinical problems of sickle cell disease by age.

HbF and HbA$_2$. The genetic factors ameliorating the disease include: the inheritance of a mild β$^+$ thalassaemia gene, coinheritance of α thalassaemia and increased γ chain production (Thein et al, 1987).

Patients with β thalassaemia intermedia grow and develop normally. The complications commonly encountered in this group are: hypersplenism, gall stones and ankle ulcers. Haemochromatosis from excess dietary iron absorption is rarely significant. Treatment consists of clinical surveillance, folic acid supplementation, periodic blood transfusions and, in iron overload, DF chelation. The treatment of leg ulcers is the most problematic. Blood transfusions, bed rest, supportive surgical stockings, zinc ointments and tablets may be of help.

THE MANAGEMENT OF SICKLE CELL DISEASE

Despite our understanding of the molecular basis of sickle cell disease (SCD) and the pathology of the sickling phenomenon the condition remains a major risk to health with a high mortality and morbidity at all ages (Grey et al, 1991). The clinical problems of SCD by age are summarized in Figure 2. In childhood the peak incidence of death is between 1 and 3 years of age, predominantly related to infection (Leikin et al, 1989). In adolescence cerebrovascular accidents are the most common cause of death and in adults deaths are most often related to respiratory complications. With active management the proportion of patients expected to survive to 20 years of age is now approximately 89% and approximately 85% for SS patients (Leikin et al, 1989). The greatest contribution to the reduction in infant mortality in SCD has been the introduction of neonatal screening programmes for the early detection of the disease and subsequent medical care with the prescription of prophylactic penicillin (Editorial, 1986; Gaston et al, 1986).

While SS patients generally have the most severe clinical course, many with Sβ^0 thalassaemia, in particular those arising from the Mediterranean region, often follow a similarly severe course. Haemoglobin SC disease usually presents fewer problems in childhood but the patients are also at risk of infection, sudden death and have a higher incidence of the proliferative retinopathy and avascular necrosis of bones.

The greatest challenge in the management of SCD is why some patients are more severely affected than others, and why some fluctuate between periods of relatively good health and frequent, severe complications.

A number of ameliorating factors are known; including the persistent production into adolescence and adult life of HbF. A level of ≥ 10% HbF offers protection against stroke and avascular necrosis while ≥ 20% HbF offers protection from episodic manifestations such as painful crises or pulmonary complications (Powars et al, 1984). Co-inheritance of α-thalassaemia has been shown to reduce the levels of haemolysis as judged by higher Hb and lower reticulocyte and serum bilirubin levels (Higgs et al, 1978). Environmental factors and poor socio-economic status can precipitate sickling. It is important that patients should be aware of, and avoid the following: infection, hypoxia, dehydration, cold and exhaustion.

Infancy

In infancy the most important clinical problems relate to infection, splenic sequestration and dactylitis. At birth infants are protected from the problems of SCD because of their high levels of HbF which interferes with the molecular gelation of the β^s. Painful vaso-occlusive crisis is therefore, rarely seen before 6 months of age and almost never before four months of age. Fulminant pneumococcal septicaemia and acute splenic sequestration crises do however, present before 6 months often in previously undiagnosed cases leading rapidly to a fatal outcome (Powars, 1989).

When children with SCD become ill they easily become dehydrated because of both the reduced fluid intake and also their inability to concentrate their urine; related to the sickle damage to the renal tubules. This *hyposthenuric defect* is evident in children by the age of 2 or 3 years. Consequently patients' clinical state can deteriorate very rapidly. It is essential that the patient's 'steady state' laboratory parameters are known and monitored for the purposes of comparison. Indications for hospital admission are as follows:

1. The vaso-occlusive pain is uncontrolled by oral analgesia.
2. There is a severe associated constitutional upset, e.g. tachycardia ≥ 100, pyrexia $\geq 38.5°C$.
3. There is any visceral involvement, e.g. tachypnoea ≥ 16 per min, absent bowel sounds.
4. Presence of any neurological signs.

The spleen is a major site of sickling because of the relative hypoxia and acidosis. This results in auto-splenectomy with *impaired immune function* in all types of SCD resulting in a high risk of the infection, in particular *Streptococcus pneumoniae* and *Salmonella* (Rogers et al, 1982). Infection with salmonella may present in unusual ways such as with hepatic sequestration, though it most commonly presents with septicaemia and/or osteomyelitis. *Meningitis* and *chest infections* are also more common in infants with SCD, affecting particularly SS children, also often caused by *Haemophilus influenzae* (Powars et al, 1983). Paradoxically the children with palpable spleens at, or before, the age of 1 year are those most prone to pneumococcal infection during the first years of life.

The necessity and efficacy of penicillin prophylaxis has been tested and proved by the American National Cooperative Study of Sickle Cell Disease (Gaston et al, 1986). It is therefore, essential that all children with any type of SCD should take oral penicillin prophylaxis, which should be commenced not later than 4 months of age; in a dose of 62.5 mg twice daily (b.i.d.) up to the age of one year, rising to 125 mg b.i.d. from one to three years and 250 mg b.i.d. thereafter until adult life. This regimen requires parental compliance which must be emphasized; a recent study has shown that only 47% of SCD children were proven to be taking penicillin (Cummins et al, 1991). Pneumococcal vaccine as discussed for pre-splenectomy under β thalassaemia major (see above) should be used as a complement to penicillin.

Doctors should be alert to the risk of infection in these children and institute prompt therapy with antibiotics in the presence of a fever. It is important to treat with benzyl penicillin, or a penicillin ester, parenterally in order to cover *Streptococcus pneumoniae*. With this treatment the rapid progression of pneumococcal infection with circulatory collapse and shock can usually be prevented.

Many children with SCD will visit areas where *malaria* may be contracted and they must receive appropriate malaria prophylaxis because they are at risk of developing severe haemolytic crises with profound anaemia and cardiac failure.

Another medical emergency is *splenic sequestration* which results from trapping of sickled red blood cells in the spleen with massive organ enlargement and a fall of Hb $\geq 2\,\mathrm{g\,dl^{-1}}$. There is severe abdominal pain and anaemia, which may become so severe that circulatory collapse results with vomiting, diarrhoea and congestive cardiac failure leading to death. Progression is generally acute and rapid over the space of 1 to 2 hours. The aetiology is uncertain although pneumococcal infection has been implicated. The children should be admitted to hospital urgently, an intravenous infusion started immediately and a replacement blood transfusion is almost always required. The high mortality can be prevented by early recognition and intervention so parents should be taught to palpate the spleen. There is at least a 30% risk of recurrent sequestration and a 37% risk of hypersplenism following an initial episode of acute splenic sequestration (Topley, 1981). It is therefore, recommended that following the presenting episode children should undergo routine splenectomy.

Painful vaso-occlusive crisis results from microvasculature obstruction causing hypoxia and pain most generally in the bones but also in joints, muscles and, on occasions, the soft tissues. In paediatric clinics we see the '*hand/foot*' *syndrome* as the earliest presentation (Davies and Brozovic, 1989). In this there is dactylitis—that is, sickle vaso-occlusion of the metacarpals or metatarsals—with overlying soft tissue involvement. It is rare before the age of 6 months or after the age of 3 years. The pain can be very severe and in cases where the diagnosis of SCD has not already been made a variety of misdiagnoses have been entertained, including non-accidental injury and insect bites. It can affect one limb or all four at the same time; it can last only a day or 3 to 4 weeks. It is essential that the syndrome should be properly recognized and treated otherwise chronic damage may occur resulting in poor bone growth and subsequent deformity (Figure 3). The treatment, which is standard for all vaso-occlusive SCD crises, is rest, warmth, increased fluids to prevent dehydration, and adequate analgesia (initially paracetamol in standard doses). This management should be applied as a first-line for all complications of SCD at all ages. In our experience it is rarely necessary to admit infants with the 'hand/foot' syndrome, but it is important to advise parents that they should not force the child to use a limb or walk whilst the pain continues. Admission is usually based on either the need for parenteral analgesia or the coexistence of constitutional upset (see list above). Hospital treatment is with the standard regimen of rest, warmth, intravenous fluids (at $80\,\mathrm{ml\,kg^{-1}\,24\,h^{-1}}$) and adequate analgesia under close

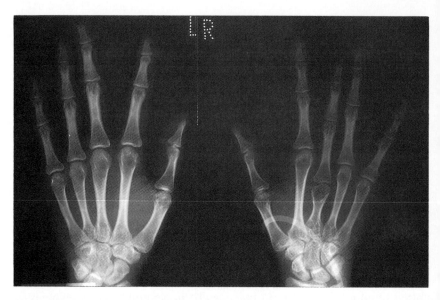

Figure 3. Hand X-ray of an adult SS patient showing a markedly shortened right 3rd metacarpal as a result of a severe dactylitis in infancy.

observation. We use continuous infusions given intravenously of either pethidine at a starting dose of $2 \, mg \, kg^{-1} \, h^{-1}$, or morphine at $10 \, \mu g \, kg^{-1} \, h^{-1}$; the respiratory rate must be carefully monitored with these regimens while the dose is titrated against the pain relief.

Pethidine is broken down into a stable metabolite, nor-pethidine, which is neuroexcitatory and on occasions causes fitting in SCD patients. It is therefore essential to monitor carefully the pain and clinical state of the patients during opiate therapy.

Preschool children (3–5 years)

The most common problems in this age group are painful vaso-occlusive crisis, aplastic crisis and upper airways obstruction. Splenic sequestration and deaths related to infection occur, but rather less commonly than in the infants.

The distribution of *pain* alters with age, most probably related to the recession of the red bone marrow. In this age group the pain is generally sited in the long bones and there may also be *sympathetic joint effusions* as a result of juxta-articular sickling. Septic arthritis is very rare, so aspiration of the joint effusions should only be undertaken in those rare cases where there is either no associated bone pain or there is proven septicaemia with one very severely affected joint. Mild painful vaso-occlusive crisis can be managed by the parents at home as above.

Aplastic crises can occur at any age in SCD and are almost invariably associated with infection. The most common cause is with the parvovirus B19 strain which, while only causing 'fifth' disease in people with normal haemopoiesis, infects the developing erythroblasts causing a transient cessation of production (Pattison, 1987). The Hb can drop precipitously over a few days as the red cell life-span in SCD is reduced to 6 to 10 days. Patients are generally admitted with signs and symptoms of anaemia, absent bone pain and, in very severe cases, congestive cardiac failure. Reticulocytes are absent from the peripheral blood. Parvovirus-specific IGM may be tested for, and in early cases the parvovirus antigen will be seen on electron microscopy. A replacement blood transfusion should be given if Hb ≤ 4 g dl^{-1} or the patient is clinically compromised.

Adenotonsillar hypertrophy giving rise to *upper airways obstruction* (UAO) can become a problem from the age of 18 months. In severe cases this can give rise to hypoxaemia at night with consequent sickling. The marked hypertrophy is probably a compensation for the loss of lymphoid tissue in the spleen. UAO occurs in at least 18% of SS children and we have also documented adolescents with HbSC who have UAO (Davies et al, 1989). Children with UAO snore while asleep. They should have their tonsils and adenoids removed in order to prevent vaso-occlusive crisis at night. This may prevent neurological events. Transfusion is not required prior to operation.

Schoolchildren (5–15 years)

In this age group the commonly encountered complications are the severe painful crisis and the 'chest' and 'girdle' syndromes. Splenic sequestration is rarely seen and infection occurs less commonly than in the infants.

In the painful crisis the site of the pain moves more centrally in the body as the children grow older and is also generally more severe. The average hospital admission for a patient in this age group with limb pain is 4.9 days as compared with 8.3 days if the pain is situated in the trunk (Brozovic et al, 1987). Treatment is with the standard regimen as previously described. Visceral complications may occur when the pain is experienced in the trunk, shoulders, spine, ribs, pelvis and hips. The most important complications are the 'sickle chest syndrome' and the acute abdomen or 'girdle syndrome'.

The *sickle chest syndrome* has now been well described (Davies et al, 1984; Yardumian and Davies, 1987). The term has been coined to describe a syndrome of pneumonic consolidation and associated hypoxaemia, which is presumed to result from vaso-occlusion of the pulmonary vasculature and in which no infective cause has been demonstrated. The clinical symptoms and signs precede the X-ray changes so it is essential to take action based on the clinical picture. Patients invariably have severe vaso-occlusive pain in the chest wall. They develop tachypnoea followed by the signs of consolidation, including crepitations on auscultation and dullness to percussion. As they become hypoxaemic central cyanosis can be seen in the mucous membranes. The best way of monitoring is by arterial blood gas estimations or trans-cutaneous oximetry; if the PaO$_2$ falls to ≤ 80 ml Hg on air, inspired oxygen is given and if it continues to fall to ≤ 60 ml Hg then exchange transfusion is carried out (see below). X-ray changes are generally those of opacities which start at the lung bases and move to the mid-zones and then upper zones (Figure 4). A few very rapidly progressive cases never develop the classic X-ray features as described but instead have hilar shadowing. The sickle chest syndrome can develop slowly, over a period of days, or rapidly which can be fatal. Any SCD patient with tachypnoea should be admitted as an emergency to hospital and monitored closely. Initial treatment is by the standard regimen but more active intervention should be considered.

The chest syndrome may occur in complete isolation, or associated with abdominal distension and discomfort if not the full-blown picture of the *sickle girdle syndrome*. In the girdle syndrome an acute abdomen develops, presumably related to sickle vaso-occlusion of the mesenteric blood supply (Figure 5). If it is uncomplicated by other visceral involvement and treated appropriately it is generally self-limiting in 24 hours to 5 days. It is essential however, to look for and be aware of other causes of an acute abdomen; in particular the rarely encountered bowel ischaemia which can develop into bowel infarction when emergency surgical resection is life-saving. In general the only treatment required for the girdle syndrome is to stop oral intake and maintain hydration. Patients can be monitored by measuring their girth measurement around the umbilicus regularly (generally hourly) and

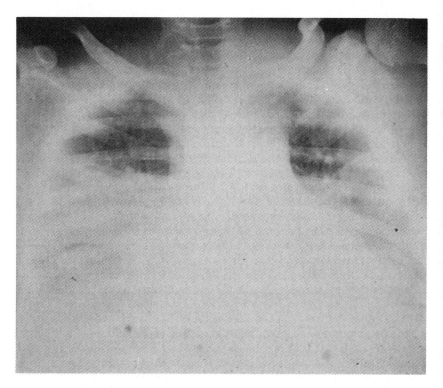

Figure 4. Chest X-ray demonstrating the lung consolidation seen in a severe sickle 'chest syndrome'.

auscultating for bowel sounds. On occasions there may be involvement of the liver which can progress to *hepatic sequestration*. In this, as with splenic sequestration, the Hb drops by $\geq 2\,\mathrm{g\,dl^{-1}}$ due to the trapping of red blood cells in the liver. The liver distends and its function is impaired. It is generally associated with septicaemia (Hatton et al, 1985), and may occur at any age once the spleen has atrophied and fibrosed.

A broad spectrum of *neurological complications* of SCD have now been described, including occlusive and haemorrhagic *cerebrovascular accidents*, transient ischaemic attacks, cranial nerve lesions, mental changes and spinal cord syndromes. The commonest presentation is an acute onset hemiplegia or hemiparesis due to cerebral infarction occurring in 7–29% of SS patients. A mean age of onset of 7.7 years and a modal age of 5 years has been reported (Hindmarsh et al, 1987). These occlusive strokes result from blockage of middle to large arteries in the brain as a result of a primary proliferation of smooth muscle and fibroblasts in the intima. The pathology

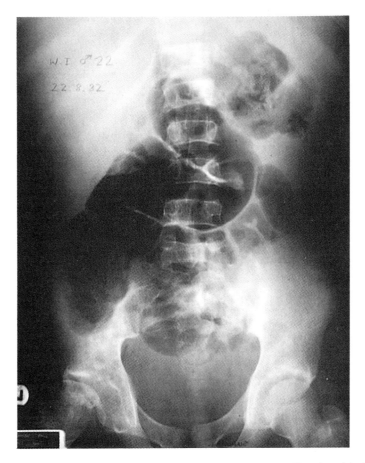

Figure 5. Abdominal X-ray during the sickle 'girdle syndrome' showing dilatation of the bowel.

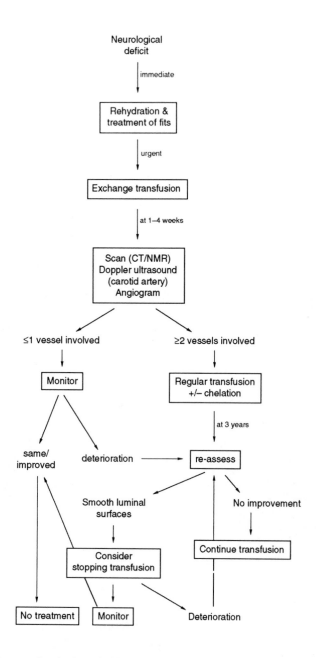

Figure 6. Strategy for the investigation and treatment of neurological deficit in sickle cell disease.

is therefore, quite unlike the sickle vaso-occlusion experienced in the small vessels elsewhere in the body. Once blockage has occurred many patients then develop a collateral circulation which is generally thin-walled and prone to rupture. The increased incidence of subarachnoid haemorrhage in late adolescence and adult life is related to these and also rupture of intracranial aneurysms in the Circle of Willis. Covert neurological damage related to SCD can also be demonstrated in patients with exhaustive investigation (Herold et al, 1986; Hindmarsh et al, 1987).

Any child who has an acute neurological event should be admitted to hospital as an emergency and the strategy shown in Figure 6 followed. There is a greater than two thirds risk of a reoccurrence, with 80% of subsequent strokes occurring before 3 years (Powars et al, 1978). Recurrence can undoubtedly be prevented by a long-term transfusion regimen (see below). It is important, however, that this regimen is closely adhered to and that the sickle haemoglobin is kept below 25%. The most important issue to be resolved at present is how long transfusion therapy should be continued in order to remove the risk of recurrence. A reasonable compromise is to reassess at 3 years. However, as with other patients who undergo long-term transfusion therapy there is the problem of transfusion-induced haemosiderosis and compliance with chelation therapy to be considered (see thalassaemia).

The *proliferative sickle retinopathy* (PSR) is now well recognized among patients with SCD and can be seen as early as 10 years. From this age monitoring on a regular yearly basis, where possible by a specialist ophthalmological clinic, should be performed because early intervention with laser or cryotherapy can prevent loss of sight. PSR is one of the more severe complications encountered in HbSC disease.

Adolescence

Trunk pain often with associated visceral involvement is the main problem in this age group. Priapism can also occur. Patients in this age group often have an increased frequency of admissions with painful crisis. Treatment is the same regardless of age, but adolescents present particular *psychological problems* related to their development and altered home environment. They no longer see themselves as children and therefore find the paediatric ward irritating, yet few hospitals have the necessary dedicated adolescent wards and adult wards are totally unsuitable for them at times of illness.

Chronic organ damage resulting from repeated sickling, in particular *avascular necrosis* of the head of the femur can be seen as early as 13 years of age in all types of SCD with up to 21% of young adults being affected (Taylor, 1985). When the femoral head is involved there is pain in the groin which may radiate to the knee. The patient limps and there is limitation of movement on external rotation. Without intervention this settles but many joints will eventually be destroyed. While hospital admission for parenteral opiates is rarely required it can interfere with daily life and work for many months or even years, requiring long-term oral opiate derivatives. The successful insertion of hip prostheses has been widely reported. In our view operation should be delayed as long as possible because of the high risk of complications postoperatively, both infective and later loosening of the joint, and the limited life-span of any prosthesis necessitating renewal anything from 5 to 20 years later. Longevity of the joint may well be improved by the insertion of non-cemented prostheses.

Priapism may occur from childhood either as recurrent, short-lived (generally 2–6 hours) stuttering attacks, as have been reported in 42% of Jamaican SS patients, or as fulminant attacks (Serjeant et al, 1985). Anti-testosterone hormones such as stilboestrol have been used to terminate attacks of stuttering priapism (Serjeant et al, 1985). Fulminant attacks must be treated as a medical emergency. If there is no improvement within a couple of hours then proceed to exchange transfusion. If there is no improvement at 24 hours following exchange transfusion then a surgical manoeuvre is probably necessary. The simplest approach is drainage and lavage using normal saline. Venous shunts should be held as a last resort. Active treatment is essential as prolonged priapism can lead to fibrosis within the corpora cavernosa and subsequent erectile impotence. Priapism becomes more frequent with age.

The classic 'sickle habbitus' is rarely encountered in the SCD patients of the Western world, although it is still seen in some patients in their native surroundings. However, it is well documented that both sexes and all types of SCD have a *reduced body weight and short stature* (Platt et al, 1981), leading to delayed growth spurt and menarche. Boys are more severely affected than girls (Phebus et al, 1984). Nasogastric nutritional supplementation has been shown to produce rapid sustained increases in growth rate; unfortunately, neither simple oral nor mineral and vitamin supplementation have shown an effect (Heyman et al, 1985).

BLOOD TRANSFUSION IN SCD

Table 5 lists indications for the use of blood transfusion in SCD. It is important to consider carefully before using transfusion in SCD because of the risks previously described of infection, iron overload and alloimmunization.

Alloimmunization is particularly important in Northern Europe and North America where the donor population is predominantly Caucasian while the affected SCD population is predominantly AfroCaribbean and West African in origin. Red cell antibodies have been reported in 17.6% of transfused patients with rhesus and Kell antibodies accounting for two thirds (Davies et al, 1986; Vichinsky et al, 1990). We therefore recommend that prior to giving a blood transfusion to an SCD patient extended red cell phenotyping should be carried out, including ABO, full rhesus, Kell, MNSs, Jk, Lewis and Js[a] and Js[b]. All S−, s− individuals should be U-typed. All R_0 individuals should be transfused with C negative, E negative blood (rr or R_0). Kell-compatible blood should always be given.

Blood for transfusion should be screened for the presence of HbS as donors with sickle cell trait often have Hb levels that are acceptable for blood donation. Other precautions, as for β thalassaemia, should be

Table 5. Indications for blood transfusion in children with sickle cell disease.

Replacement
Use when the Hb $\leq 4\,g\,dl^{-1}$, or the child is clinically compromised
Sequestration crises
Aplastic crisis
Haemolytic crises, e.g. malaria infection
Bleeding

Exchange transfusion
Use to improve the oxygen carrying capacity of blood without altering the blood viscosity
Neurological deficit
'Chest and girdle' syndromes
Priapism
Occasional patients with severe/protracted painful crisis
Severely affected patients preoperatively

Long-term transfusion
Use to maintain the haemoglobin between 10.5 and $15\,g\,dl^{-1}$, with $\leq 25\%$ HbS
Neurological deficit
Rarely to improve growth and development
Occasionally to prevent painful crisis

followed. Plasma reduced blood may be used but red cell concentrates should be avoided.

HIV infection in SCD patients is now recognized in Europe. This results most often from blood transfusions received in the high-risk areas of Africa. HIV infections in SCD should be treated actively in the standard manner (see above).

Table 5 shows the indications for exchange transfusion. The aim is to reduce HbS to less than 25% and to keep the haemoglobin level $< 15\,g\,dl^{-1}$ because of the risk of increasing the whole blood viscosity, while maintaining a steady blood volume. The total Hb and proportion of HbS should be measured prior to each exchange.

In children, this is usually achieved by exchanging approximately one and a half times the total calculated blood volume over three exchanges:

$$\text{exchange volume (ml)} = (35 \times \text{weight in kg})$$

In very sick patients, exchange transfusion may be performed as a single, continuous procedure or as two separate exchanges.

Long-term transfusion is best carried out by regular exchange transfusions. In patients with poor venous access it may be necessary to start with full exchange transfusion followed by top-up transfusions at regular intervals, generally 4-weekly, Iron chelation treatment may be required.

SCD IN THE COMMUNITY

It is essential that children and their families should understand the pathophysiology sufficiently to be aware of situations and activities that they should avoid. They should be encouraged to be open with school teachers, and health professionals should be prepared to advise the schools. The teacher should recognize the manifestations of SCD and the problems associated with living with it. Most particularly the need for frequent drinks and the children's inability to concentrate their urine so that they must have easy access to toilets. Many of the children suffer from enuresis so school trips become a problem; fortunately, most children achieve control at or before puberty.

Each child should find a level of physical activity that (s)he can undertake during that period of life. It has proved impossible to make blanket recommendations respecting sports. Most SS children cannot swim during the winter months but the few that find that swimming does not precipitate painful vaso-occlusive crisis and are prevented will be less inclined to respect other restrictions placed upon them. Unless there is overt neurological damage there is no indication for SCD children to receive special schooling apart from additional tuition to catch up on time that has been lost related to painful crisis or hospital admission.

A multidisciplinary approach from the professionals is essential as every bodily system can be involved by the sickling phenomenon. This is generally best co-ordinated by the paediatrician or haematologist.

CONCLUSION

In the 1990s every couple in the developed world who is 'at risk' of having a child with a clinically-significant haemoglobinopathy, such as homozygous β thalassaemia or sickle cell disease, should now be screened and counselled preconceptually or early in pregnancy. They should be counselled respecting the natural history, the problems of living with the disease, the improved therapies now available and the improved prognosis. Prenatal testing should be available and offered to these couples.

The greatest clinical advances over the last decade have been in the thalassaemias with the introduction of 'optimal therapy' and bone marrow transplantation. In sickle cell disease the effect of prophylactic penicillin in reducing mortality has been proven and general guidelines for clinical management are now being agreed. In this article we have discussed the contemporary management of these diseases.

Acknowledgements

The authors would like to thank Professor G. B. Arden for ophthalmological advice, Dr V. De Sanctis for help in compiling the endocrine tables, Dr C. Borgne-Pignatti for Figure 1 and Brian Dugan for typing the manuscript.

REFERENCES

Aldouri MA, Wonke B, Hoffbrand AV et al (1990) High incidence of cardiomyopathy in β thalassaemia patients receiving regular transfusion and iron chelation: reversal by intensified chelation. *Acta Haematologica* **84**(3): 113–117.
Bartlett AN, Hoffbrand AV & Kontoghiorghes GJ (1990) Long term trial with the oral chelator 1,2-dimethyl-3-hydroxypyrid-4-one (L1). *British Journal of Haematology* **76**: 301–304.

Bond LR, Hatty SR, Horn MEC et al (1987) Gall stones in sickle cell disease in the United Kingdom. *British Medical Journal* **295:** 234–236.

Bronspiegel-Weintrob N, Olivieri NF, Tyler B et al (1990) Effect of age at the start of iron chelation therapy on gonadal function in β thalassaemia major. *New England Journal of Medicine* **323:** 713–719.

Brozovic M, Davies SC & Brownell AI (1987) Acute admissions of patients with sickle cell disease who live in Britain. *British Medical Journal* **294:** 1206–1208.

Cao A, Pinto L, Lecca U et al (1984) Control of homozygous beta thalassaemia by carrier screening and antenatal diagnosis in Sardinians. *Clinical Genetics* **26:** 12–22.

Cumming P, Wallace E, Schorr J & Dodd R (1989) Exposure of patients to human immuno-deficiency virus through the transfusion of blood components that test antibody negative. *New England Journal of Medicine* **321:** 941.

Cummins D, Heuschel R & Davies SC (1991) An audit of penicillin prophylaxis in children with sickle cell disease resident in Brent. *British Medical Journal* (in press).

Davies SC & Brozovic M (1989) The presentation, management and prophylaxis of sickle cell disease. *Blood Reviews* **3:** 29–44.

Davies SC, Luce PJ, Win AA et al (1984) Acute chest syndrome in sickle cell disease. *Lancet* **i:** 36–38.

Davies SC, Stebbens VA, Samuels MP & Southall DP (1989) Upper airways obstruction and cerebrovascular accident in children with sickle cell anaemia. *Lancet* **ii:** 283–284.

Donohue M, Wonke B, Hoffbrand AV & Dusheiko J (1990) Detection of antibodies to hepatitis C virus and the use of alpha 2b interferon in the treatment of chronic non-A, non-B hepatitis in multiply transfused thalassaemia patients. *Blood* **76**(10): 1432–1433.

Editorial (1986) Penicillin prophylaxis for babies with sickle cell disease. *Lancet* **ii:** 1432–1433.

Feretis CB, Legakis NC, Apostolidis NS et al (1985) Prophylactic cholecystectomy during splenectomy for beta thalassaemia homozygous in Greece. *Surgery, Gynaecology and Obstetrics* **160:** 9–12.

Gaston MH, Verter JI, Woods G et al (1986) Prophylaxis with oral penicillin in children with sickle cell anemia. A randomized trial. *New England Journal of Medicine* **314:** 1593–1599.

Girot R (1991) European Mediterranean WHO working group on haemoglobinopathies. *Proceedings of the Cooley Care 1990 meeting, Athens, 14–15 June 1990*, (in press).

Gray A, Anionwu A, Davies SC & Brozovic M (1991) Mortality in sickle cell disease. *Journal of Clinical Pathology* (in press).

Gutteridge J & Halliwell B (1989) Iron toxicity and iron radicals. *Baillière's Clinical Haematology* **2:** 195–256.

Hatton CSR, Bunch C & Weatherall DJ (1985) Hepatic sequestration in sickle cell anaemia. *British Medical Journal* **290:** 744–745.

Herold S, Brozovic M, Gibbs J et al (1986) Measurement of regional cerebral blood flow, blood volume and oxygen metabolism in patients with sickle cell disease using positron emission tomography. *Stroke* **17:** 692–698.

Heyman MB, Vichinsky E, Katz R et al (1985) Growth retardation in sickle cell disease treated by nutritional support. *Lancet* **i:** 903–906.

Higgs DR, Aldridge BE, Lamb J et al (1978) The interaction of alpha thalassaemia and homozygous sickle cell disease. *New England Journal of Medicine* **306:** 1441–1446.

Hindmarsh PC, Brozovic M, Brook CGD & Davies SC (1987) Incidence of overt and covert neurological damage in children with sickle cell disease. *Postgraduate Medical Journal* **63:** 751–753.

Kazazian HH Jr (1990) The thalassemia syndromes: molecular basis and prenatal diagnosis in 1990. *Seminars in Hematology* **27:** 209–228.

Leikin SL, Gallagher D, Kinney TR et al (1989) Mortality in children and adolescents with sickle cell disease. *Pediatrics* **84:** 500–508.

Lucarelli G, Galimberti M, Polchi P et al (1990) Bone marrow transplantation in patients with thalassaemia. *New England Journal of Medicine* **322:** 417–421.

Marcus R, Davies S, Bantock H et al (1984) Desferrioxamine to improve cardiac function in iron overloaded patients with thalassaemia major. *Lancet* **i:** 392–393.

Modell B & Berdouskas V (1984) *The Clinical Approach to Thalassaemia*, p 171. London: Grune & Stratton.

Modell B, Petrou M, Ward R et al (1984) Effect of foetal diagnosis testing on birth rate of thalassaemia major in Britain. *Lancet* **ii:** 1383–1387.

Mok J, Underhill G, Wonke B et al (1989) Intradermal hepatitis B vaccine in thalassaemia and sickle cell disease. *Archives of Disease in Childhood* **64:** 535–540.

Moroni GA, Piacentini G, Terzoli S et al (1984) Hepatitis B or non-A, non-B virus infection in multitransfused thalassaemic patients. *Archives of Disease in Childhood* **59:** 1127–1130.

Olivieri N, Buncic R, Chew E et al (1986) Visual and auditory neurotoxicity in patients receiving subcutaneous desferrioxamine infusions. *New England Journal of Medicine* **314:** 869–873.

Pattison JR (1987) B19 virus—a pathogenic human virus. *Blood Reviews* **1:** 58–64.

Phebus CK, Gloninger MF & Maciak BJ (1984) Growth patterns by age and sex in children with sickle cell disease. *Journal of Pediatrics* **105:** 28–33.

Pintor C, Cella SG, Manso P et al (1986) Impaired growth hormone (GH) response to GH-releasing hormone in thalassaemia major. *Journal of Clinical Endocrinology and Metabolism* **62:** 263–267.

Platt OS, Rosenstock W & Espeland MA (1981) Influence of sickle hemoglobinopathies on growth and development. *New England Journal of Medicine* **311**(1): 7–12.

Politis C, Di Palma A, Fisfis M et al (1990) Social integration of the older thalassaemic patient. *Archives of Diseases in Childhood* **65:** 984–986.

Porter JB & Huehns ER (1989) The toxic effects of desferrioxamine. *Baillière's Clinical Haematology* **2:** 460.

Porter JB, Huehns ER & Hiden RC (1989) The development of iron chelating drugs. *Baillière's Clinical Haematology* **2:** 257–292.

Powars D (1989) Diagnosis at birth improves survival of children with sickle cell anemia. *Pediatrics* **83** (suppl.): 830–833.

Powars D, Wilson B, Imbus C et al (1978) The natural history of stroke in sickle cell disease. *American Journal of Medicine* **65:** 461–471.

Powars D, Overturf G & Turner E (1983) Is there an increased risk of *Haemophilus influenzae* septicemia in children with sickle cell anemia? *Pediatrics* **71:** 927–931.

Powars D, Weiss JN, Chan LS & Schroeder WA (1984) Is there a threshold level of fetal hemoglobin that ameliorates morbidity in sickle cell anemia? *Blood* **63:** 921–926.

Rogers DW, Serjeant BE & Serjeant GR (1982) Early rise in 'pitted' red cell count as a guide to susceptibility to infection in childhood sickle cell anaemia. *Archives of Disease in Childhood* **57:** 338–342.

Sabato AR, De Sanctis V, Atti G et al (1983) Primary hypothyroidism and low T3 syndrome in thalassaemia major. *Archives of Disease in Childhood* **58:** 120–127.

Saenger P, Schwartz E, Markenson AL et al (1980) Depressed serum somatomedin in β thalassaemia. *Journal of Pediatrics* **96:** 214–218.

Serjeant GR, De Ceulaer K & Maude GH (1985) Stilboestrol and stuttering priapism in homozygous sickle cell disease. *Lancet* **ii:** 1274–1276.

Shinar E & Rachmilewitz EA (1990) Oxidative denaturation of red cells in thalassaemia. *Seminars in Haematology* **27**(1): 70–82.

Swart AM & Weller T (1990) Early HIV infection: to treat or not to treat? *British Medical Journal* **301:** 825–826.

Taylor LJ (1985) Sickle cell disease in Britain: a review (Jacksonian Prize winning thesis). London: *Royal College of Surgeons*.

Thein SL, Wainscoat JS, Sampietro M et al (1987) Association of thalassaemia intermedia with a beta globin gene haplotype. *British Journal of Haematology* **65:** 367–373.

Topley JM, Rogers DW, Stevens MCG & Serjeant GR (1981) Acute splenic sequestration and hypersplenism in the first five years in homozygous sickle cell disease. *Archives of Disease in Childhood* **56:** 765–769.

Vermylen C, Fernandez-Robles E, Ninane J & Cornu G (1988) Bone marrow transplantation in five children with sickle cell anaemia. *Lancet* **ii:** 1427–1428.

Vichinsky EP, Earles A, Johnson RA et al (1990) Alloimmunization in sickle cell anemia and transfusion of racially unmatched blood. *New England Journal of Medicine* **322:** 1617–1621.

Webb DKH, Darby JS, Dunn DT, Terry SI & Serjeant GR (1989) Gall stones in Jamaican children with homozygous sickle cell disease. *Archives of Disease in Childhood* **64:** 693–696.

Wonke B & De Sanctis V (1991) Endocrine manifestations in haemoglobinopathies. *Clinical Endocrinology*. Blackwells, (in press).

Wonke B, Hoffbrand AV, Aldouri M et al (1989a) Reversal of desferrioxamine induced auditory neurotoxicity during treatment with Ca-DTPA. *Archives of Disease in Childhood* **64:** 77–82.

Wonke B, Hoffbrand AV, Aldouri M & Ward S (1989b) Cardiac complications in homozygous beta thalassaemia. *Advances and Controversies in Thalassaemia Therapy*, pp 51–56. Alan R. Liss.

Wonke B, Hoffbrand AV, Brown D & Dusheiko J (1990) Antibody to hepatitis C virus in multiply transfused patients with thalassaemia major. *Journal of Clinical Pathology* **43:** 638–640.

World Health Organization (1985) Recommendations for transfusion treatment of beta thalassaemia major. Therapy of thalassaemia. *Proceedings of the 1st Mediterranean Meeting on Blood Transfusion in Thalassaemia*, pp 237–255. Milan: WHO.

World Health Organization (1987) *The Haemoglobinopathies in Europe.* A combined report on two WHO meetings: Brussels, March 14, 1986 & Paris March 20–21, 1987. Geneva, WHO document EUR/ICP/MCH 110.

Yardumian A & Davies SC (1987) Sickle cell anaemia and the lung. *Respiratory Disease in Practice* **5:** 18–23.

5

Antenatal diagnosis

JOHN M. OLD
CHRISTOPHER A. LUDLAM

THE HAEMOGLOBINOPATHIES

The first prenatal diagnosis of haemoglobinopathies was performed in 1974 (Kan et al, 1975) by the analysis of globin chain synthesis in a fetal blood sample. Since then this approach has been adopted successfully by many thalassaemia centres and more than 10 000 cases of thalassaemia have been diagnosed to date (Alter, 1991). The methods used for the examination of fetal blood for haemoglobinopathies have been extensively reviewed (Alter 1983, 1989) and will not be discussed here as this approach has been largely replaced by the molecular analysis of fetal DNA.

DNA analysis techniques for prenatal diagnosis were first performed on amniotic fluid cell DNA: α^0-thalassaemia in 1976 (Kan et al); sickle cell anaemia in 1978 (Kan and Dozy); β-thalassaemia in 1980 (Kazazian et al). The prenatal diagnoses were usually carried out with cultured amniocytes because a 20 ml amniotic fluid sample would not provide the 20–30 µg of DNA required for gene mapping by the Southern blot techniques. In 1982 chorionic villus samples were shown to be a better source of fetal DNA for molecular analysis (Old et al, 1982); many couples soon opted for this technique for prenatal diagnosis of the haemoglobinopathies (Old et al, 1986) because it is performed at 9–11 weeks' gestation when termination can be performed more safely and with less psychological trauma.

Recently the molecular analysis of fetal DNA has been revolutionized by the discovery of the polymerase chain reaction (PCR) which amplifies enzymatically short, specific genomic DNA sequences (Saiki et al, 1985). PCR has made the analysis of fetal DNA quicker, simpler and easier to carry out using smaller quantities of fetal DNA; indeed it is possible to analyse DNA sequences in single cells (Li et al, 1988) illustrating the great sensitivity of this technique. Fetal DNA must be pure for prenatal diagnosis. PCR has also enabled the development of some new approaches to the detection of mutations, for example: the chemical cleavage method for detecting factor IX mutations (Montadon, 1989) and for analysing β-thalassaemia mutations; the amplification refractory mutation system (ARMS) using allele-specific primers (Old et al, 1990); the competitive priming technique using fluorescently-labelled primers (Chehab and Kan, 1989); the denaturing gradient gel electrophoresis technique which analyses DNA heteroduplexes containing mismatched nucleotides (Losekoot et al, 1991) and direct sequencing of amplified DNA (Wong et al, 1987).

The protocols for some of these techniques and the current strategies for diagnosing mutations are described in detail in this chapter.

DNA TECHNIQUES FOR ANTENATAL DIAGNOSIS

DNA preparation

DNA is usually made from anticoagulated blood samples, amniocytes, chorionic villi or fetal tissue samples. Although the development of PCR has allowed prenatal diagnosis to be performed directly on minute amounts of DNA from some remarkable sources (such as Guthrie spots, mouthwash cells or just a few μl of whole blood) larger scale preparations of DNA for each patient are still necessary to create a DNA bank for future reference and research.

Blood

Approximately 250 μg of DNA can be expected to be obtained from 10 ml of blood anticoagulated with EDTA or heparin. Blood samples can be sent in the post at room temperature for up to 3 days without any deterioration, and can be stored at 4°C before use for several weeks. If frozen the blood sample can be kept for at least 6 months at −20°C and probably indefinitely at −70°C. To prepare DNA, 30 ml of distilled water is added to 10 ml fresh or thawed blood to lyse the red cells and a white cell pellet is collected by centrifugation at 3000 g for 10 min. The white cell pellet is homogenized with 25 ml of 0.1% Nonidet P40 to dissolve the red and white cell membranes and a nuclei pellet collected as before. This is then lysed with 10 ml of lysis buffer (100 mM NaCl, 25 mM EDTA, 0.5% SDS and 20 mg ml^{-1} proteinase K) and incubated for 2 h at 55°C or overnight at 37°C. The protein is removed by two phenol–chloroform extractions and then the residual phenol is removed by two chloroform extractions. The DNA is then precipitated by adding a half volume of 7.5 M ammonium acetate (5 ml) and two volumes of ethanol (30 ml). Usually a large clump of DNA forms which can be removed from the ethanol, rinsed in 70% ethanol, dried briefly and finally left to dissolve in 1 ml of buffer or distilled water. If no clump of DNA forms it means the DNA concentration is very low and the solution must be cooled at −20°C for 1 h and then centrifuged. The pellet will contain both DNA and RNA and should be carefully dissolved in just 0.5 ml of distilled water. Once dissolved, the DNA can be removed from the RNA by reprecipitation without cooling with 0.25 ml of 7.5 M ammonium acetate and 1.5 ml of ethanol. If no clump of DNA forms this time then there is probably no or insufficient high molecular weight DNA present and a repeat sample should be requested.

Chorionic villi

DNA is prepared from chorionic villi by the same method as for blood except that smaller volumes are used and the extraction can be carried out in 1.5 ml Eppendorf tubes. The chorionic villus sample must be sorted free from any contaminating maternal cells by the centre performing the CVS. The villi can then be sent to the laboratory in tissue culture medium if the distance is short. If it has to be in transit for 24 h or longer it is best sent frozen on dry ice or, even better sent in the incubation volume (0.5 ml) of lysis buffer (see above) at room temperature. The chorionic villi will slowly lyse in transit and can be given a short incubation upon receipt to complete the lysis. A sample which was lost in shipment for 2 weeks survived perfectly in lysis buffer and a prenatal diagnosis was obtained without problem. After precipitation (normally as white fibrous strands) the DNA is removed as a clump or spun down if necessary with only a short 30 s spin in order to keep the precipitated RNA suspended in the supernatant. The DNA precipitate is washed with 70% ethanol and redissolved in 50 μl of distilled water or buffer.

Amniocytes

DNA can be prepared from amniotic fluid cells directly or after culturing. If 30 to 40 ml of fluid is obtained by amniocentesis, 10 ml should be used for culture and the remainder used to make DNA. The cells should be pelleted by centrifugation and the amniotic fluid removed before shipment. The pellet must be sent frozen on dry ice or in 0.5 ml of lysis buffer at room temperature. The DNA extraction procedure is the same as for chorionic villi. 20 ml of amniotic fluid will only yield between 1.5 and 7 μg of DNA. With such small amounts of DNA, it usually does not form a visible fibrous precipitate and must be collected by centrifugation after 1 h at −20°C. The pellet is dissolved in 25 μl of buffer and no attempt is made to remove the RNA by reprecipitation for fear of losing the DNA which is usually only marginally sufficient for one Southern blot analysis. Sometimes however no DNA is obtained and the back up cultures are required. Two 25 ml flasks of cells grown to confluency will yield between 30 and 90 μg of DNA similar to the amount obtained from chorionic villi samples (Old et al, 1986).

DNA concentration and purity

These are determined by measuring the absorbance at 260 and 280 nm of a 5 μl aliquot made up to 1 ml with distilled water in a quartz semi-micro cuvette. A DNA solution of $1 \, g \, dl^{-1}$ has an absorbance of 200 units at 260 nm. Therefore if a reading of 0.2 is obtained for example, this would represent a DNA concentration of $1 \, mg \, dl^{-1}$ or $10 \, \mu g \, ml^{-1}$. Thus the 5 μl aliquot contained 10 μg of DNA and the total yield if dissolved in 50 μl would be 100 μg. The purity of the DNA sample can be judged from the 260/280 ratio which should be around 1.8. Any large difference reflects impurities such as protein or phenol left in the DNA solution. Such samples should be re-extracted to clean them up before proceeding to carry out restriction enzyme mapping or PCR.

Storage of DNA

DNA solutions may be stored at 4°C, at −20°C or at 70°C. At 4°C the DNA does not undergo repetitive freeze–thaw cycles when it is used and is advised for working with very high molecular weight DNA which may be damaged by the freezing process (for example, DNA required for pulsed field gels). For Southern blot analysis or PCR, DNA does not appear to be harmed by freeze–thaw cycles and therefore DNA may be kept at −20°C or −70°C. In our laboratory DNA samples are kept for long-term storage in sectioned aluminium trays at −20°C. Although −70°C is thought to be better for long-term storage, such freezers are not so user-friendly. For a short period, until the prenatal diagnosis is complete, the DNA samples are kept at 4°C for ease of use. Longer storage at 4°C runs the risk of microbial growth in the samples unless an antimicrobial agent is added.

Southern blot analysis

The protocol for Southern blot analysis used in our laboratory has been described in detail several times (Old and Higgs, 1983; Old, 1986) and will not be presented here. The only modification we have made to the procedure is that our polaroid camera has been replaced by a video camera and thermal-paper printer for taking cheaper pictures of ethidium bromide stained gels on a UV light box. We still use nitrocellulose filters (now strengthened) in preference to nylon because the background on the auto-radiograph appears to be better than with nylon filters. We have tried using non-radioactive labelling systems such as the chemiluminescence method (with variable results) but have not adopted them for routine use as we still prefer the standard radioactive labelling technique. One improvement which looks promising but we have not yet tried in the laboratory is the replacement of heat-sealed plastic bags for hybridization of the filters with an oven containing a rotisserie arrangement of glass hybridization bottles. This device should improve the autoradiograph backgrounds by standardizing the hybridization conditions more easily as well as being easier to handle and less hazardous than plastic bags.

Polymerase chain reaction

This is carried out according to the standard conditions (Table 1) supplied by Cetus with their cloned Taq polymerase (Amplitaq). However for economy we use a quarter of the specified amounts by reducing the reaction volume from 100 μl to 25 μl. The PCR mixture is prepared with a set of dedicated automatic pipettes which are never used for pipetting amplified DNA. As few pipettings as possible are done by making up pre-mixes. A reaction mixture (4 ml) is first prepared containing 0.5 ml 10× Cetus buffer (100 mM Tris pH 8.3, 500 mM KCl, 15 mM $MgCl_2$, 0.1% gelatin), 0.8 ml of dNTP solution (1.25 mM of each) and 2.7 ml of sterile water. A 20 μl aliquot of the reaction mixture is placed in a 0.5 ml tube and then 4 μl of a primer–enzyme mixture added. The 4 μl contains 0.5 μl of Amplitaq and 5 pmol of each

Table 1. Standard PCR conditions.

---

1. 100 µl volume containing:
    50 mM KCl
    10 mM Tris–HCl (PH 8.4)
    1.5 mM MgCl$_2$*
    100 µg ml^{-1} gelatin
    0.2 µM of each primer (20 pmol)
    200 µM of each: dATP, dCTP, dGTP, dTTP†
    1 µg of sample DNA
    2.5 Units Taq polymerase
    50 µl light paraffin oil

2. 30 cycles of 94°C for 20 seconds
    55°C for 20 seconds
    72°C for 1 minute per 1000 bases

    (a) Some primers may require a higher MgCl$_2$ concentration between 1.5 and 5.0 mM
    (b) Each dNTP solution must be neutralized with NaOH and its concentration
         determined in a UV spectrophotometer before use. Ready-made neutralized
         solutions can be purchased (e.g. Boehringer Mannheim) and are recommended

---

primer. Finally, 1 µl of DNA solution is added to make the total volume to 25 µl and the mixture overlaid with 25 µl of light paraffin oil.

To amplify for restriction enzyme digestion or dot blot analysis, the tube is placed in a PCR machine programmed for 30 cycles at 93°C for 1 min, 55°C for 1 min and 72°C for 1.5 min followed by a final extension step at 72°C for 3 min. No initial denaturation step is necessary. These conditions suit most of our primers although some do require different annealing temperatures which are found by trial and error. The type of PCR machine appears to make little difference as we have successfully amplified the same DNA sample under these conditions in four different makes of machine. The amplified product may be analysed by the following methods.

Restriction enzyme digestion

RFLPs and mutations which affect restriction enzyme sites can be analysed by restriction enzyme digestion and agarose gel electrophoresis. After the PCR programme has finished 20 µl of the reaction mixture is removed to a clean Eppendorf tube. Usually 2 µl of the appropriate 10× restriction enzyme buffer (except when the enzyme requires only 50 mM salt or less which is already present from the PCR buffer) and 10–20 Units of restriction enzyme are added and the tube incubated at the appropriate temperature for 1 h. A 5 µl aliquot of ficol/bromophenol blue dye (15%/0.05%) is added and the sample loaded onto a 3% agarose gel made up of 1.5% agarose and 1.5% Nusieve agarose. After electrophoresis at 100 V for approximately 1 h the gel is stained in ethidium bromide solution and photographed by video camera on a UV light box.

Dot blot analysis

Point mutations and small nucleotide insertions or deletions can be analysed by the hybridization of labelled allele-specific oligonucleotide probes.

Five μl of the amplified product is removed and added to 100 μl of 0.4 M NaOH–25 mM EDTA to denature the DNA. The sample is then dot-blotted onto a nylon filter pre-wet with 200 μl of 2M NH_4OAc using a vacuum dot blotting apparatus. After loading the sample is washed through with 200 μl of 2M NH_4OAc and fixed to the nylon by a short exposure face down on a UV light box. The filter can be hybridized without a prehybridization step. ^{32}P-labelled oligonucleotide (prepared according to the method of Thein and Wallace, 1986) is added to 6 ml of 0.1 M Tris-HCL, pH 8.0, 6 mM EDTA, 1M NaCl, 5× Denhardts, 10% dextran sulphate, 0.5% NP-40 and 100 mg ml^{-1} single-stranded DNA at 55°C for 2 hours. The filter is washed in 6× SSC at the Tm of the probe and autoradiographed. Filters can also be washed in tetramethylammonium chloride (TMAC) at a temperature which depends on the length of the probe and not its composition (Wood et al, 1985).

Chemical cleavage

Point mutations can also be detected by chemical cleavage analysis of heteroduplexes formed between amplified mutant and wild-type DNA (Cotton et al, 1988). This approach has been used extremely successfully for carrier and antenatal diagnosis of haemophilia B (Montandon et al, 1989). Amplified wild-type DNA is end-labelled with ^{32}P and mixed with similarly amplified but unlabelled mutant DNA. The mixture is denatured and reannealed to form heteroduplexes and self-annealed homoduplexes. The heteroduplexes will contain a mismatch at the site of the mutation which can be cleaved by treatment with either osmium tetroxide or piperidine. The end-labelled DNA strand is reduced to a size characteristic for the particular mutation and can be analysed by acrylamide gel electrophoresis. However the exact nature of the mutation can only be determined by direct DNA sequencing.

ARMS analysis

Point mutations, small insertions or deletions and RFLPs can also be detected by amplification using allele specific primers. This method, developed by Newton et al (1989) and called the amplification refractory mutation system (ARMS), has been adapted for the detection of β-thalassaemia mutations (Old et al, 1990) and is described later. Amplification of DNA with ARMS primers is carried out with exactly the same reaction mixture as described above except for the fact there are four primers present in the mixture instead of two. The amplification is for 25 cycles at 93°C for 1 min, 65°C for 1 min and 72°C for 1.5 min followed by a final extension step of 72°C for 3 min. After the programme is complete, 5 μl of the ficol–blue dye mixture is added to the tube and the sample vortexed and spun for a few seconds. A 20 μl sample can then be removed and loaded onto a 1.5% agarose and 1.5% Nusieve agarose gel, electrophoresed, stained and photographed as described above.

ANTENATAL DIAGNOSIS OF THE HAEMOGLOBINOPATHIES

α-thalassaemia

The α-thalassaemias are a group of disorders which are characterized by a reduction in α-globin synthesis. They can be divided into the severe types (α°-thalassaemias), which result in the Hb Bart's hydrops fetalis syndrome in the homozygous state, and the mild types (α^+-thalassaemia) in which carriers have three out of four functional α-globin genes and homozygotes have two. In regions where both types of α-thalassaemia are common individuals can be found with the compound genotype of α^+-thalassaemia/α°-thalassaemia, i.e. with only one functional α-globin gene. Such individuals have Hb H disease and although they have a moderately severe anaemia they lead a relatively normal life and only occasionally require blood transfusion (Weatherall and Clegg, 1981). Prenatal diagnosis is therefore only usually required when both partners are carriers of α°-thalassaemia.

α^+-thalassaemia

DNA mapping is the best approach to distinguish α^+-thalassaemia from α°-thalassaemia. The carrier state for α^+-thalassaemia is phenotypically silent and the clinical phenotype of the homozygous state is similar to that of α°-thalassaemia trait. Restriction enzyme mapping has shown that at least

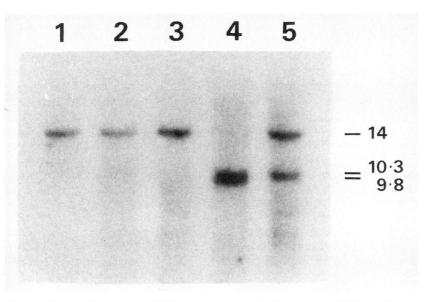

Figure 1. Southern blot analysis of DNA from patients with α-thalassaemia. DNA was digested with *Bam*H1 and hybridized to an α-globin gene probe. Lane 1, DNA from an α^+-thalassaemia trait, genotype $\alpha^T\alpha/\alpha\alpha$; lane 2, DNA from an α°-thalassaemia trait, genotype --/$\alpha\alpha$; lane 3, DNA from a normal individual, genotype $\alpha\alpha/\alpha\alpha$; lane 4, DNA from an α^+-thalassaemia homozygote, genotype $-\alpha^{3.7}/-\alpha^{4.2}$; lane 5, DNA from an α^+-thalassaemia trait, genotype $-\alpha^{3.7}/\alpha\alpha$.

six different single α-gene deletions may give rise to the −α haplotype (Higgs, 1990). All of these can be detected by *Bam*HI digestion and hybridization with an α-gene probe. The two commonest mutations are the 3.7 kb deletion ($-\alpha^{3.7}$) and the 4.2 kb deletion ($-\alpha^{4.2}$). These deletions change the normal (αα) *Bam*HI fragment of 14.0 kb to 10.3 kb and 9.8 kb respectively (Figure 1). These fragments can just about be separated in DNA from the rare case of an α^+-thalassaemia double heterozygote $-\alpha^{3.7}/-\alpha^{4.2}$ as illustrated in Figure 1, lane 4. Carriers for α^+ thalassaemia are identified by the presence of one 14 kb and one 10 kb band whereas homozygotes only have the 10 kb band. Individuals who just have the 14 kb band can have one of several genotypes. They may be completely normal (αα/αα), have a non-deletional type of α thalassaemia or be heterozygous for α°-thalassaemia with a genotype of αα/--.

Sixteen non-deletion mutations which cause α-thalassaemia have now been characterized at the molecular level (Higgs, 1990). These are single base or oligonucleotide mutations affecting either the α2 globin gene (denoted $\alpha^T\alpha$ haplotype) or the α1 gene (denoted $\alpha\alpha^T$). Mutations of the dominant α2 gene result in a more severe phenotype than those affecting the α1 gene with the result that homozygotes ($\alpha^T\alpha/\alpha^T\alpha$) for some of the forms have Hb H disease (Pressley et al, 1980). Two of the mutations are directly detectable by DNA analysis. A five nucleotide deletion at the α2 IVS-1 donor site destroys an Hph 1 site (Orkin et al, 1981) and a single base change in the α2 initiation codon destroys an *Nco*I site (Pirastu et al, 1984).

α°-thalassaemia

There are now fourteen different deletions which may account for the α°-thalassaemia haplotype (Higgs, 1990). These are most commonly seen in southeast Asia and Mediterranean countries and are best detected by a combination of two single digests, *Bam*HI and *Bgl*II, hybridized to a ζ-globin gene probe. For screening individuals for α° mutations we find it convenient to digest DNA samples with *Bam*HI and *Bgl*II and hybridize the filter first to an α-probe and then to wash and rehybridize to a ζ-gene probe. For prenatal diagnosis we usually run two gels, one for α-probe hybridization and the other for the ζ-probe. A map of the *Bgl*II sites in normal and all the common α-thalassaemia genes is shown in Figure 2a.

A typical Southern blot of *Bgl*II digested DNA hybridized to a ζ-probe is illustrated in Figure 2b. The band patterns observed are complicated by the presence of a polymorphic hypervariable region between the ζ and ψζ genes (interzeta HVR) and also within the introns of IVS-I and IVS-II of the ζ-like genes (ζ-intron HVRs). These regions are polymorphic in both normal individuals and those with α-thalassaemia and so great care should be exercised in interpreting Southern blots. A normal individual usually produces two *Bgl*II fragments of 12.6 kb and two ζ-ψζ gene fragments of varying length: 11.0 and 11.3 kb are the common sizes, plus two rarer alleles of 10.0 and 10.5 kb. The Mediterranean mutation $-(\alpha)^{20.5}$ and the Southeast Asian deletion $--^{SEA}$ both result in the 12.6 kb fragment changing to a 10.5 kb band which is the only fragment observed in a homozygote (lane

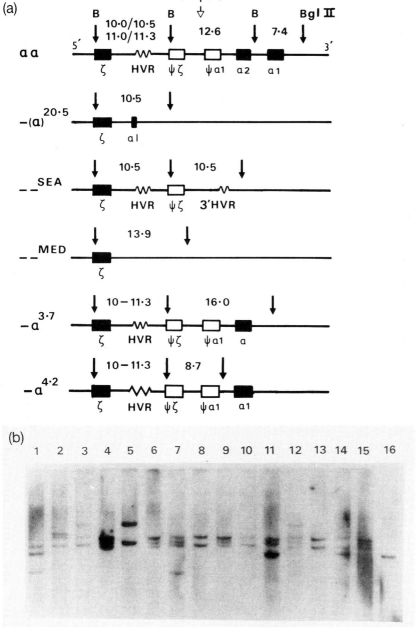

Figure 2. (a) Maps of the *Bgl*II sites in the normal α-globin gene cluster (αα) and the common α-thalassaemia genes. The polymorphic *Bgl*II site is shown by the dashed arrow. The hypervariable regions (HVRs) are represented by zigzags. (b) Southern blot analysis of DNA from patients with α-thalassaemia. DNA was digested with *Bgl*II and hybridized to a ζ-gene probe. Genotypes are as follows: lane 1, $-\alpha^{4.2}/--^{SEA}$; 2, $--^{MED}/\alpha\alpha$; 3, $-\alpha^{3.7}/\alpha\alpha$; 4, αα/αα; 5, $-\alpha^{3.7}/-\alpha^{3.7}$; 6, αα/αα; 7, $-\alpha^{4.2}/\alpha\alpha$; 8, αα/αα; 9, αα/αα; 10, αα/αα; 11, $--^{SEA}/\alpha\alpha$; 12, $-\alpha^{3.7}/\alpha\alpha$; 13, αα/αα; 14, $--^{SEA}/\alpha\alpha$, 15, αα/αα; 16, $--^{SEA}/--^{SEA}$.

16). The lack of a 12.6 kb band is diagnostically important because of the possibility of a 10.5 kb band arising from a normal α-globin complex. This is further complicated by a BglII site polymorphism inside the 12.6 kb fragment which when observed results in the splitting of the fragment into two: a 5.2 kb ψζ gene containing fragment (not seen in Figure 2b) and a 7.4 kb fragment (not detected). BamH1 digests will confirm both deletions; the $-(\alpha)^{20.5}$ mutation creates an abnormal 4 kb fragment containing some α-globin gene sequence and thus is observed on the α-gene blot; the Southeast Asian deletion $-^{SEA}$ results in a normal 10.8 kb ψζ fragment changing to an abnormal 20 kb fragment observed on the ζ-gene blot. The other common Mediterranean mutation $-^{MED}$ results in a single BglII ζ-gene fragment of 13.9 kb (lane 2). This is easily observed running just above the 12.6 kb band in heterozygotes provided the gel is electrophoresed for long enough to give a good separation of the bands.

Other points to note in interpreting BglII digests are the possibility of chromosomes containing triplicated or single ζ-globin genes (Winichagoon et al, 1982), and the abnormal fragments which result from the single α-gene deletions. The $-\alpha^{3.7}$ deletion changes the 12.6 kb fragment to 16 kb (lane 6) and the $-\alpha^{4.2}$ deletion changes it to 8.7 kb (lane 1). The 12.6 kb fragment may also vary slightly in size because of the ζ-intron HVRs.

PCR detection

Deletions may be diagnosed by the absence of a PCR product from a multiplex reaction in which other PCR products are detected as controls to the analysis. The homozygous state for α°-thalassaemia can be analysed in this manner (Chehab et al, 1987; Lebo et al, 1990). However this approach cannot be used to identify α-thalassaemia deletions in heterozygotes and is therefore of limited use. A comprehensive diagnostic PCR method requires amplification across each end of the deletion break points to generate a characteristic product for each mutation, as in the case of the 619 bp β°-thalassaemia deletion (Old et al, 1990). Such an approach for α-thalassaemia awaits development.

β-thalassaemia

There are at least 91 different point mutations or small changes of DNA sequence which produce the disorder of β-thalassaemia (Kazazian, 1990). The list has nearly doubled since the discovery of the polymerase chain reaction because of the ease of DNA sequencing of unknown mutations. It is still increasing, but fortunately, PCR has also made it easier to detect them. The first task is to identify the ethnic group to which a couple requiring prenatal diagnosis belong. The four main ethnic groups at risk for β-thalassaemia are Mediterranean, Asian Indian, Chinese and Africans. Each group has its own collection of β-thalassaemia mutations which make up more than 90% of the mutations for each group. These are listed in Table 2. β°-thalassaemia genes produce no β-globin whereas β⁺ genes produce a very much reduced amount. However most β⁺ genes are as severe as the β°

Table 2. The common β-thalassaemia mutations.

Mutation	Type	Frequency (%)	Altered site	Reference
Mediterranean				
IVSI-110 (G→A)	+	32		a
Nonsense CD39 (C→T)	O	26	+Mae 1	b
IVSI-6 (T→C)	+	10	+Sfa N1	c
IVSI-1 (G→A)	O	9	−BspM1	c
IVSII-1 (G→A)	O	7	−Hph 1	d
IVSII-745 (C→G)	+	6	+Rsa 1	c
Frameshift CD6 (−A)	O	2	−Dde 1	e
Frameshift CD8 (−AA)	O	1		b
−87 (C→G)	+	1	−Avr II	c
Asian Indian				
IVSI-5 (G→C)	+	22		f
619 bp deletion	O	21		g
Frameshift CD8/9 (+G)	O	19		f
IVSI-1 (G→T)	O	13	−BspM1	f
Frameshift CD41/42 (−TTCT)	O	11		f
Nonsense CD 15 (G→A)	O	4		f
Nonsense CD 16 (−C)	O	1		f
Chinese				
Frameshift CD 41/42 (−TTCT)	O	42		f
Nonsense CD 17 (A→T)	O	28	+Mae 1	h
IVSII-654 (C→T)	O	8		i
Frameshift CD 71–72 (+A)	O	5		i
−28 (A→G)	+	9		i
−29 (A→G)	+	6		k
African				
−29 (A→G)	+	55	+Nla III	k
−88(C→T)	+	21		l
CD 24 (T→A)	+	8	+FoK I	m

Key to references: (a) Westaway and Williamson (1981); (b) Orkin and Goff (1981); (c) Orkin et al (1982a); (d) Baird et al (1981); (e) Kazazian et al (1983); (f) Kazazian et al (1984a); (g) Orkin et al (1979); (h) Chang and Kan (1979); (i) Cheng et al (1984); (j) Orkin et al (1983); (k) Antonarakis et al (1984); (l) Orkin et al (1984); (m) Goldsmith et al (1983).

types and give rise to the condition of β⁻ thalassaemia in the homozygous form (Weatherall and Clegg, 1981). The exceptions are a few mutations which are observed in individuals with the non transfusion-dependent condition of β-thalassaemia intermedia, namely IVSI nt 6 and IVSI nt 87 mutations in Mediterraneans (Weatherall et al, 1985), IVSI nt 88 and Cap + 1 mutations in Asian Indians (Thein et al, 1988) and the IVSI nt 88 and IVSI nt 29 mutations in Africans (Antonarakis et al, 1984). However it should be noted that the association of β-thalassaemia intermedia with mild β⁺ mutations is not complete as some individuals with these mutations do not have β-thalassaemia intermedia and some β-thalassaemia intermedia patients have β° or severe β⁺ mutations which are affected by other factors such as the coinheritance of genes for α-thalassaemia or high Hb F.

The β-thalassaemia mutations may be detected directly by either hybrid-ization of allele-specific oligonucleotides (ASOs), by allele-specific priming

(ARMS method) or in particular cases by restriction enzyme digestion (see Table 2). They may also be diagnosed indirectly by linkage analysis of restriction fragment length polymorphisms (RFLPs) within the β-globin gene cluster. The best approach is to use a combination of both direct and indirect analysis whenever possible in order to eliminate mistakes through simple laboratory errors such as switched samples.

ASO's-Dot blot approach

This requires a battery of specific oligonucleotide probes synthesized in pairs; one mutant probe complementary to the mutant sequence and one normal probe complementary to the normal β gene sequence. These are usually synthesized as 19 or 20-mers with the sequence difference in the centre of the oligonucleotide. The standard approach is to 5'-end label with γ^{32}P-ATP (Saiki et al, 1986) although an alternative non-radioactive labelling method with horseradish peroxidase is just as sensitive (Saiki et al, 1988). To test for each mutation a dot blot has to be hybridized with a labelled probe and then washed at a critical temperature determined for each probe (as described by Thein and Wallace, 1986), or one filter can be hybridized for the most common mutation, stripped and then given successive hybridizations to the less common mutations. This latter method has worked very well for laboratories in Mediterranean countries such as Sardinia where one mutation accounts for the majority of cases of β-thalassaemia and most individuals are characterized in the first screening (Ristaldi et al, 1989).

However for Asian Indians there are five mutations which are more or less equally common (Thein et al, 1988). These are the 619 bp deletion, IVSI nt 5, IVSI nt 1, Frameshift 41–42 and Frameshift 8–9. To detect these quickly on newly referred couples on a week to week basis was found to be both hazardous and a logistical problem for our laboratory which also receives referrals from Mediterranean and, occasionally, Chinese ethnic groups. Therefore we have developed an alternative PCR approach for the detection of mutations which is non-radioactive and allows all the mutations for a particular ethnic group to be screened simultaneously in just 3 hours (Old et al, 1990). This approach is a development of the amplification refractory mutation system (ARMS) originally described by Newton et al (1989).

ARMS approach

Mutations are detected by ARMS primers in a similar fashion to using ASOs. Two ARMS primers are required per mutation; a mutant primer to detect the β-thalassaemia mutation and a normal primer to demonstrate its absence. Each primer is complementary to either the mutant or normal DNA sequence except for the deliberate introduction of a mismatched nucleotide four bases from the 3' end (to increase the primer specificity). The point mutation in the genomic sequence is complementary to the 3' terminal nucleotide of the mutant primer. Under carefully controlled amplification conditions over 25 cycles the mutant primer will mismatch with

Table 3. Oligonucleotide sequence of primers for Asian Indian mutations.

(a) Control and common primers

Control : A		CAA	TGT	ATC	ATG	CCT	CTT	TGC	ACC
Control : B		GAG	TCA	AGG	CTG	AGA	GAT	TGC	AGG
Common : C		ACC	TCA	CCC	TGT	GGA	GCC	AC	
Common : D		CCC	CCT	CCT	ATG	ACA	TGA	ACT	TAA

(b) ARMS primers

Primer												Used with	Fragment size
IVSI nt5	m	CTC	CTT	AAA	CCT	GTC	TTG	TAA	CCT	TGT	TAG	C	285
	n	CTC	CTT	AAA	CCT	GTC	TTG	TAA	CCT	TGT	TAC	C	285
IVSI nt1	m	TTA	AAC	CTG	TCT	TGT	AAC	CTT	GAT	ACG	AAA	C	281
	n	GAT	GAA	GTT	GGT	GGT	GAG	GCC	CTG	GGT	AGG	D	450
Fr. 41–42	m	GAG	TGG	ACA	GAT	CCC	CAA	AGG	ACT	CAA	CCT	C	439
	n	GAG	TGG	ACA	GAT	CCC	CAA	AGG	ACT	CAA	AGA	C	443
Fr. 8–9	m	CCT	TGC	CCC	ACA	GGG	CAG	TAA	CGG	CAC	ACC	C	215
	n	CCT	TGC	CCC	ACA	GGG	CAG	TAA	CGG	CAC	ACT	C	214
C15	m	TGA	GGA	GAA	GTC	TGC	CGT	TAC	TGG	CCA	GTA	D	500
	n	TGA	GGA	GAA	GTC	TGC	CGT	TAC	TGG	CCA	GTG	D	500
Fr. 16	m	TCA	CCA	CCA	ACT	TCA	TCC	ACG	TTC	ACG	TTC	C	238
	n	TCA	CCA	CCA	ACT	TCA	TCC	ACG	TTC	ACG	TTG	C	239
−88	m	TCA	CTT	AGA	CCT	CAC	CCT	GTG	GAG	CCT	CAT	D	655
	n	TCA	CTT	AGA	CCT	CAC	CCT	GTG	GAG	CCT	CAC	D	655
CAP+1	m	ATA	AGT	CAG	GGC	AGA	GCC	ACT	TAT	TGG	TTC	D	567
	n	ATA	AGT	CAG	GGC	AGA	GCC	ACT	TAT	TGG	TTA	D	567

nt, nucleotide; Fr., Frameshift; C, codon; m, mutation-specific (mutant); n, normal sequence-specific (normal).
The normal primers for mutations Fr. 16, −88, CAP+1 have not been tested due to lack of a homozygous DNA sample.

normal genomic sequence at its 3' nucleotide (and vice versa for the normal primer) and fail to prime the extension step of the polymerase chain reaction. Thus an amplified product will only be observed with the mutant primer if its 3' end is base-paired with the genomic sequence, i.e. if the mutation is present in the genomic DNA.

The ARMS primers devised to detect the Asian Indian mutations are listed in Table 3. Each ARMS primer requires a common primer with which it combines to produce an amplified product (C or D in Table 3). A second pair of primers is included in the PCR mixture to act as a control (A and B in Table 3). These primers have been designed to lie either side of the 619 bp β° deletion and therefore in addition to producing a normal control fragment of 861 bp in length the primers also detect the deletion gene by producing a characteristic smaller fragment of 242 bp. Figure 3a illustrates the results

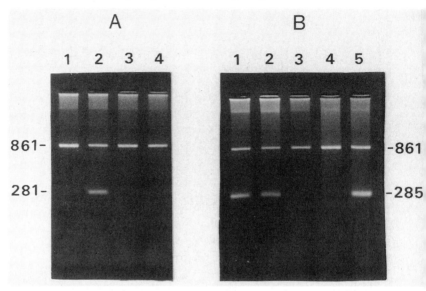

Figure 3. (A) Electrophoresis of the products from a screening of an unknown heterozygous DNA sample for the common five Indian mutations using ARMS primers. Track 1 shows the products of amplification with the mutant primer for IVSI nt 5 mutation, 2 with IVSI nt 1 mutant primer, 3 with Fr. 41–42 mutant primer, and 4 with Fr. 8–9 mutant primer. The upper band is the control band of 861 bp produced by primers A and B. If the 619 bp deletion gene was present in the sample a band of 242 bp would be observed in all four tracks. This is not the case as a lower band is only observed in track 2, which contained the primer for the IVSI nt 1 mutation. Therefore the DNA sample comes from an individual carrying the IVSI nt 1 mutation. (B) A prenatal diagnosis using ARMS primers. The pedigree shows the mother (1), father (2) (each heterozygous for IVSI nt 5 mutation), their normal child (3) and the CVS (4). The electrophoresis products in the 3% agarose gel (1.5 agarose and 1.5% Nusieve agarose) are as follows: first lane contains maternal DNA with IVSI nt 5 mutant primer; second lane contains paternal DNA with IVSI nt 5 mutant primer; third lane contains DNA from the normal child with mutant primer; fourth lane contains CVS DNA with the normal IVSI nt 5 primer; fifth lane contains CVS DNA with the mutant IVSI nt 5 primer. No amplified product was observed with the normal IVSI nt 5 ARMS primer indicating that no normal sequence was present at the IVSI nt 5 position in the CVS DNA. Therefore the diagnosis was an affected fetus, homozygous for the IVSI nt 5 β-thalassaemia mutation.

Table 4. Oligonucleotide sequences of primers for Cypriot mutations.

(a) Control and common primers

		Sequence							
Control	A:	CAA	TGT	ATC	ATG	CCT	CTT	TGC	ACC
Control	B:	GAG	TCA	AGG	CTG	AGA	GAT	TGC	AGG
Common	C:	ACC	TCA	CCC	TGT	GGA	GCC	AC	
Control	E:	AGT	GCT	GCA	AGA	AGA	ACA	ACT	
Control	F:	CTC	TGC	ATC	ATG	GGC	GAG	CTC	

(b) ARMS primers

		Sequence								Used with	Fragment size
IVSI nt 110	m	ACC	AGC	CTA	AGG	GTG	GGA	AAA	ACT	C	390
	n	ACC	AGC	CTA	AGG	GTG	GGA	AAA	ACC	C	390
IVSI nt 1	m	TTA	CTG	TCT	TGT	AAC	CTT	GAT	AAT	C	281
	n	TTA	CTG	TCT	TGT	AAC	CTT	GAT	AAC	C	281
IVSI nt 6	m	TCT	TAA	ACC	TGT	CTT	GTA	ACC	ATG	C	286
	n	TCT	TAA	ACC	TGT	CTT	GTA	ACC	ATA	C	286
C39	m	CAG	CCC	AAA	GGA	CTC	AAA	GAA	GTA	C	436
	n	CAG	CCC	AAA	GGA	CTC	AAA	GAA	GTG	C	436
C6	m	CCC	GGG	CAG	TAA	CGG	CAG	ACT	GCC	C	208
	n	CCC	GGG	CAG	TAA	CGG	CAG	ACT	GCT	C	208
IVSII nt 1	m	AAG	ACA	TCA	AGG	GTC	CCA	TAG	GAT	C	634
	n	AAG	ACA	TCA	AGG	GTC	CCA	TAG	GAC	C	634
IVSII nt 745	m	TCA	TGC	TAA	TAG	CAG	CTA	CAA	AGG	B	323
	n	TCA	TGC	TAA	TAG	CAG	CTA	CAA	AGC	B	323

Abbreviations as for Table 3.

from the simultaneous screening of an unknown carrier DNA sample for the
five common Asian Indian mutations. An amplified ARMS fragment was
produced by the IVSI nt 1 mutant primer in track 2. No product was
observed with the other three mutant primers indicating that the individual
has the IVSI nt 1 mutation. If a 242 bp fragment was observed in all four
tracks then the individual would have the 619 bp deletion gene. Figure 3b
shows a prenatal diagnosis using ARMS primers for a couple at risk for an
affected child homozygous for the IVSI nt 5 mutation. The results show that
the CVS DNA was homozygous for this mutation.

We have also developed the ARMS method for the detection of the seven
commonest Mediterranean mutations (Kazazian et al, 1984a). The ARMS
primer sequences are listed in Table 4. Their use in screening DNA from a
Greek Cypriot individual heterozygous for β-thalassaemia is illustrated in
Figure 4. A positive result was obtained in track 1 with the IVSI nt 110
mutation ARMS primer producing a 390 bp fragment. All the other mutant
ARMS primers failed to produce a band with the sample DNA (odd
numbered tracks). Note that the IVSII nt 745 ARMS primers required a
different common primer to all the others, and also a different set of control
primers. The site of the mutation lies within the usual control primers which
produce the 861 bp fragment from the 3' end of the β-globin gene. The
control primers used are those for the $^G\gamma$-globin gene HindIII RFLP (see
Table 5) which produce a 323 bp fragment.

Direct detection by restriction enzyme digestion

A small number of the 91 β-thalassaemia mutations either abolish a
restriction enzyme site or create a new one within the β-globin gene. The

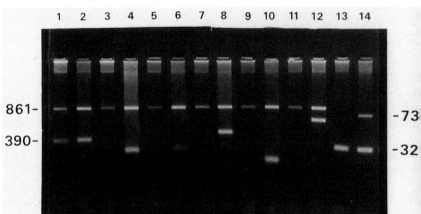

Figure 4. ARMS analysis of the seven commonest Mediterranean mutations. Odd numbered
lanes contain DNA from an unknown Cypriot β-thalassaemia heterozygote. Even numbered
lanes contain a control DNA with a known mutation. Mutant specific primers used were lane
and 2, IVSI nt 110; 3 and 4, IVSI nt 1; 5 and 6, IVSI nt 6; 7 and 8, codon 39; 9 and 10, codon 6; 1
and 12, IVSII nt 1; 13 and 14, IVSII nt 745. In tracks 1–12, the 861 bp fragment is the control
band. In tracks 13 and 14, the 323 bp fragment is the control band.

Table 5. Primers for RFLP analysis.

RFLP		Sequence (5'→3')	Size	Fragments		
				(−)	(+)	constant
*Hind*II/ε	S	TTAAGAGAGCTAGAACTGGGTGAG	158	158	86	—
	AS	AAGCCTCATATAAAGGAGCAAATC		72		
*Hind*III/$^G\gamma$	S	AGTGCTGCAAGAAGAACAACTACC	323	323	235	
	AS	CTCTGCATCATGGGCACTGAGCTC			98	—
*Hind*III/$^A\gamma$	S	GACTAGTGCTTGAAGGGGAACAAC	1004	776	681	228
	AS	CCTCTGCTGATTCATTTCTTACAC			95	
*Ava*II/ψβ	S	TCCTATCCATTACTGTTCCTTGAA	794	794	442	—
	AS	ATTGTCTTATTCTAGAGACGATTT			352	
*Hind*II/5'ψβ	S	As for *Ava*II/ψβ	795	794	687	—
	AS	As for *Ava*II/ψβ			107	
*Hind*II/3'ψβ	S	GTACTCATACTTTAAGTCCTAACT	914	914	480	—
	AS	TAAGCAAGATTATTTCTGGTCTCT			434	
*Rsa*I/β	S	AGACATAATTTATTAGCATGCATG	1152	413	331	644
	AS	ACATCAAGGGTCCCATAGAC			82	95
*Ava*II/β	S	ACTCCCAGGAGCAGGGAGGGCAGG	676	315	214	361
	AS	TTCGTCTGTTTCCCATTCTAAACT			101	
*Hinf*I/β	S	TGGATTCTGCCTAATAAAA	741	341	213	244
(= *Bam*HI)	AS	GGGCCTATGATAGGGTAAT			128	154

S = sense; AS = antisense.

mutations and their affected restriction enzyme sites are listed in Table 2. These mutations can be detected directly by amplification of the part of the β-globin gene containing the affected restriction site and then digesting the product with the appropriate enzyme. After digestion for an hour the products are run on an agarose gel and the fragment pattern observed against normal DNA controls for the presence of the mutation. The amplified product if possible should contain a second restriction site to provide an internal control against partial digestion. If this is not possible because the nearest site is too far away, a control DNA sample in which the restriction site is known to be cut should be amplified and digested under exactly the same conditions as the test sample. Although this is a useful method of detecting thalassaemia mutations once they have been identified using ASO or ARMs primers, it is not a viable screening method for unknown mutations because only some of the mutations in each ethnic group can be diagnosed in this way. Also some of the restriction enzymes required are extremely expensive (e.g. *Avr*II, *Sfa*NI, *Nla*III) and it is not cost-effective to use them for screening uncharacterized DNA samples.

RFLP linkage analysis

There are 18 known RFLPs within the β-globin gene cluster (Kazazian and Boehm, 1988). However, not all of these are useful because some have been found to be non-randomly associated with each other to produce just a handful of haplotypes (Antonarakis et al, 1982). In particular they form a 5' cluster which is 5' to the δ gene and a 3' cluster which extends downstream from the β-globin gene. In between is a 9 kb stretch of DNA containing a relative hotspot for meiotic recombination. The recombination between the two clusters has been calculated to be approximately one in 350 meioses (Chakravarti et al, 1984). ASO hybridization studies have shown that each β-thalassaemia mutation is strongly associated with just one or two haplotypes (Orkin et al, 1982a; Kazazian et al, 1984b), probably because of their recent origin compared to the haplotypes. Each haplotype normally consists of 5 RFLPs located in the 5' cluster (HindII/ε-gene; HindIII/^{G}γ-gene; HindIII^{A}γ-gene; HindII/3'ψβ; and HindII/5'γβ) and two RFLPs in the 3' cluster (AvaII/β-gene; BamHI/β-gene) (Old et al, 1983).

All of these seven RFLPs can be analysed by PCR very simply and quickly (Kulozik et al, 1988). Primers have been designed to span the RFLP site and produce easily identifiable fragments after electrophoresis of the digested products in an agarose gel usually comprising a mixture of agarose and Nusieve agarose in order to give good resolution of small fragments. The primer sequences and fragments generated are listed in Table 5. The BamHI RFLP is located within a L1 repetitive element and a HinfI RFLP located just 3' to the β-globin gene is used instead. These two RFLPs have been found to exist in linkage disequilibrium (Semenza et al, 1989). Two other RFLPs are included in Table 5. An AvaII RFLP in the ψβ-gene is extremely useful in haplotype analysis of Mediterranean β-thalassaemia heterozygotes. The ($-$) allele for this RFLP is frequently found on chromosomes carrying the IVSI nt 110 mutation while it is very rare on normal β-globin chromosomes (Wainscoat et al, 1984) and thus is a very useful informative marker for individuals heterozygous for this mutation. The second additional RFLP in the list is the RsaI RFLP located just 5' to the β-globin gene. This site is useful because it lies in the region of DNA containing the hot spot for recombination and because of the relative sequence randomization of this region it shows little association with either the 5' or 3' sequence clusters.

If a family study is possible we always use RFLPs for prenatal diagnosis of β-thalassaemia in addition to the direct detection of mutations by the ARMS technique. To obtain the linkage phase of informative RFLPs one requires DNA from either: (i) a normal or an affected child; (ii) both sets of grandparents if no children are available; or (iii) one set of grandparents if a child heterozygous for β-thalassaemia is available. It is essential that one of the grandparents on each side of the family is normal with respect to β-thalassaemia otherwise the linkage phase cannot be determined. For the correct assignment it is essential that all the individuals analysed have been correctly phenotyped and that paternity is true. Because of the non-random association of the RFLPs in the 5' cluster it is not necessary to analyse all of these RFLPs. In our laboratory we just analyse the two HindII RFLPs in the ψβ-gene. These two sites can identify the three most common 5' haplotypes in Caucasians ($+----$, $-++-+$, $-+-++$). We then analyse the 3' cluster RFLPs in the order AvaII, HinfI, RsaI until an informative RFLP is found. It is important to study these even if the 5' haplotype is informative for prenatal diagnosis because of the very slight chance of recombination between the 5' cluster and the β-globin gene.

Informative RFLPs are found in more than 80% of the families studied. Thus haplotype analysis is a very useful alternative approach to provide confirmation of a diagnosis obtained by the direct detection of mutations using ARMS primers. In our first 100 diagnoses using ARMS primers there was only one case in which RFLP linkage analysis gave a different prediction to that obtained with the ARMS primers (Old et al, 1990). Fresh blood samples were obtained from all the individuals involved in this particular case and further investigation revealed a mislabelled DNA sample in the first batch of samples. Thus a combination of the two different approaches identified one possible cause of error and misdiagnosis (switched or wrongly labelled samples). Such a strategy may also help to reveal other possible causes such as non-paternity or maternal DNA contamination.

Structural variants of haemoglobin

Hb S

The detection of sickle cell anaemia has evolved from indirect linkage analysis (Kan and Dozy, 1978) to the direct detection by restriction enzyme analysis (Orkin et al, 1982b) and finally to direct detection by oligonucleotide hybridization (Conner et al, 1983). The application of PCR technology has improved all these approaches (Saiki et al, 1986; Chehab et al, 1987), and permitted the development of new ones such as the colour complementation assay (Chehab and Kan, 1990) or the ARMS approach (see below). Thus there is no lack of choice for a method of diagnosing sickle cell anaemia.

The approaches used in our laboratory are the direct detection by the restriction enzyme DdeI and occasionally, in cases where it is necessary to distinguish between β^S and β^C mutations, the ARMS method. The enzyme MstII (now unobtainable commercially) or its isoschizomers SauI, CVnI or OxaN1, fails to cut the β^S gene at the site of the sickle mutation and was the enzyme of choice for Southern blot analysis because it produces reasonably large DNA fragments that can be detected by blot analysis. DdeI has a similar but less specific recognition site to MstII and therefore cuts genomic DNA more frequently. However, this is not a problem for PCR analysis and DdeI can be used instead of the more expensive MstII isoschizomers as illustrated in Figure 5. The primers used produce a fragment containing four constant DdeI sites which should always be completely cut in every digested sample. The sickle mutation creates a 351 bp fragment which is absent in a normal individual (AA). Similarly the two normal fragments of 150 and 201 bp on either side of the sickle mutation are absent in a sickle cell homozygote (SS).

Hb C

Although the Hb C mutation lies at the centre of the recognition site for MstII and DdeI the site for these enzymes remains intact because the middle nucleotide is non-specific. The enzymes cut both β^A and β^C genes to give the same fragment pattern and therefore a different method of detection is required; either allele-specific oligonucleotide hybridization to dot blots or the ARMS technique. We use the latter technique with the same protocol as for detecting β-thalassaemia mutations. The sequence of the mutant ARMS primer to detect Hb C is CCA CAG GGC AGT AAC GGC AGA CTT CTC GTT and is used in combination with primer C listed in Table 4.

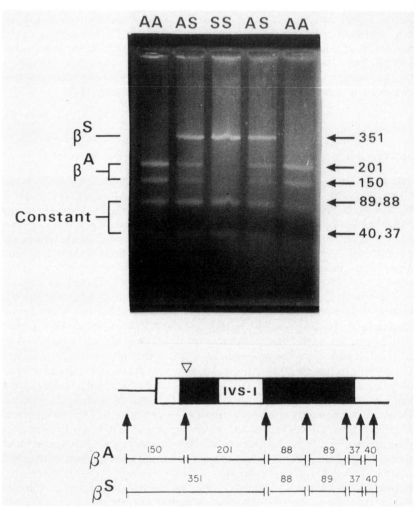

Figure 5. Diagnosis of the sickle cell mutation by PCR and digestion of the amplified product with *Dde*I. A map of the *Dde*I sites and fragment sizes produced from β^A and β^S genes is shown below the photograph of the *Dde*I digestion products in an ethidium bromide-stained gel (2% agarose/2% Nusieve agarose). The fragment sizes are indicated following *Dde*I digestion of a 665 bp fragment produced by amplification with primers GGCCAATCTACTCCCAGGAG and ACATCAAGGGTCCCATAGAC of DNA from individuals with sickle cell anaemia (SS), sickle cell trait (AS) and normal β-genes (AA).

Hb S is detected in the same way with the mutant primer sequence CCC ACA GGG CAG TAA CGG CAG ACT TCT GCA. The ARMS technique provides a quick method of distinguishing between the β^S and β^C mutations.

Hb D Punjab and Hb O Arab

The mutations for Hb D-Punjab and Hb O-Arab both abolish an *Eco*RI site in codon 121 of the β-globin gene (Trent et al, 1984). Detection of both mutations is carried out by amplifying a β-globin gene fragment containing the *Eco*RI site region and digesting with *Eco*RI. As there is no other *Eco*RI site within several kilobases of the β-globin gene no internal control site can be included in the amplified product and the only control is to amplify DNA from a normal individual at the same time.

Hb E

Although relatively harmless in the homozygous state, Hb E also results in a severe haemoglobinopathy when combined with a β-thalassaemia gene. The Hb E mutation (codon 26, G to A, Orkin et al, 1982c) affects an *Mnl*I site (Thein et al, 1987) and can be detected by amplification and restriction enzyme digestion in a similar manner to the Hb S gene. Primers C and the normal Fr. 41–42 ARMS primer (Table 4) can be used. The *Mn*1 site abolished by the β^E mutation is flanked by another located 60 bp on the 5' side and one 170 bp on the 3' side. Therefore the β^E gene produces a diagnostic *Mnl*1 fragment of 230 bp which can be identified on a 4% agarose/ Nusieve agarose gel.

Hb Lepore

The Hb Lepores are δ–β fusion globins which result from a δ to β globin gene deletion. The 7 kb deletion can be detected by an abnormal 3.8 kb *Xba* fragment on a Southern blot (Flavell et al, 1978) or by PCR using a δ gene primer and a β-gene primer to amplify across the breakpoint of the fusion gene (Camaschella et al, 1990). These primers fail to amplify normal DNA as they are more than 7 kb apart.

δβ Thalassaemia and HPFH

In these disorders no δ- and β-globin chains are synthesized in adults as a result of large DNA deletions in the β-globin gene complex (Weatherall et al, 1989). Detection of these disorders in heterozygotes is difficult because of the presence of a complete set of normal fragments from the normal β-globin chromosome masking any deleted fragments on a Southern blot. However they can be identified by using a gene probe which hybridizes to a restriction enzyme fragment which spans the breakpoint of the deleted DNA and gives a new fragment of a different size to those from the normal chromosome. For example the deletion δβ° thalassaemia Type 1 produces a characteristic 3 kb *Eco*RI fragment which hybridizes to a β-globin gene probe whereas the $\delta\beta^\circ$ thalassaemia Type 2 deletion produces an abnormal 7 kb *Bgl*II fragment which hybridizes to a γ-gene probe (Fritsch et al, 1979). Hereditary persistence of fetal haemoglobin (HPFH) deletions result in a high level of Hb F synthesis in adults which compensates for the lack of β-globin. Prenatal diagnosis for HPFH disorders is never required but they can be diagnosed in the same manner as $\delta\beta^\circ$-thalassaemia deletions. The two common deletions HPFH1 and 2 are characterized by abnormal 14 kb and 16 kb *Bam*HI fragments instead of a normal 18 kb fragment, all of which can be detected by hybridization to a γ-gene probe (Tuan et al, 1980). These are just four examples from the many deletions that have now been characterized in $\delta\beta$ thalassaemia and HPFH disorders.

SUMMARY OF PRENATAL DIAGNOSIS OF HAEMOGLOBINOPATHIES

Prenatal diagnosis of the haemoglobinopathies has evolved from globin chain biosynthesis studies through DNA analysis by Southern blotting to PCR-based diagnostic methods. Fetal blood analysis is still a useful back-up for diagnosis in the rare cases where a DNA diagnosis cannot be made for technical reasons or in late referrals of unstudied couples at risk. Southern blotting is still required for the diagnosis of α°-thalassaemia and takes from 10 days to 3 weeks to obtain a result. In contrast a diagnosis for β-thalassaemia can be made by PCR methods in as little as 3 hours but usually takes from 2 to 5 days in a routine service laboratory. Prenatal diagnosis for β-thalassaemia can be done directly without family studies. However, if children or relatives are available, RFLP linkage analysis provides a useful back up method for either confirmation of the direct approach result or in cases where the mutations could not be identified. The diagnostic error rate for both fetal blood analysis and Southern blot approach is less than 1% (Old et al, 1989). It is too early for an error rate figure for the PCR approach but a recent study of 300 cases diagnosed by both a PCR based method (ASO-dot blot) and a non-amplification method (ASO-Southern blot) showed the same result was obtained by both methods in every case (Rosatelli et al, 1990). Thus PCR methods appear to be as reliable as other DNA techniques provided that all maternal decidua is carefully dissected from the chorionic villus sample before DNA analysis.

INHERITED HAEMOSTATIC DISORDERS

Haemophilia A and B are the commonest severe congenital bleeding disorders which result from a reduction of the plasma factor VIII and IX coagulant activity (VIIIC and IXC). Both are transmitted as X-linked recessive disorders and are clinically indistinguishable. The haemorrhagic manifestations are predominantly into large joints, e.g. elbows and knees, and muscles, e.g. calf. Individuals with less than 2% normal VIIIC or IXC are classified as having a severe form of the disorder which is characterized by spontaneous bleeding. Those with more than 2% clotting activity usually only bleed after trauma and are characterized as having moderate haemophilia, whilst those with over 10% clotting activity bleed after major injury or surgery and have a mild form of the disorder. Within a single family pedigree all affected males will have haemophilia of the same degree of severity due to each inheriting the same genetic defect of the factor VIII or IX gene.

Factor VIIIC is predominantly synthesized in hepatocytes and in the circulation is non-covalently bound to its carrier protein von Willebrand factor (vWF). When activated by thrombin, it greatly accelerates the activation of factor X by IXa in the coagulation cascade. In the majority of patients with haemophilia there is a parallel reduction in the coagulant activity of the molecule (VIIIC) and its antigen (VIIIAg) concentration. Some individuals, however, have a much greater reduction of coagulant activity than antigen, and are classified as cross reacting material positive (CRM+). The mature VIIIC protein is composed of 2332 amino acids and computer analysis has revealed the peptide chain to be composed of three homologous A domains, a B domain rich in asparagine and two C domains. There is considerable homology between the A domain of factor VIII, factor V and caeruloplasmin (Church et al, 1984; Gitschier et al, 1984; Toole et al, 1984). Thrombin activates factor VIII by proteolytic cleavage; the B domain is released and appears to have no function in coagulation. The activated molecule is subsequently inactivated by further proteolysis by activated protein C as well as thrombin.

The gene for factor VIII is situated at band Xq28 close to genes for colour blindness and glucose-6-phosphate dehydrogenase. The 186 kb gene is composed of 26 exons which code for mRNA of 9 kb. The clinical disorder of haemophilia A results from a large number of different mutations of the gene and because of the size of the gene it has only been possible to characterize these in a small proportion of patients. Of the abnormalities characterized, approximately equal numbers are deletions and point mutations (Antonarakis and Kazazian, 1989; Tuddenham, 1989b; White and Shoemaker, 1989). Hot spots for mutation include CpG to TpG transitions which can result in loss of a Taq I restriction site (TCGA), these are often easy to identify because of a change in Taq I digest fragment pattern (Youssoufian et al, 1986). The CpG nucleotide is thought to be a hot spot for mutation as cytosine can be methylated and subsequently spontaneously deaminated to thymine. In several reported cases where the CGA triplet within a Taq I site is in-frame and therefore codes for an arginine residue the change of cytosine to thymidine results in the generation of a stop codon (TGA). To date most of the described genomic deletions have been large (2–210 kb) but with increasing use of PCR and analysis of amplified fragment length it will be possible to characterize much smaller deletions (Tuddenham, 1989b), as well as further point mutations.

Factor IX is also synthesizsed by hepatocytes and circulates as an inactive zymogen which is activated either by factor XIa or tissue factor–VIIa complex. The gene is small compared to factor VIII and is 33 kb in length with 8 exons. The reader is referred to excellent reviews describing the structure–function relationships of the protein (Brownlee, 1989; Giannelli, 1989). As in factor VIIIC deficiency states there may or may not be an equivalent reduction in IXC and IXAg concentration in the plasma. With the advent of PCR technology, and because the gene is small, it has become relatively straightforward to characterize most mutations of the factor IX genes and these have been reviewed elsewhere (Giannelli, 1989).

von Willebrand's Disease is an autosomal disorder due to defective synthesis of vWF by endothelial cells and megakaryocytes. As well as being the carrier protein for factor VIIIC it performs an important function in promoting primary haemostasis by promoting adhesion of platelets to subendothelial components at points of vascular injury and high shear flow of blood. In most pedigrees, vWD only causes mild haemorrhagic symptoms which usually manifest as epistaxis, easy bruising, menorrhagia and occasionally, gastrointestinal haemorrhage. Because in the majority of incidences it is a clinically mild disorder there is little call for antenatal diagnosis. Severe von Willebrand's disease is rare and results often in a severe haemorrhagic diathesis similar to severe haemophilia A; such individuals are usually double heterozygotes of parents with minimal or no bleeding symptoms resulting from each being heterozygous for a different defect in the vWF gene (Bernardi et al, 1988b; Peake et al, 1990a). Because of the clinical severity of severe vWD, facilities for antenatal diagnosis should be available (Rozmajzl, 1988; Peake et al, 1990b). The vWF 178 kb gene is located on chromosome 12 p1.2 and is complex with 52 exons (Mancuso et al, 1989; Tuddenham, 1989b). The situation is further complicated by the presence of a pseudogene on chromosome 22.

Other severe congenital haemorrhagic disorders are relatively rare; platelet abnormalities occasionally result in major haemorrhagic diathesis. The severe conditions, e.g. thrombasthenia, due to a deficiency of glycoprotein IIb/IIIa and Bernard Soulier syndrome due to a deficiency of glycoprotein Ib are best detected antenatally by fetal blood sampling even though the genes characterizing these glycoproteins have been identified. Recent reports indicate that genotypic analysis may also be informative (Bray and Shuman, 1990).

ANTENATAL DIAGNOSIS OF INHERITED HAEMOSTATIC DISORDERS

To determine whether a fetus may have haemophilia or another severe bleeding disorder it is first necessary to assess the risk of the mother carrying the mutant gene. Unlike other 'recessive' disorders e.g. thalassaemia, there is no simple technique for identifying female carriers of haemophilia. If the fetus is to be assessed phenotypically, e.g. by fetal blood sampling at 18–20 weeks gestation, the minimum information necessary is to know that the mother has a high chance of being a carrier from examination of the pedigree, e.g. sister of a haemophiliac (50% chance); it is not necessary to demonstrate unequivocally that she is a carrier. On the other hand if the fetus is to be assessed by RFLP, it is essential to demonstrate that the mother is a carrier and to know the phase of the mutant gene in relation to the restriction site alleles. Finally, if the nature of the gene mutation is identified and readily characterized, by study of an affected family member, characterization of the mother (and fetus by chorionic villus sampling (CVS) if appropriate) will assign carriership and diagnosis unequivocally.

Haemophilia carrier identification

Unlike the haemoglobinopathies where heterozygote carriers are usually easy to identify, carriers of haemophilia A and B are not readily diagnosed. This in part is due to lyonization resulting in variable expression of the normal and haemophiliac gene. In contrast to the haemoglobinopathies, haemophilia is a relatively rare disorder and due to a large variety of different mutations. It is not feasible to undertake population screening. Thus, before antenatal diagnosis, a counselee (potential carrier) must either have an antecedent family history of haemophilia or a son with the disorder. Carrier assignment is accomplished by three sequential discrete stages: review of the pedigree, phenotypic assessment and genotypic analysis.

Table 6. Obligate carriers of haemophilia.

1.   Daughter of haemophiliac.
2.   Mother of:
(a) two sons with haemophilia;
(b) dizotic male twins both with haemophilia;
(c) son with haemophilia who has another relative with haemophilia.

The prior probability that a counselee is a carrier can be assessed by reference to the pedigree. Obligate carriers are those females who must be heterozygous (or rarely homozygous) for the haemophilia gene. The criteria for obligate carriership are given in Table 6. Carriership, however, may be excluded by review of the pedigree. For the remainder of females in the pedigree, it is possible to derive a probability that each is a carrier based on simple segregation of X chromosomes. Thus the sister of a haemophiliac has a 50% chance of being a carrier. For a known carrier there is a 50% chance that each daughter will be a carrier and a 50% chance that each son will have haemophilia. In constructing a family tree for a pedigree with severe haemophilia, it is reasonable to assume that asymptomatic males are not affected, however for moderate and mild haemophilia it is essential to measure the factor VIIIC and IXC levels in asymptomatic males to ensure that they are correctly phenotyped.

It is commonly believed that the majority of haemophiliacs belong to families where the disorder has previously been known to be present. In fact approximately one third of haemophiliacs arise without any prior family history (Graham, 1989). Such sporadic cases require careful assessment because they can arise by several different mechanisms. The haemophilia gene may have been passed down several generations by female carriers without, by chance, expression in a male offspring. Alternatively the mother may be a true carrier if her father's sperm, from which she is derived, contained a new mutation of the factor VIII or IX gene (Howard et al, 1988). The mother may not be a true carrier if she is a mosaic as only a proportion of her cells contain the X chromosome possessing the mutant haemophilia gene. If in the mother only the single ovum that gave rise to her haemophilic son contained the mutant gene then subsequent sons will not be at risk of haemophilia. Thus sporadic cases can arise by several different mechanisms. It is currently estimated that the mother of a sporadic haemophiliac has a 90% chance of being a true carrier, however this estimate may well be revised in future as many mothers of sporadic haemophiliacs are assessed genetically (Graham, 1989).

Assessment of phenotype

In normal individuals the factor VIIIC concentration ranges from 50 to 150% of normal. Furthermore it is subject to marked physiological variation and particularly increases in relation to pathological processes as it is an acute phase reactant. The factor VIIIC concentration changes with age, being highest in children and older adults with a nadir at 20–30 years. Individuals of blood group O have lower factor VIII levels than those of blood group A or B (Green et al, 1986).

As a result of random inactivation of the X chromosome in early gestation (lyonization), on average the mean factor VIIIC level in carriers is 50% of normal. In practise, however, because of different degrees of lyonization and because the factor VIII level varies for other reasons (see above) the ability to assign carriership by measurement of factor VIII levels alone is limited. Very low factor VIIIC levels are highly indicative of carrier status or occasionally they represent homozygous haemophilia in the female (Pietu et al, 1988; Ingerslev et al, 1989; Randi et al, 1989). These two possibilities can now be distinguished by gene analysis (see below). The ratio of factor VIIIC to vWF provides better discrimination between carrier and normal females; the smaller the ratio the greater the risk of a given individual being a carrier. By comparing the distribution of factor VIIIC/vWF ratios in obligate carriers and normal women a likelihood ratio of carriership can be determined (Figure 6) (Peake et al, 1981). An extensive international study defined a 'universal discriminant' which took into account the observed factor VIII level in the obligate carriers in relation to age and ABO status (Graham et al, 1986).

Combining the prior probability derived from inspection of the pedigree with the likelihood ratio of carriership determined by the factor VIIIC/vWFAg ratio, allows calculation of a final probability of carriership. Except in the instance of an obligate carrier, such information merely gives an estimate of statistical chance that an individual woman is a carrier; it is estimated to be correct in approximately 80% of instances. Although this may appear a relatively high level of correct diagnosis, analysis will be incorrect in approximately 1 in 5 women counselled and therefore leaves individuals with an appreciable degree of uncertainty.

Calculation of a likelihood ratio by measuring factor IXC levels in potential carriers of haemophilia B is even less informative than the

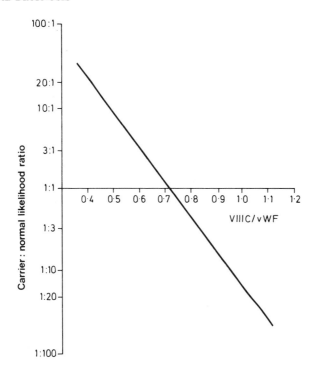

Figure 6. Carrier likelihood ratio related to VIIIC/vWF ratio. From Peake et al (1981), with permission.

equivalent measure in haemophilia A. This is partly because haemophilia B is much less prevalent and it is difficult for any one centre to collect sufficient obligate carriers to calculate a likelihood ratio. Furthermore, assessment of the factor IXC/Ag ratio does not significantly improve the calculation of risk.

A novel technique for tracking factor IX within families was described using a monoclonal antibody that distinguished between threonine (Malmo A variant) and alanine (Malmo B) which are polymorphic at the residue 148 of the factor IX peptide (Wallmark et al, 1985). It is not always possible however to detect all heterozygotes with the monoclonal antibody (Thompson et al, 1988). With the PCR, however, it is now easily possible to sequence this part of the gene and hence use the information to gene track in the pedigree (Graham et al, 1989).

Genotypic assessment

In many families it is now possible accurately to assign genotype by following the haemophilia gene in the family either by RFLP or by direct detection of the mutation.

To date, in most instances, carrier assignment and antenatal diagnosis have been made by RFLP analysis. As a large number of different genetic mutations in the factor VIII or IX gene result in the production of defective clotting proteins it is not usually possible to identify and therefore track the mutation by oligonucleotide probes or sequencing PCR amplified fragments of the relevant part of the gene. The advantage of RFLP tracking is that it is not necessary to know the site of mutation although it is necessary to know whether the enzyme restriction site is intragenic or extragenic, i.e. close by or linked to the gene. The disadvantage of extragenic restriction sites is that recombination during meiosis can occur between the gene and enzyme site leading to incorrect diagnosis. For haemophilia A probes DX13 and ST14 are closely linked to the factor VIII gene and there is a 5% chance of recombination. Fortunately there are now several intragenic RFLPs for both the factor VIII and IX genes (Tables 7 and 8) which can be used confidently to assign carriership because the chance of recombination between the intragenic probe and the site of mutation is less than 0.1%.

To gene track within a pedigree by RFLP it is necessary for appropriate females to be heterozygous for one or more of the RFLPs. The most useful probes are those that either have two alleles that are present in approximately 50% of the X chromosomes of the population or have multiple alleles. Unfortunately the utility of using two probes is not the sum of the individual heterozygote rates because of linkage disequilibrium in which there is association between two closely related alleles. Within a given population the chance of using RFLP to correctly assign the presence of a haemophilia gene within a particular family member will depend upon the allelic frequency in the population. The majority of studies have been undertaken in caucasians but recent reports indicate very marked differences when other racial groups are assessed. Thus the order in which probes are used will depend upon the geographical location (Chan et al, 1988; Suehiro et al, 1988; Inaba et al, 1990; Chan, 1990) and racial origin of the pedigree.

The results of some studies indicate that many carriers remain without a diagnosis (Lillicrap et al, 1988). Thus most information can be gained from using the probes in which the allelic frequency approaches 50%, e.g. *Xba*I within the factor VIII gene and subsequently utilizing a further probe with the allelic frequency closest to 50%, i.e. *Bcl*I or *Msp*I followed by *Bgl*I (Mibashan et al, 1989). If these probes are not informative then it may be necessary to use RFLPs that are closely linked to the factor VIII gene. The advantage of one of the linked probe, ST14, is that it detects multiple alleles and hence it is very often informative within a given pedigree. Similar constraints apply to the factor IX (Bottema et al, 1989; Mariani et al, 1990; Reiss et al, 1990), factor X (Hassan et al, 1988; MacGillivray and Fung, 1989) and vWF genes (Table 9) (Bahnak et al, 1988; Verweij et al, 1988; Bernardi et al, 1990).

The standard method of RFLP analysis, by Southern blotting is tedious, slow and the technique temperamental. By amplifying with the PCR a short section of DNA which includes the restriction enzyme site, and then digesting the product with the appropriate endonuclease, the presence or absence of the site can be detected by fragment length on electrophoresis

Table 7. Intragenic and extragenic RFLPs for the factor VIII gene. Mibashan et al (1989).

Restriction enzyme	Probe	Allelic bands (kb)	Frequency of alleles	Type	Reference
BclI	p114.12	1.1/0.8	0.29/0.71	Intragenic	Gitschier et al (1985)
BglI	Probe C	20/5	0.15/0.85	Intragenic	Antonarakis et al (1985)
XbaI (+kpnI)	p482.6	6.2/1.4 6.2/4.8	0.41/0.59	Intragenic	Wion et al (1986)
BstXI	p482.6	2.4/1.61	0.48/0.45/0.07	Intragenic	Taylor et al (1989)
MspI	p625.3	7.5/4.3	0.32/0.68	Intragenic	Youssoufian et al (1987)
HindIII					Bernardi et al (1988a)
BglII	DX13	5.8/2.8	0.5/0.5	Extragenic	Harper et al (1984)
TaqI	St14	Multiple	—	Extragenic	Oberle et al (1985)

Table 8. Intragenic and extragenic RFLPs for the factor IX gene. After Mibashan et al (1989).

Restriction enzyme	Probe	Allelic bands (kb)	Frequency of alleles	Type	Reference
TaqI	Probe VIII	1.8/1.3	0.35/0.65	Intragenic	Giannelli et al (1984)
XmnI	Probe VIII	11.5/6.5	0.29/0.71	Intragenic	Winship et al (1984)
DdeI/HinfI	Probe XIII	1.7/1.75	0.24/0.76	Intragenic	Winship et al (1984)
MspI	cDNA	5.8/2.4	0.20/0.80	Intragenic	Camerino et al (1985)
BamHI	Probe VIII	25/23	0.94/0.06	Intragenic	Hay et al (1986)
SstI	pX58dIIIc	5.9/8.8	0.43/0.57	Extragenic	Mulligan et al (1987)
BamHI	cDNA	25/16.9	0.13/0.87	Intragenic	Driscoll et al (1988)
HhaI	PCR	0.23/0.15+0.08	0.39/0.61	Extragenic	Winship et al (1989)
SacI	pX58dIIIc	5.9/8.8	0.48/0.52	Extragenic	Tanimoto et al (1989)
PuvII	oligo		0.33/0.67	Intragenic	Winship and Brownlee (1986)

Table 9. Intragenic RFLPs for von Willebrand factor gene. After Mibashan et al (1989).

Restriction enzyme	Probe	Allelic bands (kb)	Frequency of alleles	Reference
BglII	pvWF 1100	9.0/7.4	0.31/0.69	Verweij et al (1985)
BamHI	pDL34	7.8/7.2	0.18/0.82	Nishiro & Lynch (1986)
XbaI	pvWF 1210	6.9/5.2	0.13/0.87	Quadt et al (1986)
TaqI	various	See references		Bernardi et al (1987, 1988b), Inbal & Handin (1989), Lavergne et al (1988)
RsaI	pvWF 6	1.0/0.66	0.22/0.78	Iannuzzi et al (1987)
SacI	pvWF 6	14.2/10.5	0.62/0.38	Konkle et al (1987)
XbaI	pvWF 1100	3.6/10.5	0.08/0.92	Lavergne et al (1987)
EcoRI	various	See references		Lindstedt & Anvret (1989a, 1989b), Ewerhardt et al (1989), Marchetti et al (1989)

(Winship et al, 1989). This is a quick robust method but can only be utilized if the DNA sequence is known around the restriction site, so that appropriate primers can be constructed.

The alternative approach to genetic analysis is to identify precisely the nature of the mutation and then directly assign carriership or antenatal diagnosis without the necessity for tracking within a pedigree. This method may be particularly useful, compared to RFLP tracking, when essential family members are unavailable. With the factor VIII gene this has been only possible occasionally by identifying a change in the length of endo-nuclease digestion products resulting from the presence of a large deletion or insertion in the gene (Bernardi et al, 1988a; Tuddenham, 1989b; Wehnert et al, 1989; Nafa et al, 1990) or duplication (Gitschier, 1988). The ability to achieve this depends upon the sensitivity of the electrophoretic system and the length of the DNA fragments. A further way in which the haemophilia gene can be tracked through a family is if there is loss of a common endonuclease restriction site. This may not in itself be the mutation causing the haemophilia, e.g. an intron (Lillicrap et al, 1990), but if this loss of restriction site is not commonly observed in the general population, then it may serve as an informative marker within a particular family (Zhang et al, 1989). A further example of the use of a unique marker not causing the functional gene mutation is by the use of variable number of tandem repeats (VNTRs) identified within the vWF gene (Rozmajzl, 1988).

The majority of genetic defects are likely to be single base changes or small deletions. In relatively small genes, e.g. factor IX, it is readily possible to amplify and sequence each exon by PCR until the mutation is identified (Tsang et al, 1989). For large genes, e.g. factor VIII or vWF, sequencing is either very time-consuming or impossible because the gene is incompletely characterized. Screening techniques have been developed which allow the site of mutation to be localized but as yet these are not widely used (Collins et al, 1989). It is the separation of exons by long non-expressed introns which makes gene analysis difficult, however, if mRNA is readily available this greatly facilitates mutation characterization. Analysis of the complex vWF gene has been greatly facilitated by the discovery that specific mRNA can be extracted from platelets or megakaryocytes. The principal site of factor VIII synthesis is liver which is inaccessible for mRNA extraction in a haemophiliac. A recent report indicates that it is possible to amplify and sequence the minute amount of ectopic mRNA production observed in lymphocytes (Berg et al, 1991). If this is confirmed it would greatly facilitate analysis of factor VIII abnormalities as well as many other complex genes.

Timing of antenatal diagnosis

This may be requested when parents are at high risk of having a child with a severe congenital bleeding disorder, e.g. severe haemophilia A. As patients with moderate and mild disorders only bleed relatively infrequently requests for antenatal diagnosis and potential terminations are uncommon. In counselling the parents, therefore, it is crucial to know not only the diagnosis out also its severity which is usually determined from laboratory quantition of the deficiency as well as clinical evaluation.

Antenatal diagnosis can be undertaken either by phenotypic assessment at 18–20 weeks gestation by procurement of a blood sample or by genotypic analysis at 8 weeks from a CVS. It is clearly preferable, if possible, to use the latter technique which allows a decision to be made about termination prior to 12 weeks gestation.

Although fetal blood sampling at 18–20 weeks gestation may appear inappropriate when diagnosis could be made at 10–12 weeks by CVS the technique has some utility. Firstly, it is not necessary to demonstrate for certainty that the mother is a carrier of the mutant gene. For example, she might be the sister of a severe haemophiliac and if DNA is not available from him and other appropriate family members it would be impossible to diagnose her carrier status. Secondly, the appropriate intragenic RFLP probes may be uninformative perhaps because the mother is homozygous at all polymorphic restriction sites. Thirdly, gene probes may not be available if the abnormality in the coagulation or platelet disorder is rare. Fourthly, some mothers do not present for antenatal diagnosis until well into the second trimester. Finally, if a linked or extragenomic probe has been used, with a chance therefore of an incorrect diagnosis of the fetus due to recombination between the probe and gene, it would be appropriate to confirm that the fetus is normal by measurement of the plasma coagulation factor concentration or assess platelet function on a fetal blood sample.

Increasingly CVS is superceding fetal blood sampling as the preferred technique for antenatal diagnosis. The risk of the procedure at 8 weeks gestation is small (Mibashan et al, 1989) and the utility high either with RFLP analysis (Brocker-Vriends et al, 1988; Chan et al, 1989) or direct detection of the mutation.

FUTURE DEVELOPMENTS

The ability of PCR technology to detect mutations in a single DNA molecule (Li et al, 1988) has led to the development of two new approaches to the prenatal diagnosis of genetic disorders which may provide an alternative to CVS DNA diagnosis in the future. The first is the genetic testing of an embryo either before fertilization by testing the polar body (Monk and Holding, 1990) or after fertilization by testing biopsied cells from 3-day-old embryos (Handyside et al, 1989). The second development is the diagnosis of mutations in nucleated fetal cells circulating in maternal blood. This was first demonstrated by PCR of Y chromosome-specific sequences in peripheral blood of mothers with male fetuses (Lo et al, 1989); subsequently a specific paternal allele (Hb Lepore) was detected in maternal blood of mothers carrying β-thalassaemia genes at 8–10 weeks of gestation (Camaschella et al, 1990). The drawback of this approach of course is that only the paternal allele can be diagnosed and the paternal mutation must be different to the maternal one.

REFERENCES

Alter BP (1983) Antenatal diagnosis using fetal blood. In Weatherall DJ (ed.) *Methods in Haematology—The Thalassaemias*, pp 114–133. Edinburgh: Churchill Livingstone.

Alter BP (1989) Examination of fetal blood for haemoglobinopathies. In Alter BP (ed.) *Methods in Haematology—Perinatal Haematology*, pp 13–29. Edinburgh: Churchill Livingstone.

Alter BP (1991) 6th Cooley's Anemia Symposium, *Annals of the New York Academy of Sciences* (in press).

Antonarakis SE, Boehm CD, Giardina PJV & Kazazian Jr HH (1982) Non-random association of polymorphic restriction sites in the β-globin gene cluster. *Proceedings of the National Academy of Sciences, USA* **79:** 137–141.

Antonarakis SE, Orkin SH, Cheng T-C et al (1984) Thalassaemia in American Blacks: novel mutations in the TATA box and IVS-2 acceptor splice site. *Proceedings of the National Academy of Sciences, USA* **81:** 1154–1158.

Antonarakis SE & Kazazian HH (1989) Hemophilia A in man: molecular defects in the factor VIII gene. *Recent Advances in Haematology*, vol 5, p 243. Edinburgh & London: Churchill Livingstone.

Antonarakis SE, Waber PG, Kittur SD et al (1985) Hemophilia A. Detection of molecular defects and of carriers by DNA analysis. *New England Journal of Medicine* **313:** 842–848.

Bahnak BR, Lavergne JM, Verweij CL et al (1988) Carrier detection in severe (type III) von Willebrand disease using two intragenic restriction fragment length polymorphisms. *Thrombosis and Haemostasis* **60:** 178–181.

Baird M, Driscoll C, Schreiner H et al (1981) A nucleotide change at a splice junction in the human β-globin gene is associated with β⁰-thalassaemia. *Proceedings of the National Academy of Sciences, USA* **78:** 4218–4221.

Berg L, Wieland K, Millar DS et al (1991) Detection of a novel point mutation causing haemophilia A by PCR/direct sequencing of ectopically-transcribed factor VIII mRNA. *Human Genetics* (in press).

Bernardi F, Marchetti G, Bertagnolo V et al (1987) Two TaqI RFLPs in the human von Willebrand factor gene. *Nucleic Acids Research* **15:** 1347–1347.

Bernardi F, Legnani C, Volinia S et al (1988a) A HindIII RFLP and a gene lesion in the coagulation factor VIII gene. *Human Genetics* **78:** 359–362.

Bernardi F, Guerra S, Patracchini P et al (1988b) von Willebrand disease investigated by two novel RFLPs. *British Journal of Haematology* **68:** 243–248.

Bernardi F, Marchetti G, Casonato A et al (1990) Characterization of polymorphic markers in the von Willebrand factor gene and pseudogene. *British Journal of Haematology* **74:** 282–289.

Bottema CD, Koeberl DD & Sommer SS (1989) Direct carrier testing in 14 families with haemophilia B. *Lancet* **ii:** 526–529.

Bray PF & Shuman MA (1990) Identification of an abnormal gene for the GPIIIa subunit of the platelet fibrinogen receptor resulting in Glanzmann's thrombasthenia. *Blood* **75:** 881–888.

Brocker-Vriends AH, Briet E, Kanhai HH et al (1988) First trimester prenatal diagnosis of haemophilia A: two years' experience. *Prenatal Diagnosis* **8:** 411–421.

Brownlee GG (1989) Haemophilia B: a review of patient defects, diagnosis with gene probes and prospects for gene therapy. *Recent Advances in Haematology*, Vol 5, p 251. Edinburgh & London: Churchill Livingstone.

Camaschella C, Alfarano A, Gottardi E et al (1990) Prenatal diagnosis of fetal hemoglobin Lepore-Boston disease on maternal peripheral blood. *Blood* **75:** 2102–2106.

Camerino G, Oberle I, Drayna D & Mandel JL (1985) A new MspI restriction fragment length polymorphism in the hemophilia B locus. *Human Genetics* **71:** 79–81.

Chakravarti A, Buetow KH, Antonarakis SE et al (1984) Non-uniform recombination within the human β-globin gene cluster. *American Journal of Human Genetics* **36:** 1239–1258.

Chan V (1990) Prenatal diagnosis of alpha and beta thalassemias and hemophilia A: experience in Hong Kong. *Clinical Biochemistry* **23:** 79–84.

Chan V, Chan TK, Liu VW & Wong AC (1988) Restriction fragment length polymorphism associated with factor VIII:C gene in Chinese. *Human Genetics* **79:** 128–131.

Chan V, Tong TM, Chan TP et al (1989) Multiple XbaI polymorphisms for carrier detection and prenatal diagnosis of haemophilia A. *British Journal of Haematology* **73**: 497–500.

Chang JC & Kan YW (1979) β° thalassaemia, a nonsense mutation in man. *Proceedings of the National Academy of Sciences, USA* **76**: 2886–2889.

Chehab FF & Kan YW (1989) Detection of specific DNA sequences by fluorescence amplification: a color complementation assay. *Proceedings of the National Academy of Sciences, USA* **86**: 9178–9182.

Chehab FF & Kan YW (1990) Detection of sickle cell anaemia mutation by colour DNA amplification. *Lancet* **i**: 15–17.

Chehab F, Dogerty M, Cai S et al (1987) Detection of sickle cell anaemia and thalassaemias. *Nature* **329**: 293–294.

Cheng T-C, Orkin SH, Antonarakis SE et al (1984) β-thalassaemia in Chinese: Use of in vivo RNA analysis and oligonucleotide hybridisation in systematic characterisation of molecular defects. *Proceedings of the National Academy of Sciences, USA* **81**: 2821–2825.

Church WR, Jernigan RL, Toole J et al (1984) Coagulation factors V and VIII and ceruloplasmin constitute a family of structurally related proteins. *Proceedings of the National Academy of Sciences, USA* **81**: 6934–6937.

Collins M, Wolf SF, Haines LL & Mitsock L (1989) The use of denaturing gradient gel electrophoresis to screen for DNA sequence polymorphisms in the human factor VIII gene. *Electrophoresis* **10**: 390–396.

Conner BJ, Reyes AA, Morin C et al (1983) Detection of sickle cell β^S-globin allele by hybridisation with synthetic oligonucleotides. *Proceedings of the National Academy of Sciences, USA* **80**: 278–282.

Cotton RGH, Rodrigues NR & Campbell RD (1988) Reactivity of cytosine and thymine in single-base-pair mismatches with hydroxylamine and osmium tetroxide and its application to the study of mutations. *Proceedings of the National Academy of Sciences, USA* **85**: 4397–4401.

Driscoll MC, Dispenzieri A, Tobias E et al (1988) A second BamHI DNA polymorphism and haplotype association in the factor IX gene. *Blood* **72**: 61–65.

Ewerhardt B, Ludwig M, Schwaab R et al (1989) An EcoRI polymorphism in the human von Willebrand factor (vWF) gene. *Nucleic Acids Research* **17**: 5416–5416.

Flavell RA, Kooter JWQ, De Boer E et al (1978) Analysis of the β globin gene in normal and Hb Lepore DNA: Direct determination of gene linkage and intergene distance. *Cell* **15**: 25–38.

Fritsch EF, Lawn RM & Maniatis T (1979) Characterisation of deletions which affect the expression of fetal globin genes in man. *Nature* **279**: 598–603.

Giannelli F (1989) Factor IX. *Baillière's Clinical Haematology* **2**: 821–848.

Giannelli F, Anson DS, Choo KH et al (1984) Characterisation and use of an intragenic polymorphic marker for detection of carriers of haemophilia B (factor IX deficiency). *Lancet* **i**: 239–241.

Gitschier J (1988) Maternal duplication associated with gene deletion in sporadic hemophilia. *American Journal of Human Genetics* **43**: 274–279.

Gitschier J, Wood WI, Goralka TM et al (1984) Characterization of the human factor VIII gene. *Nature* **312**: 326–330.

Gitschier J, Drayna D, Tuddenham EG et al (1985) Genetic mapping and diagnosis of haemophilia A achieved through a BclI polymorphism in the factor VIII gene. *Nature* **314**: 738–740.

Goldsmith ME, Humphires RK, Ley T et al (1983) Silent substitution in β-thalassaemia gene activating a cryptic splice site in β-globin RNA coding sequence. *Proceedings of the National Academy of Sciences, USA* **80**: 5022–5024.

Graham JB (1989) Phenotypic and genotypic carrier detection in hemophilia. In Seghatchian MJ & Savidge GF (eds) *Factor VIII—von Willebrand Factor—Clinical aspects of deficiency states*, p 1. Florida: CRC Press.

Graham JB, Rizza CR, Chediak J et al (1986) Carrier detection in hemophilia A: a cooperative international study. I. The carrier phenotype. *Blood* **67**: 1554–1559.

Graham JB, Kunkel GR, Tennyson GS et al (1989) The Malmo polymorphism of factor IX: establishing the genotypes by rapid analysis of DNA. *Blood* **73**: 2104–2107.

Green PP, Mannucci PM, Briet E et al (1986) Carrier detection in hemophilia A: a cooperative international study. II. The efficacy of a universal discriminant. *Blood* **67**: 1560–1567.

Handyside AH, Pattinson JK, Penketh RJA et al (1989) Biopsy of human preimplantation embryos and sexing by DNA amplification. *Lancet* i: 347–349.

Harper K, Winter RM, Pembrey ME et al (1984) A clinically useful DNA probe closely linked to haemophilia A. *Lancet* ii: 6–8.

Hassan HJ, Guerriero R, Chelucci C et al (1988) Multiple polymorphic sites in factor X locus. *Blood* 71: 1353–1356.

Hay CW, Robertson KA, Yong SL et al (1986) Use of a BamHI polymorphism in the factor IX gene for the determination of haemophilia B carrier status. *Blood* 67: 1508–1511.

Higgs DR (1990) The molecular genetics of the α-globin gene family. *European Journal of Clinical Investigation* 20: 340–347.

Howard PL, Hoag JB, Bovill EG & Heintz NH (1988) Spontaneous mutation in the male gamete as a cause of hemophilia A: clarification of a case using DNA probes. *American Journal of Hematology* 28: 167–169.

Iannuzzi MC, Konkle BA, Ginsburg D & Collins FS (1987) RsaI RFLP in the human von Willebrand factor gene. *Nucleic Acids Research* 15: 5909–5909.

Inaba H, Fujimaki M, Kazazian HH Jr & Antonarakis SE (1990) MspI polymorphic site in intron 22 of the factor VIII gene in the Japanese population. *Human Genetics* 84: 214–215.

Inbal A & Handin RI (1989) Two TaqI polymorphisms in the 5′ region of the von Willebrand factor (vWF) gene. *Nucleic Acids Research* 17: 10 143–10 143.

Ingerslev J, Schwartz M, Lamm LU et al (1989) Female haemophilia A in a family with seeming extreme bidirectional lyonization tendency: abnormal premature X-chromosome inactivation? *Clinical Genetics* 35: 41–48.

Kan YW & Dozy AM (1978) Antenatal diagnosis of sickle-cell anaemia by DNA analysis of amniotic-fluid cells. *Lancet* ii: 910–912.

Kan YW, Golbus M, Trecartin R et al (1975) Prenatal diagnosis of homozygous β-thalassaemia. *Lancet* ii: 790–792.

Kan YW, Bolbus MS & Dozy AM (1976) Prenatal diagnosis of α-thalassaemia: clinical application of molecular hybridization. *New England Journal of Medicine* 295: 1165–1167.

Kazazian HH Jr (1991) 6th Cooley's Anemia Symposium. *Annals of the New York Academy of Sciences* (in press).

Kazazian HH & Boehm CD (1988) Molecular basis and prenatal diagnosis of β-thalassaemia. *Blood* 72: 1107–1116.

Kazazian HH Jr, Phillips III JA, Boehm CD et al (1980) Prenatal diagnosis of β-thalassaemia by amniocentesis: linkage analysis using multiple polymorphic restriction endonuclease sites. *Blood* 56: 926–930.

Kazazian HH Jr, Orkin SH, Boehm CD et al (1983) β-thalassaemia due to deletion of the nucleotide which is substituted in sickle cell anaemia. *American Journal of Human Genetics* 35: 1028–1033.

Kazazian HH Jr, Orkin SH, Markham AF et al (1984a) Quantification of the close association between DNA haplotypes and specific β-thalassaemia mutations in Mediterraneans. *Nature* 310: 152–154.

Kazazian HH Jr, Orkin SH, Antonarakis SE et al (1984b) Molecular characterisation of seven β-thalassaemia mutations in Asian Indians. *EMBO Journal* 3: 593–596.

Konkle BA, Kim S, Iannuzzi MC et al (1987) SacI RFLP in the human von Willebrand factor gene. *Nucleic Acids Research* 15: 6766–6766.

Kulozik AE, Lyons J, Kohne E et al (1988) Rapid and non-radioactive prenatal diagnosis of β-thalassaemia and sickle cell disease: application of the polymerase chain reaction (PCR). *British Journal of Haematology* 70: 455–458.

Lavergne JM, Bahnak BR, Verweij CL et al (1987) A second Xba I polymorphic site within the human von Willebrand factor (vWF) gene. *Nucleic Acids Research* 15: 9099–9099.

Lavergne JM, Bahnak BR, Assouline Z et al (1988) A Taq I polymorphism in the 5′ region of the von Willebrand factor (vWF) gene. *Nucleic Acids Research* 16: 2742–2742.

Lebo RV, Saiki RK, Swanson K et al (1990) Prenatal diagnosis of α-thalassaemia by polymerase chain reaction and dual restriction enzyme analysis. *Human Genetics* 85: 293–299.

Li H, Gyllensten UB, Cui X et al (1988) Amplification and analysis of DNA sequences in single human sperm and diploid cells. *Nature* 335: 414–417.

Lillicrap D, Holden JJ, Giles AR & White BN (1988) Carrier detection strategy in haemophilia A: the benefits of combined DNA marker analysis and coagulation testing in sporadic haemophilic families. *British Journal of Haematology* 70: 321–326.

Lillicrap DP, Taylor SA, Schuringa PC et al (1990) Variation of the non-factor VIII sequences detected by a probe from intron 22 of the factor VIII gene. *Blood* **75**: 139–143.

Lindstedt M & Anvret M (1989a) An EcoRI polymorphism of the human von Willebrand factor cDNA (VWF). *Nucleic Acids Research* **17**: 2882–2882.

Lindstedt M & Anvret M (1989b) An EcoRI polymorphism of the human von Willebrand factor cDNA (VWF). *Nucleic Acids Research* **17**: 6435–6435.

Lo YMD, Patel P, Wainscoat JS et al (1989) Prenatal sex determination by DNA amplification from maternal peripheral blood. *Lancet* **ii**: 1363–1366.

Losekoot M, Fodde R, Harteveld CL et al (1991) Denaturing gradient gel electrophoresis and direct sequencing of PCR amplified genomic DNA: a rapid and reliable diagnostic approach to beta thalassaemia. *British Journal of Haematology* **76**: 269–274.

MacGillivray RT & Fung MR (1989) Molecular biology of factor X. *Baillière's Clinical Haematology* **2**: 897–917.

Mancuso DJ, Tuely EA, Westfield LA et al (1989) Structure of the gene for human von Willebrand factor. *Journal of Biological Chemistry* **264**: 19 514–19 527.

Marchetti G, Sacchi E, Patracchini P et al (1989) Two additional TaqI RFLPs in von Willebrand factor gene (VWF) and pseudogene. *Nucleic Acids Research* **17**: 3329–3329.

Mariani G, Chistolini A, Hassan HJ et al (1990) Carrier detection for haemophilia B: evaluation of multiple polymorphic sites. *American Journal of Hematology* **33**: 1–7.

Mibashan RS, Peake IR & Nicolaides KH (1989) Prenatal diagnosis of hemostatic disorders. *Methods in Haematology—Perinatal Haematology*, Vol 21, p 64. Edinburgh & London: Churchill Livingstone.

Monk M & Holding C (1990) Amplification of a β-haemoglobin sequence in individual human oocytes and polar bodies. *Lancet* **i**: 985–988.

Montandon AJ, Green PM, Gianelli F & Bently DR (1989) Direct detection of point mutations by mismatch analysis: application to haemophilia B. *Nucleic Acids Research* **17**: 3347–3357.

Mulligan L, Holden JJ & White BN (1987) A DNA marker closely linked to the factor IX (haemophilia B) gene. *Human Genetics* **75**: 381–383.

Nafa K, Meriane F, Reghis A et al (1990) Investigation of factor VIII: C gene restriction fragment length polymorphisms and search for deletions in hemophiliac subjects in Algeria. *Human Genetics* **84**: 401–405.

Newton CR, Graham A, Heptinstall LE (1989) Analysis of any point mutation in DNA. The amplification refractory mutation system (ARMS). *Nucleic Acids Research* **17**: 2503–2516.

Nishiro K & Lynch DC (1986) A polymorphism of the human von Willebrand factor (vWF) gene with BamHI. *Nucleic Acids Research* **14**: 4697.

Oberle I, Camerino G, Heilig R et al (1985) Genetic screening for hemophilia A (classic hemophilia) with a polymorphic DNA probe. *New England Journal of Medicine* **312**: 682–686.

Old JM (1986) Fetal DNA analysis. In Davies KE (ed.) *Human genetic diseases—a practical approach*, pp 1–17. Oxford: IRL Press.

Old JM & Higgs DR (1983) Gene Analysis. In Weatherall DJ (ed.) *Methods in Haematology— The Thalassaemias*. Edinburgh: Churchill Livingstone.

Old JM, Ward RHT, Petrou M et al (1982) First trimester diagnosis for haemoglobinopathies: a report of 3 cases. *Lancet* **ii**: 1413–1416.

Old JM, Petrou M, Modell B & Weatherall DJ (1983) Feasibility of antenatal diagnosis of β-thalassaemia by DNA polymorphisms in Asian Indian and Cypriot populations. *British Journal of Haematology* **57**: 255–263.

Old JM, Fitches A, Heath C et al (1986) First-trimester fetal diagnosis for haemoglobinopathies: report on 200 cases. *Lancet* **ii**: 763–767.

Old JM, Thein SL, Weatherall DJ et al (1989) Prenatal diagnosis of the major hemoglobin disorders. *Molecular Biology and Medicine* **6**: 55–63.

Old JM, Varawalla NY & Weatherall DJ (1990) The rapid detection and prenatal diagnosis of β-thalassaemia in the Asian Indian and Cypriot populations in the UK. *Lancet* **ii**: 834–837.

Orkin SH & Goff SC (1981) Nonsense and frameshift mutations in β⁰-thalassaemia detected in cloned β-globin genes. *EMBO Journal* **3**: 593–596.

Orkin SH, Old JM, Weatherall DJ & Nathan DG (1979) Partial deletion of β-globin gene DNA in certain patients with β⁰-thalassaemia. *Proceedings of the National Academy of Sciences, USA* **76**: 2400–2404.

426   J. M. OLD AND C. A. LUDLAM

Orkin SH, Goff SC & Hechtman RL (1981) Mutation in an intervening sequence splice junction in man. *Proceedings of the National Academy of Sciences, USA* **78**: 5041–5045.
Orkin SH, Kazazian HH Jr, Antonarakis SE et al (1982a) Linkage of β-thalassaemia mutations and β-globin gene polymorphisms with DNA polymorphisms in the human β-globin gene cluster. *Nature* **296**: 627–631.
Orkin SH, Little KPFR, Kazazian HH & Boehm CD (1982b) Improved detection of the sickle mutation by DNA analysis. *New England Journal of Medicine* **307**: 30–32.
Orkin SH, Kazazian HH, Antonarakis SE et al (1982c) Abnormal RNA processing due to the exon mutation of the β^E globin gene. *Nature* **300**: 768–769.
Orkin SH, Sexton JP, Cheng T-C et al (1983) ATA box transcriptional mutation in β-thalassaemia. *Nucleic Acids Research* **11**: 4727–4734.
Orkin SH, Antonarakis SE & Kazazian HH Jr (1984) Base substitution at position -88 in a beta-thalassaemia globin gene: Further evidence for the role of distal promoter element ACACCC. *Journal of Biological Chemistry* **259**: 8679–8684.
Peake IR, Newcombe RG, Davies BL et al (1981) Carrier detection in haemophilia A by immunological measurement of factor VIII related antigen (VIIIRAg) and factor VIII clotting antigen (VIIICAg). *British Journal of Haematology* **48**: 651–660.
Peake IR, Liddell MB, Moodie P et al (1990a) Severe type III von Willebrand's disease caused by deletion of exon 42 of the von Willebrand factor gene: family studies that identify carriers of the condition and a compound heterozygous individual. *Blood* **75**: 654–661.
Peake IR, Bowen D, Bignell P et al (1990b) Family studies and prenatal diagnosis in severe von Willebrand disease by polymerase chain reaction amplification of a variable number tandem repeat region of the von Willebrand factor gene. *Blood* **76**: 555–561.
Pietu G, Thomas-Maison N, Sie P et al (1988) Haemophilia A in a female: study of a family using intragenic and extragenic restriction site polymorphisms. *Thrombosis and Haemostasis* **60**: 102–106.
Pirastu M, Saglio G, Chang JC et al (1984) Initiation codon mutation as a cause of α-thalassaemia. *Journal of Biological Chemistry* **259**: 12315–12317.
Pressley L, Higgs DR, Clegg JB et al (1980) A new genetic basis for Hemoglobin-H disease. *New England Journal of Medicine* **303**: 1383–1388.
Quadt R, Verweij CL, de Vries CJ et al (1986) A polymorphic Xba I site within the human von Willebrand factor (vWF) gene identified by a vWF cDNA clone. *Nucleic Acids Research* **14**: 7139–7139.
Randi AM, Sacchi E, Sampietro M et al (1989) Diagnosis of hemophilia A in a female subject by using restriction fragment length polymorphisms linked to the factor VIII gene. *Ricerco in Clinica e in Laboratorio* **19**: 75–79.
Reiss J, Neufeldt U, Wieland K & Zoll B (1990) Diagnosis of haemophilia B using the polymerase chain reaction. *Blut* **60**: 31–36.
Ristaldi MS, Pirastu M, Rosatelli C & Cao A (1989) Prenatal diagnosis of β-thalassaemia in Mediterranean populations by dot blot analysis with DNA amplification and allele specific oligonucleotide probes. *Prenatal Diagnosis* **9**: 629–638.
Rosatelli MC, Sardu R, Tuveri T et al (1990) Reliability of prenatal diagnosis of genetic diseases by analysis of amplified trophoblast DNA. *Journal of Medical Genetics* **27**: 249–251.
Rozmajzl B (1988) Hospital management of a patient with von Willebrand's disease and a seizure disorder: case report. *Journal of Connecticut State Dental Association* **62**: 137–137.
Saiki RK, Scharf S, Faloona F et al (1985) Enzymatic amplification of β-globin genomic sequences and restriction site analysis for diagnosis of sickle cell anaemia. *Science* **230**: 1350–1354.
Saiki RK, Bugawan TL, Horn GT et al (1986) Analysis of enzymatically amplified β-globin and HLA-DQα DNA with allele-specific oligonucleotide probes. *Nature* **324**: 163–166.
Saiki RK, Chang CA, Levenson CH et al (1988) Diagnosis of sickle cell anaemia and beta-thalassaemia with enzymatically amplified DNA and non-radioactive allele specific oligonucleotide probes. *New England Journal of Medicine* **319**: 537–541.
Semenza GL, Dowling CE & Kazazian HH Jr (1989) HinfI polymorphism 3' to the human β-globin gene detected by the polymerase chain reaction (PCR). *Nucleic Acids Research* **17**: 2376.
Suehiro K, Tanimoto M, Hamaguchi M et al (1988) Carrier detection in Japanese hemophilia A by use of three intragenic and two extragenic factor VIII DNA probes: a study of 24 kindreds. *Journal of Laboratory and Clinical Medicine* **112**: 314–318.

Tanimoto M, Kojima T, Ogata K et al (1989) Extragenic factor IX gene RFLP is useful for detecting carriers of Japanese hemophilia B. *Nippon Ketsueki Gakkai Zasshi* **52**: 774–777.

Taylor SA, Bridge PJ & Lillicrap DP (1989) A BstXI polymorphism detected by the factor VIII genomic probe p.482.6 (F8C). *Nucleic Acids Research* **17**: 6426–6426.

Thein SL & Wallace RB (1986) The use of synthetic oligonucleotides as specific hybridisation probes in the diagnosis of genetic disorders. In Davies KE (ed.) *Human Genetic Diseases— A Practical Approach*, pp 33–50. Oxford: IRL Press.

Thein SL, Lynch JR, Old J & Weatherall DJ (1987) Direct detection of haemoglobin E with Mnl 1. *Journal of Medical Genetics* **24**: 110–112.

Thein SL, Hesketh C, Wallace RB & Weatherall DJ (1988) The molecular basis of thalassaemia major and thalassaemia intermedia in Asian Indians: application to prenatal diagnosis. *British Journal of Haematology* **70**: 225–231.

Thompson AR, Chen SH & Smith KJ (1988) Diagnostic role of an immunoassay-detected polymorphism of factor IX for potential carriers of hemophilia B. *Blood* **72**: 1633–1638.

Toole JJ, Knopf JL, Wozney JM et al (1984) Molecular cloning of a cDNA encoding human antihaemophilic factor. *Nature* **312**: 342–347.

Trent RJ, Davis B, Wilkinson T & Kronenberg H (1984) Identification of β variant hemo-globins by DNA restriction endonuclease mapping. *Hemoglobin* **8**: 443–462.

Tsang TC, Bentley DR, Nilsson IM & Giannelli F (1989) The use of DNA amplification for genetic counselling related diagnosis in haemophilia B. *Thrombosis and Haemostasis* **61**: 343–347.

Tuan D, Murnane MJ, de Riel JK & Forget BG (1980) Heterogeneity in the molecular basis of hereditary persistence of fetal haemoglobin. *Nature* **285**: 335–337.

Tuddenham EGD (1989a) von Willebrand factor and its disorders: an overview of recent molecular studies. *Blood Reviews* **3**: 251–262.

Tuddenham EGD (1989b) Factor VIII and haemophilia A. *Baillière's Clinical Haematology* **2**: 849–877.

Verweij CJ, Hofker M, Quadt R, Briet E & Pannekoek H (1985) RFLP for a human von Willebrand factor (vWF) cDNA code pvWF1100. *Nucleic Acids Research* **13**: 8289.

Verweij CL, Quadt R, Briet E et al (1988) Genetic linkage of two intragenic restriction fragment length polymorphisms with von Willebrand's disease type IIA. Evidence for a defect in the von Willebrand factor gene. *Journal of Clinical Investigation* **81**: 1116–1121.

Wainscoat JS, Thein SL, Old JM & Weatherall DJ (1984) A new DNA polymorphism for prenatal diagnosis of β-thalassaemia in Mediterranean populations. *Lancet* **ii**: 1299–1301.

Wallmark A, Ljung R, Nilsson IM et al (1985) Polymorphism of normal factor IX detected by mouse monoclonal antibodies. *Proceedings of the National Academy of Sciences, USA* **82**: 3839–3843.

Weatherall DJ & Clegg JB (1981) *The Thalassaemia Syndromes*, 3rd edn. Oxford: Blackwell Scientific Publications.

Weatherall DJ, Wainscoat JS, Thein SL et al (1985) Genetic and molecular analysis of mild forms of homozygous β-thalassaemia. 5th Cooley's Anemia Symposium. *Annals of the New York Academy of Sciences* **445**: 68–80.

Weatherall DJ, Clegg JB, Higgs DR & Wood WG (1989) In Scriver CR, Beaudet AL, Sly WS & Valle D (eds) The haemoglobinopathies in the metabolic basis of inherited disease. Vol. 11, pp 2281–2340. New York: McGraw-Hill.

Wehnert M, Herrmann FH & Wulff K (1989) Partial deletions of factor VIII gene as molecular diagnostic markers in haemophilia A. *Disease Markers* **7**: 113–117.

Westaway D & Williamson R (1981) An intron nucleotide sequence variant in a cloned β⁺-thalassaemia gene. *Nature* **301**: 38–43.

White GC & Shoemaker CB (1989) Factor VIII gene and hemophilia A. *Blood* **73**: 1–12.

Winichagoon P, Higgs DR, Goodbourn SEY et al (1982) Multiple arrangements of the human embryonic zeta globin genes. *Nucleic Acids Research* **10**: 5853–5868.

Winship PR & Brownlee GG (1986) Diagnosis of haemophilia B carriers using intragenic oligonucleotide probes letter. *Lancet* **ii**: 218–219.

Winship PR, Anson DS, Rizza CR & Brownlee GG (1984) Carrier detection in haemophilia B using two further intragenic restriction fragment length polymorphisms. *Nucleic Acids Research* **12**: 8861–8872.

Winship PR, Rees DJ & Alkan M (1989) Detection of polymorphisms at cytosine phospho-guanadine dinucleotides and diagnosis of haemophilia B carriers. *Lancet* **1**: 631–634.

Wion KL, Tuddenham EG & Lawn RM (1986) A new polymorphism in the factor VIII gene for prenatal diagnosis of hemophilia A. *Nucleic Acids Research* **14**: 4535–4542.

Wong C, Dowling EE, Saiki RK et al (1987) Characterisation of β-thalassaemia mutations using direct genomic sequencing of amplified single copy DNA. *Nature* **330**: 384–386.

Wood WJ, Gitschier J, Lasky LA & Lawn RM (1985) Base composition-independent hybridization in tetramethylammonium chloride: a method for screening of highly complex gene libraries. *Proceedings of the National Academy of Sciences, USA* **82**: 1585–1588.

Youssoufian H, Kazazian HH Jr, Phillips DG et al (1986) Recurrent mutations in haemophilia A give evidence for CpG mutation hotspots. *Nature* **324**: 380–382.

Youssoufian H, Phillips DG, Kazazian HH Jr & Antonarakis SE (1987) MspI polymorphism in the 3′ flanking region of the human factor VIII gene. *Nucleic Acids Research* **15**: 6312–6312.

Zhang M, Chen SH, Scott CR & Thompson AR (1989) The factor IX BamHI polymorphism: T-to-G transversion at the nucleotide sequence −561. The BamHI/MSPI haplotypes in blacks and Caucasians. *Human Genetics* **82**: 283–284.

6

Acute leukaemias

R. F. STEVENS

In 1978, Dr Alvin Mauer reviewed the state of knowledge and experience in the treatment of childhood acute leukaemia at that time (Mauer, 1978). Eight years later, also in 'Clinics in Haematology' Judith Chessels reiterated the continuing problems associated with the treatment of paediatric leukaemia (Chessels, 1986a). Half a decade later many of these problems still remain. This is not to say that progress has not been made. In 1986 there was an emphasis on more intensive early consolidation/intensification treatment rather than continuing/maintenance therapy. Overall cure rates for acute lymphoblastic leukaemia (ALL) and acute myeloid leukaemia (AML) continue to improve, but more as a result of a gradual evolution in disease diagnosis, stratification, supportive care and long-term follow-up than a major breakthrough in understanding disease pathophysiology and treatment.

It is impossible to cover all aspects of childhood acute leukaemia in one chapter (Drs Ramsay and Davies cover the important aspect of marrow transplantation in Chapter 8). Emphasis will be given to certain areas which are of particular interest or contention. Only the next edition of 'Clinical Haematology' on childhood leukaemia will confirm their importance.

EPIDEMIOLOGY

The annual incidence of acute myeloid leukaemia in children below the age of 15 is in the region of 6 per million (Birch et al, 1988). Geographical variations have been described but are not impressive except possibly in Japan where the incidence has been reported as over 13 cases per million (Hanawa, 1975). In Baltimore, USA, the incidence of AML appears to be more common in black children within the higher socio-economic groups (Gordis et al, 1981). This may be the result of the environment associated with upward socio-economic mobility of the Baltimore black population (Neglia and Robinson, 1988).

Epidemiological studies into the causes of childhood AML are rare. This is due mainly to the low frequency of the disease. The Children's Cancer Study Group (CCSG) has carried out a study into the intrauterine and postnatal factors associated with childhood AML (Robison et al, 1987). No statistically significant increased risks were identified for a variety of

Baillière's Clinical Haematology—
Vol. 4, No. 2, April 1991
ISBN 0–7020–1532–6

intrauterine or postnatal exposures. Increased risk was associated with childhood exposure to pesticides (relative risk 1.8) and petroleum products (relative risk 1.9). Other factors include maternal exposure to drugs such as marijuana and antiemetics during pregnancy.

Congenital chromosomal abnormalities are associated with an increased susceptibility for childhood AML. These include Down's, Klinefelter's and Bloom's syndromes, ataxia telangiectasia, Fanconi's anaemia and Blackfan Diamond anaemia (Grier and Weinstein, 1985). In monozygotic twins less than 2 years old the development of AML in one sibling may be associated with up to a 20% risk of a similar disease in the other.

Acute lymphoblastic leukaemia (ALL) in children is much more common than AML. In the UK the annual incidence is in the region of 26 per million (Birch, 1983). The peak incidence in children is between the ages of 3 and 5 years after which there is a gradual decline until the later rise in the third decade. ALL below the age of 15 years is approximately 30% more common in males than females (Young and Miller, 1975) and in the case of T-cell disease the male : female ratio is nearly 4 : 1 (Kersey et al, 1973).

The list of risk factors associated with childhood ALL is substantial (Table 1). Recently, attention has centred on environmental exposures and new proposed theories on leukaemogenesis.

Much environmental and political debate has been focused on clusters of childhood leukaemia amongst communities living close to nuclear installations, in particular Sellafield (in north-west England) and Dounreay (in the north of Scotland) (Committee on Medical Aspects of Radiation in the

Table 1. Childhood ALL risk factors.

Risk factor	Approximate risk
Genetic/familial	
Sibling of leukaemic child	Up to fourfold of general population
Monozygotic twin of leukaemic child	Up to 100% during 1st year, then decreasing
Down's syndrome	Ten–fifteen-fold increase
Fanconi's anaemia	
Schwachmann's syndrome	
Neurofibromatosis	Variable risk
Klinefelter's syndrome	
Bloom's syndrome	
Ataxia telangiectasia	Up to 20% of all cases
Prenatal exposure	
Diagnostic X-rays	Up to twice non-exposed
Nuclear fallout	No definite risk factor
Maternal smoking, alcohol and oral contraceptives	Possible, but not proven risk
Interuterine viral infections	
Environmental exposure	
Nuclear fallout	Risk up to 20 times expected; youngest most at risk. AML more common in older children.
Diagnostic radiation	Risk up to twice non-exposed
Therapeutic radiation for ankylosing spondylitis	Risk up to 10 times

Environment, 1988) and also around atomic weapons research establishments (Committee on Medical Aspects of Radiation in the Environment, 1989). Recently it has been suggested that these clusters may be associated with paternal exposure to radiation prior to conception rather than increased levels of environmental radio-activity (Gardner et al, 1990).

Several theories have been proposed as to the possible causation of childhood leukaemia and ALL in particular. Knudson suggested that leukaemia may be the result of spontaneous mutation (Knudson, 1977). Ramot and Magrath (1982) have put forward the hypothesis that the pattern of lymphoid malignancy is very dependent upon the environment and relates particularly to socio-economic circumstances with B-cell leukaemia/lymphoma occurring predominantly in the socially underprivileged while common ALL has its highest frequency in the socially privileged classes.

An attempt to relate the known epidemiology of childhood ALL with current understanding of lymphocyte biology has been proposed by Greaves in a two-stage model of leukaemogenesis specific for early pre B-cell ALL (Greaves, 1988, 1989). In the first stage, spontaneous mutations occurring during genetic recombination in lymphoid progenitor cells result in the generation of a premalignant clone in utero. The second stage comprises a second genetic event, influenced by external agents which results in an expansion of this clone into clinically overt ALL. Greaves goes further to postulate that the clinical onset of ALL occurs as a result of the immune stimulation associated with a variety of common childhood infections and their timing, rather than a specific infectious agent. Other factors which may influence this second event include ionizing radiation (Boice, 1981), pesticides (Shu et al, 1988) and low frequency electromagnetic fields (Savitz et al, 1988).

There is now a strong need for carefully formulated, large, case-controlled epidemiological studies of childhood leukaemia, paying special attention to methodology (Neglia et al, 1990). Such studies are now being organized by the Children's Cancer Study Group in the USA and similar organizations in the UK and Canada. These studies will, it is hoped, help clarify the environmental contribution to childhood leukaemia and identify other aetiological postulates.

CLASSIFICATION OF ACUTE CHILDHOOD LEUKAEMIA

At first sight the classification of childhood leukaemia may appear straightforward. Improved morphology and immunology has meant that very few acute leukaemias are now labelled as 'undifferentiated'. However an increasing number of 'mixed lineage' and even 'biclonal' leukaemias are being described (see below).

Morphologies

The French American British (FAB) classification of acute leukaemia is now nearly 15 years old (Bennett et al, 1976) but remains the basis for morphological description. This classification has achieved almost universal accept-ance but various criticisms and variations have been proposed.

In the case of childhood ALL the original FAB classification (Bennett et al, 1981) requires that the distinctive morphological characteristics are evaluated in the lymphoblast population and not in the individual lympho-blasts themselves. However some investigators, the Children's Cancer Study Group (CCSG) among them, apply the FAB criteria to individual blast cells (Miller et al, 1985). Godyn (1988) has illustrated this point by quoting examples where the two different methods can result in two classifications, i.e. either L_1 or L_2 ALL depending on whether the lympho-cyte population as a whole or individual lymphoblasts are analysed.

There is room for further evolution and modification of the FAB system. Argyle et al (1989) have reviewed the interobserver variability and problems in the morphological classification of childhood AML. Concordance has improved over the years and may now be 80% but problems remain such as what constitutes 'maturation' and hence the differentiation of M_1 and M_2 subtypes. Similarly M_7 (acute megakaryoblastic leukaemia) may only be confirmed with antiplatelet antibodies (CD51 or anti-factor VIII). Hayhoe (1988) has recently suggested another classification of acute leukaemia based on cytology, cytogenetics and immunology (Table 2).

Table 2. Classification of acute leukaemia based on cytology, cytogenetics and immunology.

ALL	*(a) early B (cALL), CD 10.*
	(b) T, CD 7.
	(c) B, SmIg.
	(d) pre B (null), CD 19.
AML	Type I:
	Granulocyte and/or monocyte lineage only.
	(a) Well differentiated (>50% Sudan Black positive).
	(b) poorly differentiated (<50% Sudan Black positive).
	Type II:
	Multiple lineage granulocyte and/or monocyte and erythroblast or megakaryocyte involvement.
	(a) Well differentiated (>50% Sudan Black positive).
	(b) poorly differentiated (<50% Sudan Black positive).

Mixed ALL/AML

This approach divides the acute myeloid leukaemias into blast cell populations derived from a 'committed' clonogenic stem cell and those originating from a pluripotent stem cell. The former group (Types Ia and Ib) has only granulocytic and/or monocytic expression, while the latter (Type II) also involves erythroid and/or megakaryocytic lineages. Hayhoe (1988) suggests that such a simple classification is based (in the case of the myeloid leukaemias) primarily on cytology yet having a clearer relationship to cytogenetic variants than in the predominantly cellular approach as illustrated by the FAB classification. Only time will tell if this system proves popular.

Cytogenetics

Abnormal karyotypes can be detected in up to 80% of children with ALL (Williams et al, 1986) and AML (Progogina et al, 1986).

ALL

Over a decade ago it was realized that the ploidy of leukaemic cell karyotypes had an important prognostic influence on childhood ALL (Secker-Walker et al, 1978). The presence of more than 50 chromosomes is associated with a better prognosis irrespective of therapy (Williams et al, 1986) whereas patients in other ploidy groups (including pseudodiploid, hypodiploid or hyperdiploid 47 to 49 karyotypes) do worse (Look, 1988). This hyperdiploid group with greater than 50 chromosomes can be subdivided further into those cases also showing specific chromosomal abnormalities such as trisomies and translocations and comprises about 20% of childhood ALL (a subset of pre B-cALL).

The mechanism whereby hyperdiploidy influences response to treatment is unclear. It has been suggested that these cells may remain longer in S-phase and be more sensitive to phase-specific drugs (Look et al, 1985) or have a tendency towards 'terminal differentiation' and hence are more sensitive to steroid therapy (Smets et al, 1987).

Specific chromosomal translocations are found in karyotypes of leukaemic blasts from children with a high risk of treatment failure. Table 3 illustrates some translocations seen in childhood ALL and their association with particular immunological phenotypes.

Table 3. Chromosomal translocations in childhood ALL.

Translocation	Phenotype
t(9;22)	Variable
t(8;14)	B
t(1;19)	Pre B
t(11;14)	T
t(12;v)	Early pre B and pre B
t(4;11)	Early pre B

The translocation seen in Philadelphia positive ALL, t(9;22) is karyotypically similar to that seen in chronic myeloid leukaemia (CML). The translocation results in the fusion of the bcr (breakpoint cluster region) and c-*abl* proto-oncogene with production of a characteristic hybrid protein (p210). The p210 protein is present in only a small proportion of cases of childhood ALL whereas it is found in virtually all cases of CML (De Klein et al, 1986). Patients with the Philadelphia chromosome may fail to achieve complete remission or have a high and early relapse rate (Ribeiro et al, 1987). More intensive treatment regimens including marrow transplantation in first remission may be indicated but as Philadelphia positive ALL represents only about 4% of all childhood ALL comparative studies will be difficult.

B-cell leukaemia is invariably associated with the karyotype t(8;14) or one of the two variants t(2;8) or t(8;22) (Klein, 1983). It has been shown that in the t(8;14) translocation the c-*myc* oncogene locus is translocated into the heavy chain on chromosome 14 with reciprocal translocation of the immunoglobulin variable region to chromosome 8. In the t(2;8) and t(8;22) variants the c-*myc* gene remains on chromosome 8 and portions of the respective light-chain genes are translocated to that chromosome (Dalla-Favera et al, 1982). The c-*myc* proto-oncogene product acts as a nuclear stimulus in the transition of cells from a resting to a proliferative status (Evan and Hancock, 1985). Presumably, deregulation of c-*myc* expression as a result of one of these chromosomal translocations contributes to a malignant transformation or cellular proliferation typical of these childhood B-cell neoplasms. B-cell leukaemia is an example of a malignancy which is associated with specific cytogenetic and immunophenotypic features which contribute to its therapeutic responsiveness and where specific treatment protocols have been designed based on these characteristics (Murphy et al, 1986). Such protocols have recently resulted in success rates over 50% in childhood B-cell malignancies.

The t(1;19) translocation is specific from pre B-cell ALL and is present in approximately a third of cases of childhood ALL with this phenotype (Williams et al, 1984). At the present time the relevance of this translocation to the causation of leukaemia is unknown.

Translocation involving chromosomes 14 and 11 are frequently associated with genes encoding for the T-cell receptor in leukaemias having the T-cell phenotype (Jones et al, 1985). At present there is no evidence that t(11;14) translocation is associated with a worse prognosis than other T-cell leukaemias (Look, 1988).

The t(4;11) translocation is associated with the pre B-cell phenotype and expression of the human leukocyte HLA-DR antigen. Patients tend to present with high white cell counts, monocytic morphological features and a poor prognosis (Bloomfield et al, 1986).

The St Jude Group (Look, 1988), together with the Third International Workshop on Chromosomes in Leukaemia (Bloomfield et al, 1986), suggest that patients with the structural abnormalities t(8;14), t(9;22) and t(4;11) carry a worse prognosis necessitating intensive chemotherapy and allogeneic or autologous marrow transplantation in an attempt to reverse the high early failure rate and improve long-term remissions.

AML

A variety of specific cytogenetic abnormalities have been associated with morphological subtypes of acute myeloid leukaemia. Kalwinsky et al (1990) have provided a comprehensive chromosomal analysis of childhood AML in over 150 patients. In summary they found 20% normal, 30% miscellaneous clonal abnormalities and 50% with known cytogenetic subgroups. The translocation t(8;21) is the most common and is restricted to M_2 and to a lesser extent M_1 subtypes. The cellular oncogenes c-*mos* and c-*ets*-2 have been mapped on chromosomes 8 and 21 respectively but have not been shown to be involved in leukaemogenesis (Diaz et al, 1985; Sacchi et al, 1986). The close association between the (15;17) translocation and acute promyelocytic leukaemia (M_3) is well recognized. Kalwinsky et al (1990) identified 9 out of a total of 155 cases of childhood AML all of whom had M_3 morphology. Apart from an occasional M_3 acute blast transformation of CML (Castiagne et al, 1984), t(15;17) has not been reported in any other malignancy other than M_3 AML.

Translocations involving chromosome 11 and in particular t(9;11) are associated with M_5 leukaemia (Pui et al, 1987). Kalwinsky et al (1990) found that infants with M_5 disease and t(9;11) did significantly better than others within the M_5 group.

Children with AML frequently show karyotypes in the near dipolid range. The most common trisomy involves chromosome 8 which is found in approximately 10% of patients (Look, 1988). Monosomy 7 is frequently associated with pre-leukaemia and a difficulty in achieving complete remission (Woods et al, 1985). Deletions or monosomy of chromosomes 5 and 7 are frequently associated with secondary leukaemias suggesting a mutagenic effect of chemoradiotherapy.

TREATMENT

Treatment of childhood leukaemia is a growth industry, not due to a marked increase in the number of diagnosed cases, rather to the ever increasing number of patients who show a response to the new treatment regimens available. It is more than 40 years since remissions were described (Farber et al, 1948) and since then various treatment strategies have been used which have subsequently been incorporated in the treatment of other malignancies, both childhood and adult. Before discussing these strategies further it is pertinent to clarify some aspects of therapy.

The principle of remission induction therapy is well established and applies to both ALL and AML. The presence of less than 5% of morpho-logical blast cells in the bone marrow has become the arbitrary definition of remission. In the UK at least this is sufficient to make a diagnosis of a complete remission (CR) in ALL whereas in the case of AML other marrow cellular elements should have returned to normal. It is estimated that achieving CR in leukaemia is associated with a reduction in malignant cell load from 10^{12} to 10^9 cells.

More and more treatment regimens are using intensive chemotherapy modules once CR has been achieved. These may be termed consolidation/ intensification. Consolidation is best considered as a further course of treatment using essentially the same drugs in similar doses as were used to achieve CR on the understanding that the leukaemia cell mass has already shown some responsiveness. This approach is used particularly in treating AML. Intensification implies the use of different drugs in different doses (usually higher) in the hope of eliminating resistant leukaemia clones and residual disease in sanctuary sites (e.g. central nervous system and testes). Autologous and allogeneic marrow transplantation are also examples of intensification regimens although the latter almost certainly has added immunological implications (graft versus leukaemia effect).

So-called maintenance therapy is well established in the treatment of childhood ALL. There are few other situations in both adult or childhood malignancy where such treatment is considered to be imperative. The term 'maintenance' is not entirely appropriate; 'continuing' therapy is a better reflection of this aspect of treatment as the intent is not that of maintaining the status quo (i.e. remission) but the continuing elimination of the leukaemic clone and long-term cure.

ALL TREATMENT

Oral prednisolone, intravenous vincristine and intramuscular or sub-cutaneous L-asparaginase will result in CR in about 95% of children with ALL (Ortega et al, 1977). This combination was well established and substantiated by various collaberative groups including the Medical Research Council (MRC), Berlin–Frankfurt–Münster group (BFM) and the Children's Cancer Study Group (USCCSG) from the USA. Treatment was well tolerated, was not associated with severe neutropenia and hence infective complications and did not involve excessive hospital inpatient stay. The addition of central nervous system (CNS)-directed therapy (Aur et al, 1971) and 'maintenance' therapy resulted in long-term disease free survivals approaching 50%.

It has been more difficult to show dramatic improvements in these results over the past decade. The MRC showed no improvement in their childhood ALL studies from 1972 to 1979 but the adoption of the eighth UK study (UKALL VIII) resulted in a 15–20% improvement in disease-free survival, comparable to the USCCSG (Coccia, 1983; Medical Research Council, 1986). UKALL VIII involved a 3- or 4-drug randomized remission induction regimen, the latter showing an improved disease-free survival (DFS) despite an expected acceptable increase in complications. Other factors possibly contributing to the improved survival included continuing therapy without interrupting drug induction, a long course of intramuscular asparaginase over 3 weeks, full-dose mercaptopurine and co-trimoxazole during CNS prophylaxis, and the use of sustained maximum tolerated doses of mercaptopurine and methotrexate during continuing therapy.

ALL risk groups

Over the past decade the recognition that certain clinical and laboratory features evident at diagnosis have prognostic value allowing the assignment of patients to groups with relatively favourable or unfavourable prognoses, has altered the therapeutic approach to this disease. However differences remain in the importance of prognostic factors given by individual collaborative groups.

Table 4. Established prognostic factors in childhood ALL.

Presenting white cell count
Sex
Mediastinal mass
Speed of achieving CR
Age (i.e. <1 year or >15 years)
FAB type (i.e. L_3 B-cell disease)

The initial pre-treatment total white cell count (WBC) is probably the most important prognostic factor but other features are listed in Table 4. The CCSG at present divide their patients into five groups; good, average and poor risk (on the basis of age, WBC and FAB subtype), together with infants and children with leukaemia/lymphomatous features (Hammond et al, 1987). The German BFM group of recent years have defined four groups (high, medium and two standard risk groups) on the basis of a calculation for each patient which takes into account the initial peripheral blood blast cell count, and the sizes of the liver and spleen (Riehm et al, 1987).

The MRC have adopted a more simplistic approach in using prognostic factors to influence ALL study design. The power of any study to show differences in any treatment strategy in a randomized study is heavily dependent upon the number of patients entered into any treatment arm. The greater the number of differing treatments the larger the overall patient recruitment (and hence the larger the trial). With ever-differing approaches to patient supportive care the MRC maintains its enthusiasm for randomized studies, wherever possible, rather than those based on historical controls. With this in mind the present MRC ALL trial (UKALL X) defines only one differing risk group (i.e. those with a WBC > $100 \times 10^9 \, l^{-1}$) although patients with CNS disease at presentation do have slightly modified therapy (B-cell ALL is also excluded).

A recent analysis of prognostic features on remission and survival in childhood ALL, at the Royal Manchester Children's Hospital over a 10-year period (1979–89) is presented in Table 5 (Carr, 1990). This is based on 286 patients.

Table 5. Influence of prognostic features on remission and survival in childhood ALL (RMCH 1979–89).

Prognostic feature	Remission (p value)	Survival (p value)
WBC	0.0003	0.0002
Immunophenotype	<0.0001	<0.0001
Chromosomes	<0.0003	<0.0002
Remission at 2 weeks	<0.0001	<0.0001
Morphology (L_1 vs L_2)	0.0200	0.0040
Age 2, 2–10, 10 yr +	NS	NS
Hepatomegaly	NS	NS
Splenomegaly	NS	NS

NS, not significant.

It can be seen that WBC and FAB type (L_1 vs L_2) are confirmed as prognostic variables but age (excluding infants < 1 year) and organomegaly are not. Whilst not concentrating on the prognostic parameters of any particular study it should be remembered that the segregation of patients and therapy into particular groups will reduce the analytic power of any study. At the present time there is a strong temptation to define treatment on the basis of cytogenetic features. The difficulty in defining cytogenetics on the one hand must be balanced against the probability, but as yet unproven, that chromosomal subtypes have a major effect on disease outcome.

ALL intensification therapy

Intensification chemotherapy offers a rational approach to curative treatment of ALL. Factors potentially responsible for treatment failure in ALL include inadequate initial reduction in the leukaemic load, the development of resistant leukaemic clones and the presence of 'sanctuary' sites of resistant disease. In 1976 the BFM group introduced an element of early intensification in their high-risk patients (based on a calculated risk score) and showed an improvement in survival which they have confirmed in subsequent studies (Riehm et al, 1987). Similar encouragement in the use of intensification has come from the CCSG (Hammond et al, 1987), the Boston Group (Clavell et al, 1986) and the group from St Jude Children's Hospital USA (Rivera et al, 1987).

The present Medical Research Council UKALL X trial also hopes to address the question whether short pulses of intensification chemotherapy will reduce the risk of relapse. UKALL X does have some differences in that the great majority of patients will be randomized to either early or late (or both) courses of intensification and not just children considered to be at high risk of relapse. At the time of last analysis there is suggestive evidence from UKALL X of the benefit of at least one block of additional intensification. These results are supported by those (as yet unpublished) of the America CCSG study 105. Careful analysis is being made of the mortality and morbidity (particularly in terms of infection) associated with this treatment as emphasized by the St Jude group (Rivera et al, 1987). This study will not however indicate a preference for intermittent courses of short-term intensive treatment (as in UKALL X) as compared with a more continuous but lower-dose drug approach (as in the BFM studies).

Continuing (maintenance) therapy for ALL

To be effective in reducing the likelihood of relapse, ongoing therapy must not only suppress the growth of leukaemic cells, but must also provide continuing leukaemic cytoreduction whilst preventing the emergence of a drug-resistant clone.

Early studies involved the use of vincristine and prednisolone but it was not until the addition of mercaptopurine and methotrexate that there was any advantage to survival (Simone, 1976). The optimal duration of maintenance chemotherapy has not yet been defined. The CCSG group showed that 5 years offered no additional benefit to 3 years (Nesbit et al, 1983) and recent evaluation of the MRC UKALL VIII study showed no difference between 2 and 3 years of maintenance (Eden, personal communication).

The MRC UKALL VIII trial also emphasizes the importance of drug dosage in continuing therapy. The considerable improvement in survival (around 20%) compared with previous studies was due in no small part to the persistence of ongoing therapy even in the presence of moderate neutropenia. Drug dosages were only reduced when absolute neutrophil counts fell below $1.0 \times 10^9 \, l^{-1}$. Myelosuppression during standard continuing treatment of 'standard risk' ALL has been shown to be associated with increased toxicity but reduced risk of relapse (Dolan et al, 1989). Other studies have suggested that continual rather than interrupted continuing therapy is preferable (Gaynon et al, 1987).

The dose of oral continuing chemotherapy and its bioavailability are probably important factors in the effectiveness of continuing therapy. The pharmacology of oral methotrexate and mercaptopurine are very variable suggesting a possible reason for failure (Poplack et al, 1986). It has been suggested that there is a difference in mercaptopurine metabolism between boys and girls with the former tolerating significantly more drug and having less myelosuppression (Hale and Lilleyman, 1990). This may in part explain the improved survival figures for ALL in girls. Other workers have suggested that the dose of mercaptopurine should be tailored to the individual prior to the onset of continuing treatment (Koren et al, 1990). In a recent study Whitehead et al (1990) have studied the accumulation of methotrexate and methotrexate polyglutamates in lymphoblasts. Children whose lymphoblasts incorporated higher levels had a superior event free survival. They suggest that the inherent ability of lymphoblasts to accumulate methotrexate may be important, particularly in good risk patients and that in such children inherent rather than acquired drug resistance may be an important event leading to treatment failure.

AML TREATMENT

For many years the treatment of childhood AML lagged behind that of ALL. For example, data taken from the Manchester Children's Tumour Registry indicates that whilst there has been a progressive improvement in survival for ALL over the past three decades, in the case of AML this has only occurred in the past 10 to 20 years (Birch et al, 1988). However this improvement has been dramatic and probably outstrips that of any other advance in paediatric oncology.

AML risk groups

With the improved survival for childhood AML there has come a need to predict at the time of diagnosis those patients who carry a superior or inferior prognosis. AML in children is however a rare condition and therefore prognostic factors in relation to therapeutic strategies are difficult to define. Many suggested factors have not been consistently described and some factors may exert their influence on different stages of the disease such as remission induction, or the risk of relapse. For example, Grier et al (1987) have suggested that age less than 2 years at diagnosis, a high presenting WBC ($> 100 \times 19^9 l^{-1}$) and M_4/M_5 morphology are associated with a poor prognosis.

The largest study correlating cytogenetic findings and prognosis has been provided by the CCSG (Woods et al, 1985). Patients with normal karyotypes had the same remission rate as those with chromosomal abnormalities. However t(8;21) was associated with a high CR rate, monosomy 7 carried a low CR rate, and t(15;17) was associated with a high risk of haemorrhage during remission induction. Patients with myelodysplastic syndromes have an increased frequency of abnormalities associated with chromosomes 7 or 5. They may also be associated with leukaemia secondary to previous therapy or environmental exposure.

The BFM group have recently suggested the identification of two risk groups in childhood AML (Creutzig et al, 1990). On the basis of event-free interval they have suggested a low-risk group comprising 37% of all children achieving CR made up of the following criteria: FAB M_1 with Auer rods; FAB M_2 with WBC $< 20 \times 10^9 l^{-1}$; all FAB M_3 types; and FAB M_4 with eosinophilia. They go further to suggest that bone marrow transplantation should be mandatory only for the high-risk group.

Controversy remains over prognostic groups in AML particularly in relation to therapy. In the present Medical Research Council study (AML 10), all children below the age of 16 are eligible, as any 'stratification' on the basis of prognostic groups would reduce patient numbers and the ultimate power of any randomized analysis. Only time will tell if this approach is more relevant than that of the German BFM group.

At the present time there is however broad agreement that adverse prognostic factors include a high presenting WBC, FAB monocytic varieties, previous myelodysplasia or secondary leukaemia, monosomy 7, blast crisis of chronic myeloid leukaemia and a longer time to achieve complete remission.

AML treatment regimens

The considerable improvement in treatment results in childhood AML are due to a variety of factors. One important advance has been in the quality of patient supportive care. This includes the brisk and energetic treatment of haemorrhage, infection and metabolic complications including leukostasis. Hann (1990) has recently summarized the supportive care necessary for the treatment of AML patients.

Another important advance in the treatment of AML has been the advent of more aggressive therapeutic protocols. However it remains unclear as to what is the ideal drug combination or the exact way these drugs should be combined. At the present time, the treatment for all children with AML is very intensive. Experience shows that remission induction invariably follows a period of severe marrow hypoplasia and stable remission must be associated with less than 5% of bone marrow blasts and evidence of recovery of normal cellular elements.

Remission induction

The present tendency is to use combination chemotherapy using a variety of drugs (usually 3 or 4) but cytosine arabinoside, daunorubicin or adriamycin, with or without etoposide or thioguanine are the most frequently used. Complete remission rates for the majority of paediatric studies have been in the region of 70–90% (Table 6). Patients who fail to achieve CR can be divided roughly into non-responders (resistant disease), haemorrhagic/infective deaths, and early deaths before the onset of treatment. It is particularly important not to exclude this latter group from any analysis.

It can be seen from Table 6 that CR rates vary from approximately 70 to 90%. Differences depend on several factors including the number of patients entered into the study but the more recent studies suggest CR rates approaching 90%. The ongoing Medical Research Council's 10th AML trial has over 100 paediatric entrants and the remission induction rate is running at 90%.

Continuing therapy

Included under this heading are both consolidation and intensification treatment. In AML, terminating treatment once CR has been achieved leads to a more than 90% chance of relapse within 12 months. The exact nature of continuing treatment remains controversial. For example some groups have advocated consolidation (second induction) therapy (e.g. VAPA, Boston 80-035, UK, AIEOP-8204; Table 6) whereas others have used intensification (e.g. VAPA, St Judes 80, Boston 80-035, UK, AIEOP-8204 and BFM-83; Table 6) whereby different drugs at different doses are introduced, once CR has been achieved. Maintenance (on-going treatment) has been used by some groups (BFM-78, CCSG-251, St Judes-80, AIEOP-8204 and BFM-83; Table 6) lasting from 6 months to 2 years. Whereas other groups (VAPA, Boston 80-035, UK; Table 6) have not used any ongoing therapy.

This complexity of approaches to intensification/maintenance therapy only goes to show that this phase of treatment for AML remains undefined. As yet there are no large randomized studies in children which have shown an advantage for maintenance or stopping therapy post intensification. Any such analysis would be difficult to perform as the influence of different remission induction/consolidation therapy must always be taken into account. Nevertheless the studies summarized in Table 6 indicate that between 25 and 50% of children treated with chemotherapy alone can be expected to be surviving free of disease at least 2 years after diagnosis and this represents a major advance over results of 10 to 20 years ago.

Table 6. Summary of paediatric AML trials.

Study	VAPA	BFM-78	CCSG-251	St Jude-80	Boston 80-035	UK	AIEOP-8204	BFM-83
Study period	1976–80	1978–82	1979–83	1980–83	1980–84	1982–85	1982–86	1982–86
Patients entered	61	151	508	87	64	66	133	182
CR	74%	80%	68%	75%	70%	91%	80%	80%
EF survival	33%	37%	25%	20%	29%	42%	33%	49%

References: VAPA, Weinstein et al (1983); BFM-78, Creutzig et al (1987); CCSG-251, Nesbit et al (1987); St Jude-80, Dahl et al (1987); Boston 80-035, Weinstein et al (1987); UK, Marcus et al (1987); AIEOP-8204, Amadori et al (1987); BFM-83, Creutzig et al (1990).

Therapeutic philosophy

There are many important therapeutic questions which need to be answered in childhood AML. These include the role of intensification, the place of maintenance therapy and the need for bone marrow transplantation either allogeneic or autologous. Two different approaches seen to be crystallizing as exemplified by the German BFM group and the UK Medical Research Council. The BFM group feel confident that they can define low- and high-risk groups for childhood AML based on certain prognostic factors. The low-risk group (37% of patients entered) included FAB types with granulocytic differentiation and the additional features: M_1 with Auer rods, M_2 with WBC $20 \times 10^9 l^{-1}$, all M_3 patients and M_4 with eosinophilia. The high-risk group comprises the remaining patients. They suggest further that bone marrow transplantation should be mandatory only for children of the high-risk group (Creutzig et al, 1990).

The British MRC group would contend that such patient stratification is not justified because of low patient numbers. Their philosophy is one of randomized studies with a minimum of exclusions. In the present AML 10 study all children with AML (FAB M_1 to M_7) below the age of 16 are eligible. All patients receive four courses of intensive chemotherapy. The main therapeutic question in this study is the place of allogeneic or autologous transplantation as patients with a matched sibling donor receive an allograft as of right, whereas the remainder (approximately 70%) are randomized between an autologous BMT or stopping chemotherapy.

It would be obtuse to exclude either approach out of hand. Hopefully valuable information will be obtained from both these, and many other studies. However great care is required to avoid further clouding of what is already a rather confusing subject. The non-trial controlled introduction of treatment strategies such as etoposide and cranial irradiation for monocytic varieties or retinoids for M_3 should be avoided.

INFANT LEUKAEMIA

The clinical and biological features of acute leukaemia in infants below the age of 1 year are different from those of older children. In ALL, over 50% of infants have a high leukocyte count ($> 100 \times 10^9 l^{-1}$) as compared to 13% of those overall in the MRC UKALL X trial (Chessells, personal communication). Most have organomegaly and CNS disease at diagnosis is relatively common. Immunological classification shows a higher frequency than expected of mixed immunological phenotype with a preponderance of early B-cell disease whereas T-cell ALL is very rare. Some infants appear to have common ALL but a significant number show cytoplasmic immunoglobulin and are a pre B-cell variant. Table 7 shows a breakdown of 43 cases of infant ALL as regards immunological phenotype.

Cytogenetic analysis shows a higher proportion of abnormalities than seen in older children with the specific translocations t(4;11)(q21;q23) and t(11;19)(q23;p13) being particularly common (Bloomfield et al, 1986; Gibbons et al, 1990).

Table 7. Immunological phenotype in infant ALL (courtesy of
J Chessells, 1990).

Null ALL	28
Common ALL	7
Pre B-ALL	4
T-ALL	1
Mixed	3

Infants with acute myeloid leukaemia generally have acute monoblastic (M_5) or myelomonocytic (M_4) subtypes and hyperleukocytosis and extra-medullary (particularly the skin) involvement are common. These variants are particularly common in congenital leukaemia. Erythroid (M_6) and megakaryoblastic (M_7) varieties have been described but there is a relatively low incidence of typical myeloid subtypes (M_1 and M_2) compared with older children (Pui et al, 1988).

Infants with ALL have a significantly worse prognosis than older children even after adjustment for other presenting prognostic factors (Crist et al, 1986). On the other hand, infants with AML, although more susceptible to the complications of treatment, do seem to achieve remission at a rate not significantly different from that of older children and have a similar chance of long-term survival (Pui et al, 1988). More intensive treatment may be required however to prevent CNS leukaemic relapse and bone marrow transplantation may offer an even greater chance of cure (Johnson et al, 1987) although the long-term side-effects are likely to be quite profound in this age group.

In the case of infant ALL in the UK, it is suggested that having achieved complete remission using standard childhood ALL induction therapy, further intensification is given using epipodophyllotoxin, cytarabine and moderate dose methotrexate in an attempt to prevent overt CNS disease. In the absence of an allogeneic sibling donor, autologous marrow transplantation should be considered, particularly in children with a high presenting white cell count (Chessells, personal communication). The long-term effects of treatment in this group of young children remains a matter of considerable concern.

MIXED LINEAGE LEUKAEMIA

Most contemporary models of leukaemia differentiation adhere to the principle of 'lineage fidelity' whereby leukaemic blast cells originate from the clonal expansion of a single transformed progenitor cell with specific myeloid or lymphoid characteristics (Greaves, 1982). With the introduction of techniques (e.g. immunophenotyping and cytogenetics) for analysis of phenotypic and genotypic lineage-associated characteristics of leukaemic blasts cases of acute leukaemia have been described which contradict this principle and have led to the concept of 'lineage infidelity'.

The term 'lineage infidelity' (also known as 'biphenotypic leukaemia', 'mixed-lineage' and 'hybrid leukaemia') is meant to indicate the situation where leukaemia blast cell populations express both lymphoid and myeloid characteristics. 'Biclonal leukaemia' is where the leukaemia is made up of two separate blast cell populations, one with myeloid and one with lymphoid characteristics.

Two theories have been suggested to explain this infidelity. Smith et al (1983) have suggested that leukaemogenesis may be the result of aberrant genetic programming rather than the conventional theory that lineage gene expression is maintained in leukaemia. Greaves et al (1986) prefer the concept that rather than genetic misprogramming there is a transient phase of limited gene expression occurring in normal bipotential or multipotential progenitors.

It is clear that a proportion of cases of otherwise typical AML may express lymphoid markers, TdT and CD7 (an early T lymphocyte marker) in particular (Bradstock et al, 1981; Vodinelich et al, 1983). Mirro et al (1985) have suggested that approximately 25% of cases of AML will exhibit lymphocyte-associated surface markers and that 13% of cases of typical ALL will show surface markers common to the myeloid lineage.

The clinical significance of mixed lineage leukaemia remains unclear. It has been suggested that AML in children with T-cell markers may have a reduced response to cytarabine and daunorubicin (Mirro et al, 1985) and an increased incidence of CNS relapse. Patient numbers are however too small and analysis of multicentre co-operative trials using standard reagents is required.

Reports of biclonal leukaemias indicate that the two cellular populations can be demonstrated either simultaneously or they appear sequentially in an individual patient, in the latter case in a relatively short period of time so as to differentiate from a therapy-related secondary leukaemia. Biclonal leukaemia in children is very uncommon with only a few cases having been reported (Creutzig et al, 1981; Perentesis et al, 1983; Schmitt-Graff et al, 1988).

The clinical significance of mixed lineage and biphenotypic leukaemia remains unclear. Further studies to clarify the regulation of lineage associated gene expression are required to expand our knowledge of these leukaemias and to help unravel the disruption of genetic control that occurs during leukaemogenesis.

CENTRAL NERVOUS SYSTEM LEUKAEMIA

Preventative therapy for ALL

Prior to the onset of CNS preventative therapy (also erroneously known as prophylaxis) the CNS was the commonest site of leukaemic relapse in childhood ALL with relapse rates of up to 75% (Evans et al, 1970). The introduction of CNS-directed radiotherapy (and later chemotherapy) demonstrated that symptomatic CNS leukaemia could be prevented in the majority of patients. Studies from the St Jude Children's Research Hospital provided a breakthrough in the treatment of childhood ALL (Aur et al, 1971; Simone, 1974).

Because craniospinal irradiation may retard spinal growth and cause excessive myelosuppression, cranial irradiation (24 Gy) plus intrathecal methotrexate became the standard form of preventative treatment and has been extensively adopted since the 1970s. However concerns were raised over adverse effects including neuroendocrine dysfunction, CT brain scan abnormalities, altered psychomotor and intellectual function (see section on late effects). A reduction in the dose of irradiation to 18 Gy appears to be equally effective however it is not yet evident if this dose is associated with fewer side-effects (Bleyer and Poplack, 1985; Tamaroff et al, 1985). A variety of other methods have been used in an attempt to avoid cranial irradiation. These include triple intrathecal therapy (methotrexate, cytarabine and hydrocortisone) alone, intermediate-dose methotrexate (with or without intrathecal methotrexate), intrathecal methotrexate alone, and high-dose systemic methotrexate (Poplack, 1988).

The incidence of CNS leukaemia is dependent upon a variety of prognostic factors (such as presenting WBC and age) and there is now evidence that cranial irradiation can be withheld from children with a good prognosis (Littman et al, 1987). The Children's Cancer Study Group (CCSG Protocol 105 Preliminary results, unpublished data) have randomized average risk patients to receive cranial irradiation or long-term intrathecal methotrexate. Likewise the forthcoming Medical Research Council UKALL XI study intends to omit cranial irradiation for children with a WBC less than $50 \times 10^9 \, l^{-1}$. These patients will be randomized to receive (a) continuing intrathecal methotrexate or (b) this, together with three high dose intravenous infusions of methotrexate. A vital element of this study is a long-term evaluation of CNS toxicity in terms of learning and neuropsychological effects.

Overt CNS lymphoblastic leukaemia

Although CNS preventative therapy is effective in the majority of patients, CNS relapse remains a significant cause of treatment failure. The incidence of CNS relapse in most studies is reported to be less than 10%. Subsequent second remissions can be induced in more than 90% of patients but long-term survival is uncommon with a medium survival of 1 to 2 years (Bleyer and Poplack, 1985). The most successful therapy for CNS relapse to date has been based on initial intrathecal chemotherapy followed by either craniospinal irradiation or maintenance chemotherapy (Willoughby, 1976; Kun et al, 1984; Land et al, 1985).

The choice of CNS therapy for relapse is partly dependent upon the initial preventative treatment. If cranial irradiation was absent in initial therapy up to a third of patients will achieve prolonged survival following CNS relapse if craniospinal irradiation and intrathecal chemotherapy are used (Willoughby, 1983). If the patient has already received irradiation then the place of further craniospinal prophylaxis is less clear and is likely to be associated with increased neurotoxicity (Kun et al, 1984).

Other approaches have been used in the treatment of CNS relapse. These include 'triple' intrathecal cytotoxics (Bleyer and Poplack, 1985), intraventricular chemotherapy (via a ventricular subcutaneous reservoir) (Bleyer and Poplack, 1979), high-dose intravenous methotrexate (Borsi and Moe, 1987), and high-dose systemic cytarabine (Frick et al, 1984). The use of radiolabelled (I^{131}) monoclonal antibodies directed against CSF leukaemic blasts and injected via the intraventricular or lumbar routes is being evaluated (Pizer, personal communication). This approach remains experimental.

In summary, patients who relapse in the CNS having previously completed first line therapy have a better prognosis than those who relapse on therapy. Patients who have not received prior cranial irradiation also have a better outlook. Systemic re-induction and craniospinal radiotherapy does appear to cure a small number of children, primarily those with low WBC 'common' ALL who had a long first remission. Toxicity is nevertheless considerable with over 50% of long-term survivors being limited neurologically, educationally or both. The younger the child at diagnosis, the closer the two courses of irradiation, the worse the toxicity. An isolated CNS relapse often heralds a marrow relapse and concurrent systemic chemotherapy is mandatory (Nesbit et al, 1981).

CNS disease in AML

Although CNS leukaemia is more common in ALL, the frequency of this complication of AML appears to be increasing with improved survival times (Pui et al, 1985a). However the role and optimal method of CNS prophylaxis in AML remains controversial. An early St Jude Children's Research Hospital study suggested that craniospinal irradiation was an effective method of preventing meningeal leukaemia (Dahl et al, 1978), but such treatment had no apparent effect on the quality or duration of subsequent survival. CNS leukaemia is more commonly seen in those with monoblastic (M_5) disease (Grier et al, 1987) with CNS relapse (either single or combined) accounting for about 10–20% of all relapses. Although there is no data from randomized trials of CNS-directed therapy versus none, and there is no convincing data showing benefit to overall survival when this therapy is given, most investigators believe that the morbidity of CNS relapse is such that it is best avoided (Lampkin et al, 1988). Effective CNS therapy can be accomplished with intrathecal cytarabine or methotrexate but this may be insufficient for children with high-risk factors for a CNS relapse (Pui et al, 1985a).

LEUKAEMIC RELAPSE

Bone marrow relapse in ALL

The most common site of relapse in ALL is the bone marrow. A second remission can be achieved in the majority of patients. The longer the time period until the time of relapse the greater the chance of achieving a second remission (Chessells, 1986b). Patients who relapse whilst on treatment or shortly after its discontinuation have a particularly bad prognosis (Bleyer et al, 1986). In children with multiple relapses, the re-induction rate declines with each successive relapse, presumably due to the development of resistant leukaemic clones.

Similar factors apply to long-term survival in relapsed childhood ALL. The overall survival of patients who relapse off therapy is better than those who relapse on treatment (Bleyer et al, 1986). The prognosis for patients who relapse off treatment is inversely proportional to the time period from the time of completing continuation therapy to the time of relapse. A review of 600 children with ALL in second remission treated with chemotherapy reported prolonged second remissions in less than 5% of children who relapsed within 18 months of achieving first remission. This compared with prolonged second remissions in 25% of children who relapsed more than 18 months after first CR (Butturine et al, 1987). The results of recent studies suggest that remissions of longer than 2 years can be obtained with aggressive chemotherapy in between 10% and 25% of patients who relapse on therapy and up to a third of children relapsing after completion of continuing therapy (Rivera et al, 1986; Henze et al, 1987).

The majority of treatment centres feel that allogeneic bone marrow transplantation is the treatment of choice for those with matched sibling donors (Brockstein et al, 1987). The place of autologous transplantation (with or without bone marrow purging) as compared with high-dose re-induction, intensification and continuing therapy has not yet been defined. A forthcoming Medical Research Council relapsed ALL study hopes to address this issue in a randomized way.

Testicular relapse

Testicular relapse is a major cause of late treatment failure and occurs in approximately 10% of boys although there have been reports as high as 16% (Eden et al, 1978, 1983). Overt testicular relapse usually presents as painless testicular enlargement. Bilateral wedge biopsies are usually necessary to confirm the diagnosis but the incidence of false negatives may be as high as 10% (Chessells, 1986b). Routine testicular biopsies performed at the completion of chemotherapy have little value in predicting residual disease and subsequent relapse and have been largely abandoned by the MRC and other groups (Pui et al, 1985b).

The presence of a blood–testis barrier analagous to the blood–brain barrier has been suggested as the reason why the testis frequently represents a leukaemic sanctuary site. However it is more likely that 'isolated' testicular relapse reflects the fact that the testes are a relatively easier anatomic site in which to detect clinical relapse (Poplack and Reaman, 1988).

Optimal treatment for testicular relapse includes bilateral testicular irradiation and systemic chemotherapy. Isolated testicular disease often heralds systemic relapse hence the need for further systemic therapy. The prognosis is better when the relapse is occult or occurs as an isolated event. The need for bone marrow transplantation for isolated testicular relapse remains undecided. This should be seriously considered for relapses in children either on, or within 6 months of completing chemotherapy. In any event the effects of gonadal irradiation on sterility and testicular endocrine function must not be forgotten.

AML relapse

Once a child with AML relapses, the long-term prognosis becomes very precarious. Proponents of restricting allogeneic transplantation to patients in second CR would then advocate this line of therapy but results remain inconclusive. Approximately 50% of children will achieve a second CR using high-dose chemotherapy although remissions are usually short (Lampkin et al, 1988). At present, the best chance of cure is to improve initial therapy rather than concentrate on trying to salvage the child with resistant or relapsing disease.

LATE EFFECTS OF ANTILEUKAEMIA TREATMENT

It is a reflection of treatment success that the better the long-term survival the fewer the patient events. The fewer the events the larger (in patient numbers) and the longer (in time) any study in order to reach significance. It may well be that the time will come where the emphasis should change from improving still further questions of therapeutic success to the evaluation of long-term treatment and disease-related complications. It is now estimated that one in every 2000 children who reach the age of 20 will be a survivor of ALL (Meadows et al, 1980), and this is a good example of a childhood malignancy where the cure rate for many children (but not all) is reaching levels where further consideration should be given to the long-term effects of therapy. In the case of AML however, this situation has not yet been reached and the present philosophy is still that of increasing attempts at achieving more long-term survivors. New drugs, more intensive forms of chemotherapy, and chemoradiotherapy combinations should be applied to those subgroups of each malignancy that have a poorer prognosis and in whom the risks are more than justified.

There are three main physical areas of concern in long-term survivors of childhood ALL: CNS structural changes, endocrine effects, and second malignancies.

Central nervous system structural damage

Acute CNS toxicity associated with combined cranial irradiation and intrathecal radiotherapy is relatively uncommon. An occasional child may experience seizures or thrombotic problems associated with intrathecal therapy or L-asparaginase (Ochs et al, 1980; Clavell et al, 1986). Ventricular dilation, calcifications and focal areas of white-matter hypodensity seen on CT scan have been reported (see review of Ochs and Mulhern, 1988) although the frequency and degree of changes seen is very variable, reflecting varying methods of systemic therapy and cranial prophylaxis. In general the incidence of ventricular dilation (up to 16%), intracranial calcification (up to 9%) and white-matter hypodensity (up to 4%) occurs in patients receiving 24 Gy of cranial irradiation plus continuation intrathecal therapy (Poplack and Brouwers, 1985). The more frequent use of intravenous and intrathecal methotrexate and the omission of cranial irradiation may be associated with reduced intracranial calcification. Children under the age of two are particularly associated with neurological toxicity (Leiper and Chessells, 1986).

Endocrine effects

Endocrine abnormalities involving the hypothalamic–pituitary axis are probably secondary to cranial irradiation whereas gonadal dysfunction is probably secondary to chemotherapy (Ochs and Mulhern, 1988). The main abnormality is reduced secretion of growth hormone to provocative stimuli which occurs in between 25 and 50% of children (Shalet et al, 1976). Nevertheless the majority of children show reasonable growth curves after stopping therapy (Shalet et al, 1979; Clayton et al, 1988). Children receiving a second course of cranial irradiation are particularly at risk of growth failure with the threshold for hypothalamic–pituitary damage being in excess of 24 Gy (Shalet, 1976). Growth hormone is the first pituitary hormone to be affected by radiation damage but larger radiation doses may result in panhypopituitarism. In many patients the damage appears to be at the hypothalamic level resulting in a deficiency of endogenous growth hormone releasing factor (GRF). Treatment with synthetic GRF may provide an alternative to growth hormone therapy (Shalet, 1986).

About 3% of long-term survivors of ALL have primary hypothyroidism, 6% compensated hypothyroidism and the majority are euthyroid. Thyroid problems are more common in girls (Robison et al, 1985).

Anxieties over infertility secondary to leukaemia treatment are frequently expressed by long-term survivors and their families. Unfortunately this late effect of therapy has not been well defined. Biochemical measurements of gonadal function (e.g. FSH levels) are of little help in predicting gonadal function in the prepubertal child (Shalet et al, 1979). Boys who receive testicular irradiation will be sterile and if irradiated at a young age may well have reduced Leydig function (Leiper et al, 1983). In the case of girls it is thought that ova are more resistant to the effects of chemotherapy than are spermatozoa (Ochs and Mulhern, 1988).

Second malignancies

Retinoblastoma, CNS tumours and leukaemia itself are amongst the commonest primary neoplasms associated with secondary malignancies (Kingston et al, 1987). It is estimated that the overall 20-year incidence of secondary malignancies is in the region of 8% (Meadows, 1988). In the case of acute leukaemia, intracranial neoplasms appear to have a particular association (Kingston et al, 1987). Radiation is not the prerequisite to the development of secondary CNS tumours. Secondary haematological tumours include AML, non-Hodgkin's lymphoma and chronic myeloid leukaemia (Ochs and Mulhern, 1988). Both genetic and therapy-related factors have been implicated in the high incidence of second neoplasms.

Psychological outcome

The psychological status of long-term survivors of ALL is becoming an area of increasing interest and concern. The majority of studies comparing long-term survivors with suitable control populations have demonstrated some degree of intellectual impairment but firm generalizations as to the nature and magnitude of these defects are hard to make. The two risk factors most often implicated are the nature of the prophylactic CNS therapy and the age of the child (Ochs and Mulhern, 1988). Children treated with cranial irradiation have three to four times the risk of school problems relative to those who are not irradiated (Mulhern et al, 1988). Other problems can include behavioural problems, lower levels of satisfaction and impaired attainment of social skills (Sawyer et al, 1986). Children receiving cranial irradiation and intrathecal therapy who are less than 3 years of age are more severely affected than their older peers (Jannoun, 1983). Children who suffer a CNS leukaemic relapse appear more severely affected. A second course of cranial irradiation, a younger age at relapse and abnormal CT scan findings are predictive of lower neuropsychological performance (Ochs and Mulhern, 1988).

CONSIDERATIONS FOR THE FUTURE

Despite the dramatic improvement in prospects for the child with acute leukaemia over the past two to three decades there is still a great need for improvement.

The major challenge remains to improve therapy for the high-risk patient. There is increasing evidence that intensification of treatment has increased event-free survival but this has been associated with increased myelosuppression and its associated problems. The introduction of recombinant growth factors may shorten the periods of myelosuppression but a question mark remains over how such cytokines may affect the growth of myeloblasts in AML.

There is a need for further definition of the biological heterogeneity of childhood leukaemia. This may allow further understanding of risk groups, drug resistance and biological variability in the response of individual patients to chemotherapy and the causes of treatment failure. The recent interest in molecular genetic techniques may improve our understanding of leukaemic processes and detection of resistant or residual disease.

Leukaemic relapse remains a major problem, particularly in AML. Prevention of a relapse is better than cure. However, until high-risk groups can be defined with some certainty there remains the likelihood of overtreatment in some patients and under-treatment in others. Nevertheless, very intensive relapse regimens often involving marrow transplantation will continue to be used for some time to come. In this regard, the place of autologous transplants, marrow purging and matched unrelated donors remains open.

New antileukaemic agents are required. This includes not only cytotoxic drugs but other modes of action such as the use of 'targeting' vectors such as monoclonal antibodies and aggregates susceptible to phagocytosis by bone marrow macrophages. Radiolabelled monoclonal antibodies may also be used against CNS leukaemic blasts and hence offer the potential of therapy directed at sanctuary sites.

Finally, as the number of long-term survivors increases we are faced with the increasing task of identifying and following the long-term effects of treatment so that the future treatment-related side-effects of leukaemia treatment can be kept to a minimum.

REFERENCES

Amadori S, Ceci A, Comelli A et al (1987) Treatment of acute myelogenous leukaemia in children: Results of the Italian Cooperative Study AIEOP/LAM 8204. *Journal of Clinical Oncology* **5:** 1356–1363.

Argyle JC, Benjamin DR, Lamptein B & Hammond D (1989) Acute non-lymphoblastic leukaemias of childhood. Inter-observer variability and problems in the use of the FAB classification. *Cancer* **63:** 295–301.

Aur RJA, Simone JV, Hustu HO et al (1971) Central nervous therapy and combination chemotherapy of childhood lymphocytic leukaemia. *Blood* **37:** 272–281.

Bennett JM, Catorsky D, Daniel MT et al (1976) Proposals for the classification of the acute leukaemias. *British Journal of Haematology* **33:** 451–458.

Bennett JM, Catorsky D, Daniel MT et al (1981) The morphological classification of acute lymphoblastic leukaemia: concordance among observers and clinical correlations. *British Journal of Haematology* **47:** 553–561.

Birch JM (1983) Epidemiology of paediatric cancer. In Duncan W (ed.) *Paediatric Oncology*, pp 1–10. Berlin: Springer-Verlag.

Birch JM, Marsden HB, Morris-Jones PH et al (1988) Improvements in survival from childhood cancer: results of a population based survey over 30 years. *British Medical Journal* **296:** 1372–1376.

Bleyer WA & Poplack DG (1979) Interventricular versus intralumbar methotrexate for central nervous system leukaemia. *Medical and Paediatric Oncology* **6:** 207–213.

Bleyer WA & Poplack DG (1985) Prophylaxis and treatment of leukaemia in the central nervous system and other sanctuaries (1985). *Seminars in Oncology* **12:** 1131–1148.

Bleyer WA, Sather H & Hammond GD (1986) Prognosis and treatment after relapse of acute lymphoblastic leukaemia and non-Hodgkin's lymphoma. *Cancer* **58:** 590–594.

Bloomfield CD, Goldman AI, Alimena G et al (1986) Chromosomal abnormalities identify high risk and low risk patients with acute lymphoblastic leukaemia. *Blood* **67:** 415–440.

Boice JD (1981) Cancer following medical irradiation. *Cancer* **47:** 1081–1090.

Borsi JD & Moe PJ (1987) Comparative study of the pharmokinetics of methotrexate in a dose range of 0.5 g to 33.6 g/m^2 in children with acute lymphoblastic leukaemia. *Cancer* **60:** 5–13.

Bradstock KF, Hoffbrand AV, Ganeshaguri K et al (1981) Terminal deoxynucleotidyl transferase expression in acute non-lymphoid leukaemia: An analysis by immunofluorescence. *British Journal of Haematology* **47:** 133–143.

Brockstein JA, Kernan NA, Groshen S et al (1987) Allogenic bone marrow transplantation after hyperfractionated total body irradiation and cyclophosphamide in children with acute leukaemia. *New England Journal of Medicine* **317:** 1618–1624.

Butturine A, Rivera GK, Bortin MM & Gale RP (1987) Which treatment for childhood acute lymphoblastic leukaemia in second remission? *Lancet* **i:** 429–432.

Carr TC (1990) The evaluation of tumour markers in childhood malignancy. PhD Thesis submitted to the University of Manchester.

Castiagne S, Berger A, Jolly V et al (1984) Promyelocytic blast crisis of chronic myeloid leukaemia with both + (9;22) and + (15;17) in M_3 cells. *Cancer* **54:** 2409–2413.

Chessells JM (1986a) Acute leukaemia in children. *Clinics in Haematology* **15:** 727–753.

Chessells JM (1986b) Diagnostic value of testicular biopsy in acute lymphoblastic leukaemia. *Journal of Paediatrics* **108:** 331–332.

Clavell LA, Gelber RD, Cohen HJ et al (1986) Four-agent induction and intensive asparaginase therapy for treatment of childhood acute lymphoblastic leukaemia. *New England Journal of Medicine* **315:** 657–663.

Clayton PE, Shalet SM, Morris Jones PH & Price DA (1988) Growth in children treated for acute lymphoblastic leukaemia. *Lancet* **i:** 460–462.

Coccia PF (1983) Development and preliminary findings of Children's Cancer Study Group protocols (161, 162 and 163) for low, average and high risk acute lymphoblastic leukaemia in children. In Murphy SB & Gilbert JR (eds) *Leukaemia Research: Advances in cell biology and treatment*, pp 241–250. Amsterdam: Elsevier.

Committee on Medical Aspects of Radiation in the Environment (1988) Second report. *Investigation of the possible increased incidence of leukaemia in young people near Dounreay Nuclear Establishment, Caithness, Scotland.* London: HMSO.

Committee on Medical Aspects of Radiation in the Environment (1989) Third report. *Report of the incidence of childhood cancer in West Berkshire and North Hampshire area, in which are situated the Atomic Weapons Research Establishments, Aldermaston and the Royal Ordnance Factory, Birghfield.* London: HMSO.

Creutzig U, Eschenbach C & Ritter J (1981) Akute leukaemia bei einem 13-jahrgen jungen mist gleichzeitigen auftretan von lymphoblasten und monoblasten. *Klinic Paediat* **193:** 162–167.

Creutzig U, Ritter J, Reihm H et al (1987) The childhood AML studies BFM-78 and -83: Treatment results and risk factor analysis. In Buchner T, Schellong G & Hiddeman W (eds) *Acute Leukaemias Haematology and Blood Transfusion.* Berlin: Springer-Verlag.

Creutzig U, Ritter J & Schellong G (1990) Identification of two risk groups in childhood acute myeloid leukaemia after therapy intensification in Study AML-BFM-83 as compared with Study AML-BFM-78. *Blood* **75:** 1932–1940.

Crist W, Pullan J, Boyett J et al (1986) Clinical and biological features predict a poor prognosis in acute lymphoid leukaemias in infants: A Paediatric Oncology Group Study. *Blood* **67:** 135–140.

Dahl GV, Simone JV, Hust NHO & Mason C (1978) Preventative central nervous system irradiation in children with acute non lymphocytic leukaemia *Cancer* **42:** 2187–2191.

Dahl GV, Kalwinsky DK & Mirro J (1987) A comparison of cytokinetically based versus intensive chemotherapy for childhood acute myelogenous leukaemia. In Budner T, Schellong G & Hiddermann W (eds) *Acute leukaemias.* Haematology and Blood Transfusion, pp 83–87. Berlin: Springer-Verlag.

Dalla-Favera R, Bregni M, Erikson J et al (1982) Human c-myc onc gene is located on the region of chromosome 8 that is translocated in Birkitt lymphoma. *Proceedings of the National Academy of Sciences USA* **79:** 7824–7828.

De Klein A, Hagemeijer A, Bartram CR et al (1986) bcr rearrangement and translocation of the c-abl oncogene in Philadelphia positive acute lymphoblastic leukaemia. *Blood* **68:** 1369–1375.

Diaz MO, LeBeau MM, Rowley JD et al (1985) The role of the c-mos gene in the 8;21 translocation in human acute myeloblastic leukaemia. *Science* **229:** 767–769.

Dolan G, Lilleymann JS & Richards SM (1989) Prognostic importance of myelosuppression during maintenance treatment of lymphoblastic leukaemia. *Archives of Disease in Childhood* **64:** 1231–1234.

Eden OB, Hardisty RM, Innes EM et al (1978) Testicular disease in acute lymphoblastic leukaemia in childhood. *British Medical Journal* **1:** 334–338.

Eden OB, Rankin A & Kay HEM (1983) Isolated testicular relapse in acute lymphoblastic leukaemia of childhood. *Archives of Disease of Childhood* **58:** 128–132.

Evan GI & Hancock DC (1985) Studies on the interaction of the human c-myc protein with cell nuclei: p62 c-myc as a member of a discrete subset nuclear proteins. *Cell* **43:** 253–255.

Evans AE, Gilbert ES & Zandstra R (1970) The increasing incidence of central nervous system leukaemia in children. *Cancer* **26:** 404–409.

Farber S, Diamond LK, Mercer RD et al (1948) Temporary remissions in acute leukaemia in children produced by folic acid antagonist 4-aemthopteroylglutamic acid (aminopterin). *New England Journal of Medicine* **238:** 787–793.

Frick J, Ritch PS, Hansen RM et al (1984) Successful treatment of meningeal leukaemia using systemic high dose cytosine arabinoside. *Journal of Clinical Oncology* **1:** 365–368.

Gardner MJ, Snee MP, Hall AJ et al (1990) Results of a case control study of leukaemia and lymphoma among young people near Sellafield nuclear plant in West Cumbria. *British Medical Journal* **300:** 423–429.

Gaynon P, Bleyer WA, Steinherz P et al (1987) Impact of treatment dose and delay on the disease free survival (DFS) of children with acute lymphoblastic leukaemia (ALL) and unfavourable prognostic features. *Proceedings of the American Society of Clinical Oncology* **6:** 156.

Gibbons B, Katz FE, Ganly P & Chessells JM (1990) Infant acute lymphoblastic leukaemia with t(11;19). *British Journal of Haematology* **74:** 264–269.

Godyn J (1988) Two different classification systems of acute lymphoblastic leukaemia. *British Journal of Haematology* **69:** 100–102.

Gordis L, Zklo M, Thompson B et al (1981) An apparent increase in the incidence of acute non-lymphocytic leukaemia in black children. *Cancer* **47:** 2763–2768.

Greaves MF (1982) 'Target' cells, cellular phenotypes, and lineage fidelity in human leukaemia. *Journal of Cell Physiology* **1:** 113–115.

Greaves MF (1988) Speculations on the cause of childhood acute lymphoblastic leukaemia. *Leukaemia* **2:** 120–125.

Greaves MF (1989) Etiology of childhood acute lymphoblastic leukaemia: a soluble problem? In Gale RP, Hoelzer D (eds) *Acute lymphoblastic leukaemia*. UCLA Symposium on Molecular and Cellular Biology, New Series vol. 108. New York: Alan R Liss.

Greaves MF, Chan LC, Furley AJW et al (1986) Lineage promiscuity in haemopoietic differentiation and leukaemia. *Blood* **67:** 1–11.

Grier HE & Weinstein HJ (1985) Acute non lymphoblastic leukaemia. *The Pediatric Clinics of North America* **32:** 653–668.

Grier HE, Gelber RD, Camitten BM et al (1987) Prognostic factors in childhood acute myelogenous leukaemia. *Journal of Clinical Oncology* **5:** 1026–1032.

Hale JP & Lilleymann JS (1990) 6-mercaptopurine dose and prognosis in lymphoblastic leukaemia (abstract). *British Paediatric Association 1990*, 86.

Hammond GD, Sather H, Bleyer WA et al (1987) Stratification by prognostic factors in the design and analysis of clinical trials for acute lymphoblastic leukaemia. In Büchner T, Schellong G & Hidderman W (eds) *Acute Leukaemias* Haematology and Blood Transfusion, pp 161–166. Berlin: Springer-Verlag.

Hanawa Y (1975) *All Japan's Childrens Cancer Registration, 1969–1973*. Tokyo: Children's Cancer Association of Japan.

Hann IM (1990) Acute Myeloid Leukaemia. In Lilleyman JS & Hann IM (eds) *Paediatric Haematology* Churchill-Livingstone (in press).

Hayhoe FGJ (1988) Classification of acute leukaemias. *Blood Reviews* **2:** 5–10.

Henze G, Buchmann S, Fengler R & Hartmann R (1987) The BFM relapse studies in childhood ALL. In Büchner T, Schallong G & Hiddemann W (eds) *Acute Leukaemias*. Haematology and Blood Transfusion, pp 147–155. Berlin: Springer-Verlag.

Jannoun L (1983) Are congenital and educational development affected by age at which prophylactic therapy is given in acute lymphoblastic leukaemia? *Archives of Diseases in Childhood* **58:** 953–958.

Johnson FL, Sanders JE, Ruggiero M et al (1987) Bone marrow transplantation for the treatment of acute non-lymphoblastic leukaemia (ALL) in children aged less than two years. *Proceedings of the American Society of Clinical Oncology* **6:** 161.

Jones C, Morse HG, Kas F-T et al (1985) Human T-cell receptor x-chain genes: Location on chromosome 14. *Science* **228:** 83.

Kalwinsky DK, Raimondi SC, Schell MJ et al (1990) Prognostic importance of cytogenetic subgroups in de novo pediatric nonlymphocytic leukaemia. *Journal of Clinical Oncology* **8:** 75–83.

Kersey JH, Sabad A, Gajl-Peczalska K et al (1973) Acute lymphoblastic leukaemia with T (thymus derived) lymphocyte markers. *Science* **182:** 1355–1356.

Kingston JE, Hawkins MM, Draper GJ et al (1987) Patterns of multiple primary tumours in patients treated for cancer during childhood. *British Journal of Cancer* **56:** 331–338.

Klein G (1983) Specific chromosomal translocation and the genesis of B-cell derived tumour in mice and man. *Cell* **32:** 311–318.

Knudson AG (1977) Genetics of etiology of human cancer. *Advances in Human Genetics* **8:** 1–66.

Koren G, Ferrazini G, Sulli H et al (1990) Systemic exposure to mercaptopurine as a prognostic factor in acute lymphocytic leukaemia in children. *New England Journal of Medicine* **323:** 17–21.

Kun LE, Camitta, Mulhearn RK et al (1984) Treatment of meningeal relapse in childhood acute lymphoblastic leukaemia. Results of craniospinal irradiation. *Journal of Clinical Oncology* **2:** 357–364.

Lampkin BC, Large B, Bernstein et al (1988) Biologic characteristics and treatment of acute non-lymphocytic leukaemia in children: Report of the ANLL Strategy Group of the Childrens Cancer Study Group. *Pediatric Clinics of North America* **35:** 743–764.

Land VJ, Thomas PRN, Boyett JM et al (1985) Comparison of maintenance treatment regimes for first central nervous system relapse in children with acute lymphoblastic leukaemia. A Pediatric Oncology Group Study. *Cancer* **56:** 81–87.

Leiper AD & Chessells JM (1986) Acute lymphoblastic leukaemia under 2 years. *Archives of Diseases of Childhood* **61:** 1007–1012.

Leiper AD, Grant DB & Chessells JM (1983) The effect of testicular irradiation on Leydig cell function in prepubertal boys with acute lymphoblastic leukaemia. *Archives of Diseases of Childhood* **58:** 906–910.

Littmann P, Coccia P, Blayer WA et al (1987) Central nervous system (CNS) prophylaxis in children with low risk acute lymphoblastic leukaemia (ALL). *International Journal of Radiation, Oncology, Biology and Physics* **13:** 1443–1449.

Look AT (1988) The cytogenetics of childhood leukaemia: clinical and biologic implications. *Pediatric Clinics of North America* **35:** 723–741.

Look AT, Robertson PK & Williams DL (1985) Prognostic importance of blast cell DNA content in childhood acute lymphoblastic leukaemia. *Blood* **65:** 1079–1083.

Marcus RE, Catorsky D & Prentice G (1987) Intensive induction and consolidation chemotherapy for adults and children with acute myeloid leukaemia—Joint AML Trial 1982–1985. In Buchner T, Schellong G & Hiddeman W (eds) *Acute Leukaemia. Hematology and Blood Transfusion*, pp 346–351. Berlin: Springer-Verlag.

Mauer AM (1978) Treatment of acute leukaemia in children. *Clinics in Haematology* **7:** 245–258.

Meadows AT (1988) Risk factors for second malignant neoplasms. Report from the late effects study group. *Bulletin Cancer* **75:** 125–130.

Meadows AT, Kreimas NL & Belasco JB (1980) The medical cost of cure: Sequelae in survivors of childhood cancer. In Sullivan MP, Van Eys J (eds): *Status of the curability of childhood cancers*, pp 263–276. New York: Raven Press.

Medical Research Council (1986) Improvement in treatment for children with acute lymphoblastic leukaemia. *The Medical Research Councils UKALL Trials 1972–84. Lancet* **i:** 408–411.

Miller DR, Krails M, Bleyer WA et al (1985) Prognostic implications of blast cell morphology in childhood acute lymphoblastic leukaemia: a report from the Childrens Cancer Study Group. *Cancer Treatment Reports* **69:** 1211–1221.

Mirro J, Antoun GR, Zipf TF et al (1985a) The E-rosette associated antigen of T cells can be identified on blasts from patients with acute myeloblastic leukaemia. *Blood* **65:** 363–367.

Mirro J, Zipf TF, Piu C-H et al (1985b) Acute mixed lineage leukaemia: clinicopathologic correlations and prognostic significance. *Blood* **66:** 1115–1123.

Mulhearn RK, Friedman AG & Stone PA (1988) Acute lymphoblastic leukaemia: long-term psychological outcome. *Biomedical Pharmacotherapeutics* **42:** 243–246.

Murphy SB, Bowman WP, Abomovitch M et al (1986) Results of treatment of advanced-stage Burkitts lymphoma and B-cell (S Ig +) acute lymphoblastic leukaemia with high dose fractionated cyclophosphamide and coordinated high dose methotrexate and cytovaline. *Journal of Clinical Oncology* **4:** 1732–1735.

Neglia JP & Robinson LL (1988) Epidemiology of the childhood acute leukaemias. *The Pediatric Clinics of North America* **35:** 675–692.

Neglia JP, Severson RK & Linet MA (1990) A reply to MF Greaves: Toward a testable etiology of childhood acute lymphoblastic leukaemia. *Leukaemia* **4:** 517–521.

Nesbit ME, Sather H, Ortega J et al (1981) Effect of isolated central nervous system leukaemia on bone marrow remission and survival in childhood acute lymphoblastic leukaemia. *Lancet* **i:** 1386–1389.

Nesbit ME, Sather H, Robinson LL et al (1983) Randomised study of 3 years versus 5 years of chemotherapy in childhood acute lymphoblastic leukaemia. *Journal of Clinical Oncology* **1:** 308–316.

Nesbit ME, Buckley J, Lampkin B et al (1987) Comparison of allogeneic bone marrow transplantation with maintenance chemotherapy in previously untreated childhood acute non-lymphocytic leukaemia. *Proceedings of the American Society of Clinical Oncology* **6:** 163–166.

Ochs J & Mulhern RK (1988) Late effects of antileukaemic treatment. *Pediatric Clinics of North America* **35:** 815–833.

Ochs J, Berger P, Brecker ML et al (1980) Computed tomography brain scans in children with acute lymphocytic leukaemia receiving methotrexate alone as central nervous system prophylaxis. *Cancer* **45:** 2274–2278.

Ortega JA, Nesbit ME, Donaldson MH et al (1977) L-asparaginase, vincristine and prednisolone for induction of first remission in acute lymphocytic leukaemia. *Cancer Research* **37:** 535–540.

Perentesis J, Ramsay NKC, Brunning R et al (1983) Biphenotypic leukaemia: evidence for a common lymphoid-myeloid progenitor in humans. *Journal of Pediatrics* **102:** 63–67.

Poplack DG (1988) Acute lymphoblastic leukaemia. In Pizzo PA & Poplack DG (eds) *Pediatric Oncology*, pp 323–366. Philadelphia: Lippincott.

Poplack DG & Brouwers P (1985) Adverse sequelae of central nervous system therapy. *Clinical Oncology* **4:** 263–265.

Poplack DG & Reaman G (1988) Acute lymphoblastic leukaemia in childhood. *Pediatric Clinics of North America* **35:** 903–932.

Poplack DG, Balis FM & Zimm S (1986) The pharmacology of orally administered chemotherapy. A re-appraisal. *Cancer* **58:** 473–480.

Progogina EL, Fleischman EW, Puckkova GP et al (1986) Chromosomes in acute non-lymphocytic leukaemia. *Human Genetics* **73:** 137–146.

Pui C-H, Dahl GB, Kalwinsky DK et al (1985a) Central nervous system leukaemia in children with acute non lymphoblastic leukaemia. *Blood* **66:** 1062–1066.

Pui C-H, Dahl GB, Bowman WP et al (1985b) Elective testicular biopsy during chemotherapy for childhood leukaemia is of no clinical value. *Lancet* **ii:** 410–412.

Pui C-H, Raimondi SC & Murphy SB (1987). An analysis of leukaemic cell chromosomal features in infants. *Blood* **69:** 1289–1292.

Pui C-H, Kalwinsky DK, Schell MJ et al (1988) Acute nonlymphoblastic leukaemia in infants: clinical presentation and outcome. *Journal of Clinical Oncology* **6:** 1008–1013.

Ramot B & Magrath I (1982) Hypothesis: The environment is a major determinant in the immunological sub-type of lymphoma and acute lymphoblastic leukaemia in children. *British Journal of Haematology* **52:** 183–189.

Ribeiro RC, Abromovitch M, Raimondi SC et al (1987) Clinical and biologic hallmarks of the Philadelphia chromosome in acute lymphoblastic leukaemia. *Blood* **70:** 948–953.

Riehm M, Feickert H-J, Schrappe M et al (1987) Therapy results in five ALL-BFM studies since 1970: Implications of risk factors for prognosis. In Büchner T, Schellong G & Hiddemann W (eds) *Acute Leukaemias. Haematology and Blood Transfusion*, pp 139–146. Berlin: Springer-Verlag.

Rivera GK, Buchanan G, Boyett JM et al (1986) Intensive re-treatment of childhood acute lymphoblastic leukaemia in first bone marrow relapse: A Pediatric Oncology Group Study. *New England Journal of Medicine* **315:** 273–278.

Rivera GK, Kovnar E, Pui C-H et al (1987) Limiting toxicities during intensification remission induction chemotherapy for childhood acute lymphoblastic leukaemia. In Buchner T, Schellong G & Hiddeman W (eds) *Acute Leukaemias. Haematology and Blood Transfusion*, pp 156–160. Berlin: Springer-Verlag.

Robison LL, Nesbit ME, Sather HN et al (1985) Thyroid abnormalities in long term survivors of childhood acute lymphoblastic leukaemia. *Pediatric Research* **19:** 226–232.

Robison LL, Buckley J, Daigle A et al (1987) Environmental exposures as risk factors for childhood acute non-lymphocytic leukaemia (ANLL). *Proceedings of the American Associate for Cancer Research* **28:** 249–252.

Sacchi N, Watson DK, Geurts van Kessel AHM et al (1986) Hu-ets-1 and hu-ets-2 are transported in acute leukaemias with (4;11) and (8;21) translocations. *Science* **231:** 379–383.

Savitz DA, Wachtel H, Barnes FA et al (1988) Case control study of childhood cancer and exposure to 60-H$_3$ magnetic fields. *American Journal of Epidemiology* **128:** 21–38.

Sawyer M, Crettenden A & Toogood I (1986) Psychological adjustment of families of children and adolescents treated for leukaemia. *American Journal of Pediatric Hematology and Oncology* **8:** 200–207.

Schmitt-Graff A, Jurgens H, Reifenhauser MD et al (1988) Childhood biphenotypic leukaemia: Detection of mixed lymphoid and myeloid populations in bone marrow specimens. *Human Pathology* **19:** 651–656.

Secker-Walker LM, Lawler SD & Hardisty RM (1978) Prognostic implications of chromosomal findings in acute lymphoblastic leukaemia at diagnosis. *British Medical Journal* **2:** 1529–1530.

Shalet SM (1986) Irradiation induced growth failure. *Clinical Endocrinology and Metabolism* **15:** 591–606.

Shalet SM, Beardwell CG, Morris Jones PH et al (1976) Growth hormone deficiency after treatment of acute leukaemia in children. *Archives of Disease in Childhood* **51:** 489–493.

Shalet SM, Price DA, Beardwell CG et al (1979) Normal growth despite abnormalities of growth hormone secretion in children treated with acute leukaemias. *Journal of Paediatrics* **94:** 719–722.

Shalet SM, Hann IM, Lendon M et al (1981) Testicular function after combination chemotherapy in childhood for acute lymphoblastic leukaemia. *Archives of Disease in Childhood* **56:** 275–278.

Shu XO, Gao YT, Britton LA et al (1988) A population-based, case-control study of childhood leukaemia in Shanghai. *Cancer* **62:** 635–644.

Simone JV (1974) Acute lymphoblastic leukaemia in childhood. *Seminars in Haematology* **2:** 25.

Simone JV (1976) Factors that influence haematological remission during an acute lymphocytic leukaemia. *British Journal of Haematology* **32:** 465–472.

Smets LA, Homan-Blok J & Hart A (1987) Prognostic implications of hyperdiploidy as based on DNA flow cytometric measurement in childhood acute lymphoblastic leukaemia. *Leukaemia* **1:** 163–166.

Smith LJ, Curtis JE, Messner HA et al (1983) Lineage infidelity in acute leukaemia. *Blood* **61:** 1138–1145.

Tamaroff M, Salwen R, Miller DR et al (1985) Neuropsychological sequelae in irradiated and non-irradiated children with acute lymphoblastic leukaemia (ALL). *Proceedings of the American Society of Clinical Oncology* **4:** 165–171.

Vodinelich L, Tax W, Bai Y et al (1983) A monoclonal antibody (WYI) for detecting leukaemias of T cell precursors. *Blood* **63:** 1108–1113.

Weinstein HJ, Mayer RJ, Rosenthal DS et al (1983) Chemotherapy for acute myelogenous leukaemia in children and adults: VAPA update. *Blood* **62:** 315–319.

Weinstein HJ, Grier H, Gelber RD et al (1987) Post remission induction intensive sequential chemotherapy for children with AML. Treatment results and prognostic factors. In Buchner T, Schellong G & Holdemann W (eds) *Acute Leukaemias. Haematology and Blood Transfusion*, pp 399–410. Berlin: Springer-Verlag.

Whitehead VM, Rosenblatt DS, Vuchich M-J et al (1990) Accumulation of methotrexate and methotrexate polyglutamates in lymphoblasts at diagnosis of childhood acute lymphoblastic leukaemia. A pilot prognostic factor analysis. *Blood* **76:** 44–49.

Williams DK, Look AT, Melvin SL et al (1984) New chromosomal translocations correlate with specific immunophenotypes of childhood acute lymphoblastic leukaemia. *Cell* **36:** 101–106.

Williams DL, Harber J, Murphy SB et al (1986) Chromosomal translocations play a unique role in influencing prognosis in childhood acute lymphoblastic leukaemia. *Blood* **68:** 205–212.

Willoughby MLN (1976) Treatment of overt meningeal leukaemia in children: Results of the second MRC meningeal leukaemia trial. *British Medical Journal* **1:** 864–867.

Willoughby MLN (1983) Treatment of over CNS leukaemia. In Mastrangelo R, Poplack DG &

Riccardi R (eds) *Central Nervous System Leukaemia: Prevention and Treatment*, pp 113–122. Boston: Martinus-Nijhoff.

Woods WG, Nesbit ME, Buckley J et al (1985) Correlation of chromosome abnormalities with patient characteristics, histologic subtype and induction success in children with acute non-lymphocytic leukaemia. *Journal of Clinical Oncology* **3:** 3–11.

Young JL & Miller RW (1975) Incidence of malignant tumours in US children. *Journal of Pediatrics* **86:** 254–257.

7

Myelodysplasia

J. M. CHESSELLS

Paediatric myelodysplasia is a confusing topic which has received scant attention in the haematological literature. There are two probable reasons for this neglect: first, the rarity of all chronic myeloid disorders in childhood; and second, the tendency for paediatricians to produce clinical descriptions of syndromes in parallel, but not in collaboration with their haematological colleagues.

There are no population based statistics to determine the prevalence of myelodysplasia (MDS) in childhood. A report from Philadelphia (Blank and Lange, 1981) suggested that 17% of cases of paediatric acute myeloid leukaemia (AML) had a preleukaemic phase, but this type of analysis is obviously biased towards ascertainment of more aggressive forms of MDS. It seems unlikely that these conditions represent more than 3% of haematological malignancies.

WHAT CONDITIONS SHOULD BE CLASSED AS MYELODYSPLASIA?

The myelodysplasias are a group of disorders characterized by a cellular bone marrow but ineffective haemopoiesis; this is demonstrated by morphological and functional abnormalities of one or more cell lines and/or pancytopenia. The term myelodysplastic syndrome was coined to include conditions previously described as refractory anaemia, smouldering leukaemia and preleukaemia. All were relatively common in the elderly and all shared a predilection to the development of AML, albeit at a variable pace. The impetus to improve the definition of MDS was provided by the need to distinguish it from AML because the intensive therapy being introduced for AML might be ineffective in MDS and might shorten survival, particularly in elderly patients.

The first systematic attempt at morphological classification of MDS was provided by the Franco–American–British (FAB) group (Bennett et al, 1982). Further refinements have been provided by the addition of cytogenetic analysis as reviewed by the MIC Cooperative Study Group (Third MIC Cooperative Study Group, 1988). The recognition that many genes involved in haemopoiesis are located on chromosomes 5 and 7 in

Table 1. Classification of paediatric myelodysplasia.

Primary myelodysplasia
    Juvenile Chronic Myeloid Leukaemia (JCML)
    Infantile monosomy 7 syndrome
    Refractory anaemia (RA)
    Refractory anaemia with ringed sideroblasts (RARS)
    Refractory anaemia with excess blasts (RAEB)
    Refractory anaemia with excess blasts in transformation (RAEB-t)

Proliferative MDS
    Down's syndrome
    MDS with eosinophilia
    Atypical CML
    Familial MDS
    Miscellaneous

Secondary myelodysplasia
    Familial
    Therapy-induced

regions commonly involved in cytogenetic abnormalities has provided an exciting impetus to improve understanding of these disorders.

The conventional classification of chronic myeloid malignancies distinguishes myeloproliferative disorders from myelodysplasia. Thus chronic (Ph' positive) granulocytic leukaemia (CGL), essential thrombocythaemia, polycythaemia rubra vera and myelofibrosis would be considered myeloproliferative disorders. The distinction is perhaps somewhat artificial since all are clonal proliferations and all may evolve to a frank acute leukaemia.

The author has therefore arbitrarily chosen to use a broad definition of myelodysplasia and to include in this category all the conditions listed in Table 1. The table includes most of the chronic conditions of childhood, the most notable exception being chronic granulocytic leukaemia, amply described elsewhere and the subject of a whole issue of this series 3 years ago (Goldman, 1987). The so-called non-leukaemic myeloproliferative disorders have also been omitted; essential thrombocythaemia and polycythaemia rubra vera are both excessively rare in childhood and the authenticated cases were recently reviewed (Schwartz and Cohen, 1988). Malignant myelofibrosis as described in adults is not seen in childhood and cases of primary myelofibrosis when studied by modern techniques have proved to have megakaryoblastic leukaemia.

There are, however, a number of other rare conditions in childhood which a purist might describe as myeloproliferative. These have been included, with apologies to the FAB group, as proliferative MDS.

CLINICAL FEATURES OF MDS

The symptoms of MDS may be more non-specific than those of acute leukaemia. The diagnosis may be made after clinical examination shows an enlarged spleen or a routine blood count shows abnormalities. The symptoms may include anaemia or bruising and a history of recurrent infections is not uncommon; recurrent suppurative infections are common in juvenile chronic myeloid leukaemia and the infantile monosomy 7 syndrome. These infections may reflect neutropenia, disordered neutrophil function or both and may even be a manifestation of secondary immunodeficiency. Physical examination may be unrewarding or show hepatosplenomegaly. Lymph node enlargement is rare except in juvenile chronic myeloid leukaemia (JCML). A characteristic skin rash mimicking Langerhan's cell histiocytosis with a butterfly distribution is characteristic of JCML and, more rarely, infantile monosomy 7. During examination particular attention should be paid to features suggestive of an underlying genetic disorder such as Fanconi's anaemia.

INVESTIGATION OF SUSPECTED MDS

Blood and marrow findings

A systematic approach to investigation of paediatric MDS is essential and a list of suggested investigations is shown in Table 2. It is impossible to overemphasize the importance of proper examination of the blood film, a step too often by-passed in the diagnosis of childhood acute leukaemia. The blood film is often more helpful in diagnosis than the marrow; it is essential to note both morphological abnormalities and the presence of unusual numbers of leukocyte subtypes, monocytes, basophils and eosinophils. A list of noteworthy features is shown in Table 3 (from Mufti and Galton, 1986). Examination of the bone marrow must include an iron stain, again frequently omitted in diagnosing childhood leukaemia, in addition to the routine cytochemistry. Trephine biopsy of the bone marrow is essential and an attempt should be made to describe the findings, systematically noting cellularity and relative proportion of all cell lines, presence of fibrosis and reticulin, and localization of immature precursors.

Table 2. Investigation of myelodysplasia.

Blood
  Hb and red cell indices
  WBC and differential: absolute monocytes, basophils, eosinophils
  Blood film
  Fetal haemoglobin
  Leukocyte alkaline phosphatase
  Immunoglobulins

Bone marrow
  Aspirate and trephine biopsy
  Cytochemistry including iron stain
  Cytogenetics

Additional investigations
  Neutrophil function
  Platelet function
  Lymphocyte subsets and autoantibodies
  Colony assays

Table 3. Morphological abnormalities in myelodysplastic syndromes. From Mufti and Galton (1986).

Cell line	Peripheral blood	Bone marrow
Erythroid	Macrocytes, dimorphic picture anisopoikilocytosis; polychromatic cells; punctate basophilia; normoblasts (often dyserythropoietic)	Erythroid hyperplasia common; ring sideroblasts; dyserythropoiesis; megaloblasts; cytoplasmic vacuolation
Megakaryocytic	Giant platelets; megakaryocyte fragments	Small megakaryocytes with one or two small round nuclei; larger forms with single large round ovoid or slightly irregular nucleus; polynuclear forms
Granulocytes	Hypergranular or agranular neutrophils; 'Pelger' cells (round or bilobed forms); grossly hypersegmented neutrophils	Promyelocytes with sparse azurophilic granules; hypo- or agranularity of myelocytes, metamyelocytes and neutrophils
Monocytes	Mature forms sometimes with multiple elongated lobes, some with fine azurophilic granules (promonocytes)	Promonocytes sometimes present
Blasts	Usually small mononuclear blasts with scanty agranular (type I) or sparsely granular (type II) blasts	

Further investigations which may be helpful in diagnosis and management are included in Table 2 and in general reflect abnormal development of one or more cell lines.

The FAB classification and its relevance to paediatrics

The FAB group described five subtypes of myelodysplasia (see Table 4).

Table 4. FAB classification of myelodysplastic syndromes. From Mufti and Galton (1986).

Type	Peripheral blood	Bone marrow
Refractory anaemia (RA)*	Blasts <1%	Blasts <5%
RA with ring sideroblasts (RARS)	As RA	As RA with ring sideroblasts ≥15% of erythroblasts
RA with excess of blasts (RAEB)	Blasts <5%	Blasts 5–20%
RAEB in transformation (RAEB-t)	Blasts >5%	Blasts 20–30% or Auer rods
CMML	As any of the above with ≥1 × 10 9/1 of monocytes	As any of the above ± promonocytes

* In about 5% of cases of neutropenia, thrombocytopenia, or both with hyperplastic bone marrow, the patients are not anaemic. The term 'refractory cytopenia' is sometimes used to describe these cases.

The designations of refractory anaemia (RA), refractory anaemia with ringed sideroblasts (RARS) and refractory anaemia with excess of blasts, with and without transformation (RAEB and RAEB-t, respectively), are all appropriate to the paediatric age group and the author has seen examples of all these categories. Chronic myelomonocytic leukaemia (CMML) comprises about 16% of most MDS series and is characterized by the presence of an absolute monocytosis in blood and bone marrow, in association with dysplasia of the red cell and granulocyte precursors. The paediatric counterpart of CMML, albeit with some distinctive features, is juvenile chronic myeloid leukaemia (JCML), for many years referred to with Gallic logic in the European literature as chronic myelomonocytic leukaemia of childhood. It appears that apart from JCML there are no other forms of chronic myelomonocytic leukaemia in childhood.

Differential diagnosis of MDS

The differential diagnosis will depend on the morphological subtype but RARS must be distinguished from congenital sideroblastic anaemia, in which a low mean corpuscular volume (MCV) is usual and there are no abnormalities of other cell lines. Megaloblastic anaemia is rare in childhood but abnormalities of folate and vitamin B_{12} transport or metabolism producing a severely megaloblastic marrow with thrombocytopenia and abnormal maturation of all cell lines may mimic MDS or even acute leukaemia.

Cytogenetic analysis in MDS

Cytogenetic analysis of the bone marrow is essential in all cases of suspected MDS and analysis of the blood lymphocytes and/or fibroblasts may be needed to confirm genetic disorders such as Fanconi's anaemia or trisomy of chromosome 21. The MIC Co-operative Study Group reviewed the data on cytogenetic findings in MDS (Third MIC Cooperative Study Group, 1988) and confirmed that an abnormal karyotype is found in 60% of patients with primary MDS and in over 90% with secondary MDS. The most common abnormal findings are listed in Table 5 which is based on the data reported by the MIC group.

Cytogenetic abnormalities in MDS, unlike those in de novo AML, are not specific to any morphological subtype. The chief exception to this rule appears in adult practice and is the 5q- syndrome (Bunn, 1986). This distinct haematological disorder occurs predominantly in elderly females with macrocytic anaemia and a normal or raised platelet count. The morphology is that of refractory anaemia with or without ringed sideroblasts and hypolobulated megakaryocytes. Provided the cytogenetic abnormality is restricted to chromosome 5 patients may have a long survival. This was certainly true of the author's only experience of 5q-, a boy with refractory anaemia who survived over 10 years from diagnosis, eventually succumbing to AML.

Table 5. Chromosome changes in myelodysplasia. Modified from Third MIC Study Group (1988).

Primary MDS	Secondary MDS
−7	Single chromosome changes
+8	del(5q)
del(5)(q12–q34) and translocations involving 5q	del(7q)
del(7q)	−5
del(11q)	−7
del(12)(p11p13)	del(12p)
del(13q)	t(1;7)(p11;p11)
del(20)(q11q13)	
	Multiple chromosome changes
t(1;3)(p36;q21)	Any of the above plus:
t(2;11)(p21;q23)	+8
t(6;9)(p23;q34)	+21
t(11;21)(q24;q11.2)	3p(del or t)
i(17q)	17q (del or t), 17p (del or t), −17
	6p (del or t)
	19p or q (t)
	Xq13 (t or dup)
	Xp11 (t)

BIOLOGY OF MDS

Investigation of the myelodysplasias using G6PD, cytogenetics or, more recently, X-linked restriction fragment polymorphisms (Tefferi et al, 1990) confirms that the myelodysplasias are a group of clonal disorders arising in a multipotent or pluripotent stem cell. There is heterogeneity in the penetrance of different cell lineages in different patients with variable involvement of granulocyte, monocyte and lymphoid cell lines (Kere et al, 1987; Tefferi et al, 1990). The blood cells produced by the abnormal clone may have abnormal function and shortened survival. Progression of the disease is associated with expansion of the abnormal clone, deteriorating blood count, and/or development of acute myeloid leukaemia.

Abnormal maturation of the clonal population is accompanied by marked morphological abnormalities in one or more cell lines and abnormal function readily demonstrated in studies of granulocyte or platelet function. These abnormalities are frequently associated with immunological aberrations (particularly in elderly patients), which have been reviewed elsewhere (List et al, 1990). Defects of cellular immunity include reduced numbers of natural killer cells and an abnormal helper/suppressor ratio; such findings may reflect lymphoid involvement or be secondary to transfusion. Immunoglobulin production is usually unimpaired, but raised levels of immunoglobulins and autoantibodies are common, particularly in CMML.

Bone marrow culture studies show reduced numbers of multipotent progenitor cells CFU-GEMM, but the pattern of cultures of committed progenitors varies with the blood picture. Adult CMML is characterized by spontaneous growth of CFU-GM, and in a study of marrow culture in paediatric patients with MDS this was a frequent finding, while some patients also exhibited spontaneous growth of erythroid colonies (Brandwein et al, 1990).

There have been many enthusiastic attempts to investigate factors involved in progression towards AML including the study of serial colony assays and that of oncogene mutations, particularly in the *ras* gene family (Jacobs, 1989). The *ras* group of genes has been implicated in the control of cell proliferation, and activation of these genes has been demonstrated in MDS with a possible higher frequency in patients developing AML. It remains unclear at present whether these mutations are a primary or secondary event in the progression of MDS.

The frequent involvement of chromosomes 5 and 7 in both primary and secondary MDS is a source of intense speculation and interest. The region 5q 23–31 contains the genes for GM-CSF, IL3, CD 14, M-CSF and c-fms (the M-CSF receptor) among others. Similarly the chromosome region 7q is the site of the erythropoietin gene, the *met* proto-oncogene, and the MDR1 gene (Jacobs, 1989). The role of the genes in these regions in the genesis of MDS and secondary AML is not known, but many have found it tempting to speculate that these regions may contain repressor gene(s), and that loss of the normal allele unmasks a recessive mutant allele on the remaining normal chromosome, as in the model of retinoblastoma.

PROGNOSTIC FACTORS IN MDS

There have been several attempts to assess prognosis in MDS; these are usually based on FAB morphology and indices of bone marrow failure such as the blood count and proportion of blasts in the blood and marrow. A notable example of this approach is the so-called Bournemouth score (Mufti et al, 1985), which is reviewed with other variants by Mufti and Galton (1986). These scores are of dubious relevance considering that the mean age of affected patients may be in the region of 70 years and that many may be expected to die of unrelated causes; however, the observed rate of conversion to AML may be relevant, since treatment is more likely to be effective before the development of AML. Features associated with short survival include pancytopenia, more than 5% blasts in the blood, abnormal localization of immature precursors on trephine biopsy and a karyotype showing complex chromosomal abnormalities (Mufti and Galton, 1986). It is also generally agreed that the risk of progression to AML is greater in RAEB and RAEB-t than in refractory anaemia, with or without sideroblasts. The MIC Cooperative Study Group estimated the proportion of cases with leukaemic progression to be 12% for RA, 8% for RARS, 44% for RAEB and 60% for RAEB-t (Third MIC Cooperative Study Group, 1988). Clearly a higher proportion of paediatric cases might be expected to progress because they have longer life expectancy and few complicating medical problems.

TREATMENT OPTIONS IN MDS

There is little information about the treatment of MDS in childhood, with the exception of the two widely recognized subtypes, JCML and monosomy 7. However, a number of articles about this subject in adults are applicable to the management of children and are reviewed here with more specific comments below.

Bone marrow transplantation

Allogeneic bone marrow transplantation (BMT) is the only curative treatment for most patients with MDS. A recent review from Seattle has described the outcome in 59 patients with MDS who received BMT; the actuarial 3-year event-free survival was 45% (Applebaum et al, 1990). The patients all received preparative treatment with cyclophosphamide and total body irradiation (TBI), and 45 of 59 donors were HLA identical. The causes of failure of treatment were interstitial pneumonitis, graft failure and graft versus host disease. Factors independently predictive of good survival were young age, karyotypic abnormalities and a low proportion of blasts in the bone marrow.

The European Bone Marrow Transplant Group (EBMTG) has recently reviewed the members' experience of BMT in 78 patients with MDS and secondary AML (De Witte et al, 1990). Actuarial 2-year survival was over 50% for patients with MDS. There is scant information about paediatric BMT and the recent report from Boston only involved eight children of whom four remained well in remission (Guinan et al, 1989). However, despite the lack of specifically paediatric reports it seems safe to infer that BMT is the most effective form of therapy available at present for myelodysplasia in children, as well as in adults.

Most of the published literature on BMT for MDS has involved the use of total body irradiation. An alternative approach is the use of chemotherapy alone, usually busulphan and cyclophosphamide, as pioneered by the Baltimore group. This combination has been used with some success in CGL (Tutschka et al, 1987) and it would seem a reasonable approach in MDS particularly in the young child, to avoid the late effects of total body irradiation. There have been several recent reports about the late effects of total body irradiation (Sanders et al, 1986; Leiper et al, 1987), which vary in severity depending on the age of the patient and the dose and fractionation of the regimen. However, the late effects are considerable and include: growth failure due to spinal shortening and hypothalamic pituitary failure, delayed puberty, gonadal failure, hypothyroidism, development of cataracts and learning problems. There have as yet been no reviews of the long-term morbidity of preparative regimens containing chemotherapy alone, but these are unlikely to have such adverse effects on growth and neuro-psychological function as radiation alone.

The choice of method to prevent graft-versus-host disease lies between immunosuppression of the recipient and T-cell depletion of the donor bone marrow and there is no published information on the relative merits of these two approaches in MDS. However, recent analysis of results in CGL shows that T-cell depletion reduces the risk of graft-versus-host disease at the expense of a greater risk of graft rejection and leukaemic relapse; thus at present in CGL the risks outweigh the benefits (Apperley et al, 1988).

Thus BMT from an HLA compatible sibling may be expected to yield good results in children with MDS and at present immunosuppression of the recipient would appear to be the best method of prevention of graft-versus-host disease. The choice between chemotherapy alone or chemotherapy and radiotherapy may be influenced by the precise diagnosis (see below) and the age of the patient. Sadly, however, only one in three children in the UK has an HLA compatible sibling donor. There are two approaches in such patients: the use of haploidentical family members; and use of the matched unrelated (MUD) donor. Most of the scanty literature on this topic has involved the use of matched unrelated donor and the state of donor panels has been recently reviewed (Hows and Bradley, 1990). The chance of finding a suitable donor depends on the patient's HLA type, the size of the panel and the ethnic group of the patient and the panel; the waiting time is 3–10 months, adequate for some cases of MDS perhaps, but not for most children with JCML.

The results of BMT with a matched unrelated donor are only just being reported and it is only in the last few years that this form of treatment has become feasible for any other than a small number of patients. A recent analysis of the results of matched unrelated transplantation in 102 patients with CGL has been published by McGlave et al (1990). The actuarial event-free survival was 29% at 30 months, the major causes of death being failure of engraftment and acute and chronic graft-versus-host disease.

Intensive chemotherapy

Cheson has recently reviewed approaches to treatment in MDS and his report included an analysis of the results of intensive chemotherapy as given in AML (Cheson, 1990). A series of five published papers involved a total of 115 cases with remission rates ranging from 13% to 51%. Many of these cases were identified in retrospect from the review of trials of treatment of AML. The main obstacles to achieving remission seemed to be prolonged hypoplasia and clinical drug resistance. This view is confirmed by De Witte et al (1990) who compared the response to similar treatment in 126 patients with AML, 22 with secondary AML and 14 with MDS (RAEB and RAEB-t). The duration of hypoplasia following chemotherapy was longer in secondary AML and MDS and thrombocytopenia was significantly prolonged. Complete remission rates were similar in the three groups, and was found to be over 70% for all patients under 45 years. However, long-lasting remissions were only obtained in patients with secondary AML or MDS who subsequently underwent BMT.

Differentiating agents and cytokines

A number of agents can induce differentiation of leukaemic cells in culture, including low-dose cytarabine, retinoids and vitamin D3. The literature on this topic has been recently reviewed by Cheson (1990) who has concluded that cytarabine in vivo is acting as a cytotoxic agent rather than as an inducer of differentiation and that there is no defined role for low-dose cytarabine therapy in MDS. There have been a few randomized trials on the use of retinoic acid and vitamin D3 in the treatment of MDS, neither of which have shown to be of any benefit. Thus there is no evidence at present to support the use of any of these agents in the treatment of MDS in the paediatric patient.

The most fashionable form of treatment at present, and one that is undergoing numerous trials in these as in many other disorders, is cytokine therapy, usually with granulocyte-colony stimulating factor (G-CSF) or granulocyte-macrophage colony stimulating factor (GM-CSF). Cheson reviewed data from 95 patients treated with either of these two cytokines and found that an improvement in neutrophil count was noted in 81% and platelet count in 11% of cases. However, continued treatment was needed to sustain this improvement. It remains unclear at present whether the abnormality of neutrophil function, which is a feature of MDS, is improved by cytokine therapy. A major concern is the risk of acceleration of development of leukaemia. Most studies have excluded patients with excess marrow blasts from treatment. Nevertheless, review of a total of 82 adult patients treated with granulocyte-colony stimulating factor or granulocyte-macrophage colony stimulating factor showed that marrow blasts had increased in 22 patients, often with rapid progression to leukaemia. The results of randomized trials are eagerly awaited and the next few years should see a clearer indication of which, if any, patients with MDS will benefit from these and other growth factors now becoming available.

JUVENILE CHRONIC MYELOID LEUKAEMIA (JCML)

Clinical and laboratory features

Almost 30 years have passed since Hardisty, Speed and Till (Hardisty et al, 1964) distinguished two types of chronic myeloid leukaemia in childhood: the adult type, associated with the then newly described Philadelphia chromosome; and the juvenile type, consistently and correctly referred to in the French literature as myelomonocytic leukaemia. The great fascination of JCML lies in the reversal, or persistence, of characteristics of fetal haemopoiesis, a feature recognised for many years since the description of a raised level of fetal haemoglobin (Weatherall et al, 1968).

There are no clues as to the cause of this rare disorder, but there does seem to be a real association between JCML and neurofibromatosis. Review of the distribution of cases of childhood leukaemia in association with neurofibromatosis showed a disproportionate number of cases of chronic myeloid leukaemia (Bader and Miller, 1978) and in more recent reports there seems to be a more specific association with JCML (Mays et al, 1980; Kaneko et al, 1989).

Juvenile chronic myeloid leukaemia appears to be more common in boys and usually presents with pallor, splenomegaly and bleeding due to thrombocytopenia. A facial rash with a butterfly distribution which may also involve the trunk is a common but not invariable finding; it may precede other abnormalities by months. Biopsy of the rash shows non-specific infiltration with lymphocytes and histiocytes and is non-diagnostic. Cutaneous xanthomata have been noted in some patients (Mays et al, 1980). Progression of the disease is accompanied by wasting, enlargement of lymph nodes, which may become suppurative, and progressive splenomegaly, anaemia and bleeding.

An analysis of 38 cases of JCML seen at the Hôpital St-Louis (Castro-Malaspina et al, 1984) confirms that examination of the blood film is more helpful in diagnosis than the bone marrow. The leukocyte count was only moderately raised, being under $50 \times 10^9 \text{l}^{-1}$ in most children, anaemia was common, the platelet count was reduced and the blood film showed monocytes, eosinophils, abnormal granulocytes and some blast cells. The bone marrow showed some increase in blast cells, monocytes and myelodysplasia.

Blood and bone marrow appearances in JCML frequently resemble those of infantile monosomy 7 syndrome, and a recent report from Vancouver (Brandwein et al, 1990) has emphasized that these two conditions may be indistinguishable. However, it has been consistently found that the platelet count is lower in JCML and the fetal haemoglobin is usually greater than 10% (Sieff et al, 1981). These distinctions are of more than academic interest in view of the somewhat different natural history and response to treatment of the two conditions. The author has also seen two children with clinical features of JCML including the skin rash and progressive rise in fetal haemoglobin, in whom there was a prominent increase in normoblasts in blood and marrow; the evolution of the disease in both cases was typical of JCML rather than of an erythroleukaemia.

Cytogenetic analysis of the bone marrow in JCML may show various abnormalities or be normal; there are no pathognomonic findings (Kaneko et al, 1989). The classification as chronic myelomonocytic leukaemia is supported by the presence of monocyte specific antigens on the surface of mononuclear cells (Shannon et al, 1986) and by the results of bone marrow culture when there may be spontaneous growth of macrophage colonies without the addition of GM-CSF (Freedman et al, 1988). The growth of such colonies may be inhibited by the addition of neutralizing antisera to GM-CSF (Gualtieri et al, 1989).

However, JCML is truly a trilineage MDS and numerous publications have investigated the pattern of erythropoiesis since the observation of raised fetal haemoglobin (HbF). Examination of the red cells shows a fetal pattern of enzymes (Travis, 1983). A recent report compared the pattern of growth and globin synthesis of erythroid colony cultures in fetal and neonatal blood, blood from patients with raised fetal haemoglobin associated with stress erythropoiesis, and a child with JCML. The child's blood contained a low level of epsilon globin chains, which normally disappear by 3 months of age, and the pattern of colony growth and of gamma chain synthesis resembled that seen in fetal blood (Weinberg et al, 1990). Adult

CMML is associated with immunological abnormalities and raised serum immunoglobulins, a high incidence of antinuclear antibodies, and anti-human IgG antibodies were noted many years ago in JCML (Cannat and Seligmann, 1973).

Natural history and prognosis

The large French study of JCML (Castro-Malaspina et al, 1984) included a multivariate analysis of factors influencing prognosis; the most important variables were age, platelet count and presence of bleeding. The median survival for children in the study over 2 years of age at diagnosis was 12 months whereas younger children had a median survival of over 4 years. At the Hospital for Sick Children, Great Ormond St, we have classified children as having JCML only in the presence of a fetal haemoglobin of greater than 10% and progressive thrombocytopenia. Fourteen children have been seen with JCML at Great Ormond St over the last 20 years (11 male), with a median age of 3 years at diagnosis; the median survival was 6 months.

Some authors have referred to a terminal blast crisis in JCML; in the author's experience these patients do not develop a new leukaemia but their deterioration may be marked by weight loss, nodal enlargement and appearance of more blast cells and sometimes normoblasts in the blood. A frank blast crisis as seen in Ph' positive CGL does not occur.

Management

Following the report of Lilleyman and colleagues (1977) of the benefits of cytarabine and mercaptopurine there have been several reports suggesting that intensive chemotherapy is of value in JCML (Chan et al, 1987; Festa et al, 1990). Close analysis of these reports suggests that a true remission is not achieved and that intensive treatment at best produces a reduction in bulk disease. In view of reports of abnormal cytokine production and regulation in JCML it is possible that treatment with inhibitors or regulators of cytokines may be possible if and when these become available. The treatment of choice is allogeneic BMT and this should be pursued in all patients unless there is a clear contraindication. The only exception would be the young child, under one and possibly under two, in whom the disease appears to have a slower pace. A period of observation would appear to be reasonable, especially if there is no histocompatible sibling donor.

Analysis of the results of BMT in JCML published by the Seattle group (Sanders et al, 1988) showed that three of six children who received BMT from an HLA compatible sibling and three of eight using a donor with a 1–antigen mismatch were alive and in remission after a conditioning regimen of cyclophosphamide and total body irradiation. Leukaemia recurred after BMT in three of the 14 children. There is little information about the results of regimens involving chemotherapy alone but this may not be effective in view of the refractory nature of the disease; a recent case report demonstrated that the combination of busulphan and cyclophosphamide did not eradicate the malignant clone (Urban et al, 1990).

In view of the very poor prognosis a search for alternative donors would seem justifiable in cases without a sibling donor. If the pace of progression precludes a search for a matched unrelated donor then an attempt at haploidentical BMT would appear reasonable.

MONOSOMY 7 AND THE INFANTILE MYELODYSPLASTIC SYNDROME

The significance of chromosome 7 abnormalities

Monosomy and partial deletion of chromosome 7 are common cytogenetic findings in primary MDS, AML arising de novo, and secondary MDS and AML. All these conditions are characterized by a particular susceptibility to bacterial infection associated with defective neutrophil chemotaxis and killing (Ruutu et al, 1977), presumably because of deletion of gene(s) essential for this function. These abnormalities of chromosome 7 are normally found only in myeloid leukaemias but there have been reports of this finding in de novo acute lymphoblastic leukaemia with subsequent relapse as AML and in biphenotypic leukaemia (Chan et al, 1985). Such observations suggest that, like Ph' positive leukaemia, monosomy 7 is associated with transformation of a common lymphoid–myeloid progenitor cell.

The variability of clinical features in association with abnormalities of chromosome 7 has been recently emphasized (Baranger et al, 1990) and is illustrated by Table 6 which shows our updated experience at Great Ormond

Table 6. Clinical features and outcome in children with monosomy 7 seen at Great Ormond St.

Diagnosis	Number of patients	Treatment	Outcome
Acute myeloid leukaemia	4	Intensive chemotherapy	3 remissions—all relapsed within 9 months
Secondary AML	1	Supportive care	Survived 6 months
Myelofibrosis with myelodysplasia	1	No response to chemo-therapy. Cyclophos-phamide/TBI and allogeneic BMT when pancytopenic	Well 4½ years later
REAB in transformation	1	No response to chemo-therapy. Cyclophos-phamide/TBI and allogeneic BMT when pancytopenic	Full engraftment; relapse 8 months later
Myeloproliferative syndrome	13	BMT in chronic phase at 4 years from diagnosis (1)	Well 8½ years since BMT
		Intensive chemotherapy (6)	3 remissions; 2 alive and well at 5½ and 6½ years
		Supportive care (4)	Survival from 3 months to 4 years
		Early follow-up (2)	

St of the clinical picture in children with this finding (Evans et al, 1988). It can be seen that this is associated with AML, secondary AML, subacute AML with myelofibrosis and the infantile monosomy 7 syndrome. The diagnosis, as previously emphasized (Gyger et al, 1982), should also be considered in children presenting with repeated infections in whom there are any haematological findings suggestive of myelodysplasia. Table 6 also illustrates the importance of considering the haematological diagnosis in evaluating the treatment response in this group of conditions. The same caveats apply when considering the possible recurrence risk of monosomy 7. There have been a number of familial cases of AML or MDS with this cytogenetic abnormality (Carroll et al, 1985) and it has been suggested that as many as one third of cases of infantile MDS may be familial, although at Great Ormond St we have not yet encountered such cases. It is important to recognise that there are families with an apparent predilection to the development of AML or MDS; for example, a family from Newcastle where AML with monosomy 7 evolved during marrow hypoplasia (Paul et al, 1987), and two of the siblings described from Vancouver with monosomy 7 (Brandwein et al, 1990). It should be noted that these do not necessarily represent the same genetic condition as infantile MDS.

The infantile myelodysplastic syndrome with monosomy 7

This condition was first described by Teasdale and colleagues (Teasdale et al, 1970) as a myeloproliferative disorder occurring in three children with a missing C group chromosome. Subsequently we (Sieff et al, 1981) reviewed the published cases of this disorder and found that it was primarily one of young children. We suggest that the term MDS with monosomy 7 should be restricted to this group.

We have now seen a total of 13 children (11 boys) with this syndrome. They presented at a median age of 10 months, although our most recent patient, diagnosed at the age of 8 years, had a 6-year history of recurrent infections, hypogammaglobulinaemia and monocytosis.

Blood and bone marrow appearances are those of RA, RAEB or resemble those of JCML, monocytosis and eosinophilia being common. Thrombocytopenia and bleeding are not a dominant feature, in contrast to JCML, and the fetal haemoglobin is rarely in excess of 10%. Cytogenetic analysis of the bone marrow shows a variable number of cells lacking chromosome 7 but these usually predominate. Bone marrow culture studies (Brandwein et al, 1990) show autonomous growth of macrophage colonies and sometimes of erythroid progenitors.

Natural history and prognosis

Three of our patients with infantile MDS and five of eight from the St Jude series (Weiss et al, 1987) developed frank AML and one in each series developed massive splenomegaly and marrow fibrosis. The time to evolution of AML varied from 3 months to 2 years and in our original survey of published cases we found that three of nine with a primary disease and chronic phase survived more than 2 years. Thus infantile monosomy 7 is associated with longer survival than JCML and the patients have a specific predilection to the development of AML.

Management of infantile monosomy 7

Patients with AML and monosomy 7 are less likely to respond to remission induction (Woods et al, 1985) and our original experience with chemotherapy of infantile MDS was not encouraging. We have now treated a total of six children with this disorder with combination chemotherapy as used at Great Ormond St for AML (Phillips et al, 1991) and three achieved clinical and cytogenetic remission; two remain in remission 4 and 5 years from diagnosis. Chemotherapy after the development of AML is less likely to be successful.

The role of bone marrow transplantation has yet to be established although it would appear to be the treatment of choice. The timing of BMT is difficult and it is clearly important to avoid total body irradiation in view of the young age of the patients. One of the boys in our original series who had been in a stable state for 4 years following diagnosis was treated with cytarabine, cyclophosphamide, total body irradiation and BMT from a histocompatible sibling; he remains well and in remission at the age of 10, 5 years on from transplantation.

It would seem to be appropriate to look for a compatible donor in these patients. The optimum timing of BMT and the real place of intensive chemotherapy remain to be clarified.

OTHER PRIMARY MYELODYSPLASIAS

The paucity of reports about other forms of paediatric MDS makes it extremely difficult to determine the optimum management and the risk of progression to AML. Most of the papers on this topic involve extremely small numbers and/or a literature review. Thus Wegelius (1986) in a review of 26 cases commented on the rarity of refractory anaemia with ringed sideroblasts and the high rate of progression to AML: 23 of the cases developing leukaemia in a median time of 12 months from diagnosis. In a joint report from Germany and Italy of 21 cases more aggressive forms of MDS predominated, 20 having RAEB or RAEB-t (Creutzig et al, 1987). We have seen two cases of refractory anaemia with ringed sideroblasts, both with a chronic course, but have no idea of its prevalence. There is understandably scant information about response to treatment. Eleven patients in the series reported by Creutzig received intensive chemotherapy with six remissions of which only two were prolonged. Six children received low-dose cytarabine with unsurprising lack of response and two received BMT with one long-term survivor. The poor overall results in this group of patients with a 5-year survival of 20% is consistent with reports from the adult literature and would certainly justify BMT in this group of children. The difficult issue is whether or not this should be preceded by an attempt at remission induction. Guinan et al (1989) reported four of eight long-term survivors after BMT; none received intensive chemotherapy prior to cyclophosphamide and total body irradiation.

There are no reports yet of the use of cytokines in MDS in children but this form of therapy must await proper trials in adults and seems unlikely to be indicated in view of the aggressive nature and high rate of leukaemic transformation in most paediatric series.

PROLIFERATIVE MDS

There are a number of conditions in infancy and childhood that do not fit into the classical categories of myelodysplasia or myeloproliferative disorders. The most obvious abnormality may be proliferation of one or more cell lines but this is frequently accompanied by morphological abnormalities; it seems appropriate to include them in this review.

Down's syndrome, transient myeloproliferation and leukaemia

Children with Down's syndrome have a 10–20 fold increased risk of develop ment of acute leukaemia. About 1–2% of children with acute lymphoblastic leukaemia have Down's syndrome; the leukaemia is almost invariably the common (early pre-B) type of acute lymphoblastic leukaemia (Levitt et al 1990). The myeloid leukaemia is usually the otherwise uncommon mega karyoblastic (M7) variant, occurring in the first 3 years of life. However it has been known for many years that children with Down's syndrome are also at risk of a neonatal myeloproliferative syndrome, transient abnormal myelopoiesis (TAM) resembling acute leukaemia, which usually undergoes spontaneous remission.

The relationship between TAM and the subsequent development of AML is not yet clear, but there are now over 20 reports in the literature of infants with TAM who later developed acute leukaemia after an interval ranging from 6 months to 3 years (Bain, 1991). A number of children with AML have a prodromal myelodysplastic phase; two of the seven children with Down's syndrome and AML seen at Great Ormond St during the last 4 years had a prodromal phase with blasts in the blood over several months before treatment was initiated and review of the literature shows several similar cases (Bain, 1991). There is urgent need for a prospective study of babies with Down's syndrome to determine the true incidence of TAM, the risk of subsequent AML and whether TAM also predisposes to lymphoblastic leukaemia.

The clinical picture of TAM resembles that of congenital leukaemia with enlargement of the liver and spleen, although the skin infiltration character istic of neonatal leukaemia does not seem to be a feature (Barnett et al 1990). The blood count shows an invariable leukocytosis with many blast cells and symptoms of hyperviscosity may occur. Anaemia is moderate and the platelet count may be normal, raised or decreased. The film may show myelodysplastic features. These infants do not develop progressive marrow failure although treatment may be needed for anaemia or thrombocytopenia.

Intriguingly the blast cell in TAM is predominantly a megakaryoblast (Eguchi et al, 1989). Eguchi et al (1989) recently attempted to distinguish the blast cells in TAM from those from children with Down's syndrome who had developed AML; both reacted with platelet peroxidase and with monoclonal antibodies to megakaryocytes but the blasts in TAM showed positivity with myeloperoxidase on electron microscopy and differentiated on culture. They concluded that these blasts were in fact multipotent stem cells.

The role of trisomy of chromosome 21 in the genesis of TAM and leukaemia in these babies is unknown at present. TAM has been described in phenotypically normal children but they have been mosaic for trisomy 21 and it is this clone of cells which proliferates. Additional clonal cytogenetic abnormalities have been described in some patients with TAM although Eguchi et al have claimed that such abnormalities occur only once frank leukaemia develops. Clearly serial cytogenetic studies will be extremely important in future in such patients.

The management of TAM is conservative with supportive care only. Cytotoxic therapy is not indicated but careful follow up is essential and may improve understanding of this condition.

Eosinophilic syndromes

We have reported two infants with hepatosplenomegaly, marked eosinophilia, some myelodysplasia and chromosome analysis showing a t(1;5)(q23;q33); one was refractory to chemotherapy while the other had a more prolonged course responding to oral drugs (Derbyshire et al, 1987). We have since heard of two more similar cases in infancy.

The author has also recently seen a young boy with a prolonged history of infiltrative skin lesions and eosinophilia in association with a t(5;5)(q11.2;q31). It is of interest that the gene for IL-5, a selective eosinophilopoietic cytokine, has been mapped to this region (Sutherland et al, 1988).

Ph' negative CML and other rare conditions

There has been a recent description of two cases of chronic myeloproliferative disease in childhood in association with translocations involving 11p15 (Inaba et al, 1988). Inaba et al found four similar cases in a literature search and suggested that this is a nonrandom finding in chronic myeloproliferative disease.

The diagnosis of Ph' negative CML includes a variety of conditions. Some patients with typical morphological and clinical features of CGL in whom cytogenetic analysis is normal will prove on molecular investigation to have the bcr-abl rearrangement characteristic of CGL (Ganesan et al, 1986). The others represent a mixed group. Careful morphological reappraisal in one series of such patients (Pugh et al, 1985) showed that they all probably had some other form of myeloproliferative disorder or MDS, most notably chronic myelomonocytic leukaemia. Galton and Mufti have distinguished between atypical (Ph' negative) CML and chronic myelomonocytic leukaemia, particularly in the younger adult, on the basis that patients with the former have a large number of immature granulocytes in the blood. The prognosis of atypical CML is poor; our two patients with this condition unfortunately both died from complications of BMT.

Familial myelodysplasia

The risk of recurrence of haematological malignancy in a sibling of an otherwise healthy child is usually negligible, but anxiety about such risks is understandable. It is important to exclude an underlying genetic disorder in any child with myelodysplasia, particularly variants of Fanconi's anaemia (Nowell et al, 1984) and neurofibromatosis in which the clinical features may not be readily apparent.

There are however a number of families in which the haematological abnormality is the only problem. The most common of these is the monosomy 7 syndrome where, as discussed previously, there is evidence of a familial occurrence in some cases. There are also a number of case reports in the literature, usually of single families, of a myeloproliferative or dysplastic disorder, often imperfectly studied with modern techniques; for example, a large family described by Randall et al (1965) where children up to 4 years of age presented with splenomegaly, anaemia, leukocytosis and a leuko-erythroblastic blood film. The affected children had a variable outcome, some dying, some improving and some apparently responding to splenectomy. The basis for this type of condition and the other familial ones described in surveys of chronic myeloid disorders in childhood (Nix and Fernbach, 1981) is unknown.

SECONDARY MYELODYSPLASIA

Familial disorders

The risk of AML in patients with congenital bone marrow disorders is well recognized but these patients may also develop MDS as a prelude to AML or as a chronic entity. Patients with Fanconi's anaemia may actually present with MDS or AML rather than with progressive primary marrow failure (Auerbach et al, 1982) and treatment with chemotherapy is unlikely to be effective. Similarly patients with Schwachman's syndrome, which is associated with an increased risk of development of acute leukaemia, may also develop MDS (Woods et al, 1981); we have encountered two such patients at Great Ormond St. Ideally children with Fanconi's anaemia should be treated by BMT with an appropriate modified preparative regimen (Gluckman, 1989) before the development of leukaemia or MDS. Such treatment may prevent the onset of leukaemia but presumably not that of other cancers. The results of treatment of patients with Schwachman's syndrome with G-CSF will no doubt soon be available, but it remains to be seen whether this form of therapy will achieve the remarkable results seen in other types of congenital neutropenia or whether it will increase the risk of leukaemic progression. The many other problems encountered by these children render them largely unsuitable candidates for BMT.

Therapy-induced MDS

Risks and clinical features

The last few years have seen an increasing number of reports of secondary AML and MDS, most commonly in patients previously treated for Hodgkin's disease, but also after non-Hodgkin's lymphoma (NHL), myeloma and a variety of non-haematological solid tumours. A genetic association between the two malignancies cannot be confidently excluded in all cases but there is a strong association between the type of treatment given and the risk of AML/MDS. An extensive review of the published literature (Levine and Bloomfield, 1986) concluded that the alkylating agents were most clearly implicated, with procarbazine most frequently involved and cyclophosphamide appearing to be less leukaemogenic than other alkylating agents. The duration of treatment was an important predisposing factor and there was little evidence for synergism between radiotherapy and chemotherapy. There is some evidence that patients over 40 may be more at risk than those under 40, but whether children are less at risk than adults is not yet clear. The median time to development of AML/MDS was 48–71 months.

Hodgkin's disease is the commonest primary diagnosis in the paediatric context. The risks of secondary AML/MDS in Hodgkin's disease were more recently evaluated in a large multi-centre case control study (Kaldor et al, 1990). The risk of AML/MDS was increased by a factor of 9 in patients receiving chemotherapy; this risk was related to drug dosage and was not increased further by radiotherapy. The benefits of treatment of Hodgkin's disease clearly outweigh the risks but there is obviously a need for exploration of less toxic treatment schedules. The first UK study for paediatric non-Hodgkin's lymphoma conducted by the United Kingdom Children's Cancer Study Group using a protocol containing nitrosoureas in addition to cyclophosphamide was complicated by an actuarial risk of secondary AML/MDS of 7.8% at 7 years (Ingram et al, 1987).

The risk of secondary leukaemia after treatment of acute lymphoblastic leukaemia is not clear. There have been a small number (single figures) of cases of secondary AML/MDS with monosomy 7 in the UK after treatment of acute lymphoblastic leukaemia, but a more unusual pattern was recently reported from the St Jude Children's Research Hospital, where an actuarial risk of 4.7% at 6 years following treatment was recorded. The risk was higher in patients with T-ALL. The authors had no explanation for the incidence of secondary leukaemia but speculated that this might be related to the fact that the protocol contained repeated doses of epipodophyllotoxins (Pui et al, 1989).

The symptoms of secondary MDS are as those of bone marrow failure.

The evolution to AML in one group of patients occurred in a median time of three months. The morphological characteristics of secondary AML do not always conform readily to a FAB subtype. Basophilia may be a feature and the proportion of blasts at diagnosis may be relatively low in the presence of marked morphological abnormalities in all cell lines; bone marrow fibrosis may result in the finding of rather a dilute aspirate (Third MIC Cooperative Study Group, 1988).

Cytogenetics

Cytogenetic abnormalities, frequently multiple, are found in over 90% of cases of secondary AML/MDS and the majority of cases include abnormalities of chromosome 5 and/or 7. Other chromosomes frequently involved are 3 and 17 (see Table 5). It is of interest that chromosomes 5 and 7 are also involved in the development of leukaemia after exposure to toxins. Le Beau et al (1986) have shown that the abnormalities of chromosome 5 always involve a critical region between 5q23–32, a region that contains the genes for several growth factors and receptors. An exception to these findings is the report from St Jude Children's Hospital (Pui et al, 1989) where the secondary AML was associated with deletion of 11q23, a region frequently involved in monocytic and mixed lineage leukaemias of infancy.

Treatment

There is little paediatric experience in this difficult field. Levine and Bloomfield summarized the published literature on secondary myelodysplasia in their 1986 review. The remission rate in a number of studies varied from 30 to 80%. Not surprisingly, the lower rates were achieved in the largest studies. Most patients had received cytarabine in conventional or high doses, with or without an anthracycline. Remission was unlikely in the presence of an abnormality of chromosome 5, irrespective of other cytogenetic findings, and patients whose previous treatment had comprised radiotherapy alone, together with those whose first malignancy was a solid tumour, were most likely to achieve remission. Duration of remission was extremely short in most patients.

The only prospect for cure of secondary AML/MDS at present lies with BMT. A recent, retrospective survey of data from the European Bone Marrow Transplantation Group identified 78 patients with secondary AML or with MDS (De Witte et al, 1990). Twelve of 65 patients with MDS had received previous therapy for malignant disease, most commonly Hodgkin's disease. The disease-free survival at 2 years for the whole group of patients with MDS was over 50% but the authors did not identify the outcome in those with secondary MDS. Two of the cases reported by Guinan et al (1989) had secondary MDS and one survived. Despite the lack of published information it seems that this approach should be pursued in patients in whom there is no contraindication.

CONCLUSIONS

There is a cle.ir need for studies designed to determine the real incidence and prognosis of MDS in childhood. Such studies should help to reveal the frequency of an associated genetic disorder such as Fanconi's anaemia or its variants and the frequency of familial cases. Meanwhile an attempt should be made to fully investigate every patient in whom MDS is suspected using the investigations suggested and by applying the FAB classification systematically to all cases. No doubt the FAB scheme will undergo further modifications in the near future, hopefully rendering it more valuable in paediatrics. Only in this way can a truly informed opinion be given to families about management and prognosis of MDS, an exercise of increasing importance as treatment becomes more possible. The next few years will see a better definition of the role of BMT in the management of MDS and possibly the introduction of treatment with cytokines or other regulators of haemopoiesis. At a more fundamental level investigation of these rare conditions may lead to increased understanding of leukaemogenesis and even of the factors influencing the change from fetal to adult haemopoiesis.

REFERENCES

Appelbaum FR, Barrall J, Storb R et al (1990) Bone marrow transplantation for patients with myelodysplasia. Pretreatment variables and outcome. *Annals of Internal Medicine* **112:** 590–597.

Apperley JF, Mauro FR, Goldman JM et al (1988) Bone marrow transplantation for chronic myeloid leukaemia in first chronic phase: importance of a graft-versus-leukaemia effect. *British Journal of Haematology* **69:** 239–245.

Auerbach AD, Weiner MA & Warburton D (1982) Acute myeloid leukemia as the first hematologic manifestation of Fanconi anemia. *American Journal of Hematology* **12:** 289.

Bader JL & Miller RW (1978) Neurofibromatosis and childhood leukemia. *Journal of Pediatrics* **92:** 925–929.

Bain B (1991) Down's syndrome—transient abnormal myelopoiesis and acute leukaemia. *Leukemia and Lymphoma* **3:** 309–317.

Baranger L, Baruchel A, Leverger G et al (1990) Monosomy-7 in childhood hemopoietic disorders. *Leukemia* **4:** 345–349.

Barnett PLJ, Clark ACL & Garson OM (1990) Acute nonlymphocytic leukemia after transient myeloproliferative disorder in a patient with Down's syndrome. *Medical and Pediatric Oncology* **18:** 347–353.

Bennett JM, Catovsky D, Daniel MT et al (1982) Proposals for the classification of the myelodysplastic syndromes. *British Journal of Haematology* **51:** 189–199.

Blank J & Lange B (1981) Preleukemia in children. *Journal of Pediatrics* **98:** 565–568.

Brandwein JM, Horsman DE, Eaves AC et al (1990) Childhood myelodysplasia: suggested classification as myelodysplastic syndromes based on laboratory and clinical findings. *American Journal of Pediatric Hematology/Oncology* **12:** 63–70.

Bunn HF (1986) 5q- and disordered haematopoiesis. *Clinics in Haematology* **15:** 1023–1035.

Cannat A & Seligmann M (1973) Immunological abnormalities in juvenile myelomonocytic leukaemia. *British Medical Journal* **1:** 71–74.

Carroll WL, Morgan R & Glader BE (1985) Childhood bone marrow monosomy 7 syndrome: a familial disorder? *Journal of Pediatrics* **107:** 578–580.

Castro-Malaspina H, Schaison G, Passe S et al (1984) Subacute and chronic myelomonocytic leukemia in children (juvenile CML). *Cancer* **54:** 675–686.

Chan HSL, Estrov Z, Weitzman SS & Freedman MH (1987) The value of intensive combination chemotherapy for juvenile chronic myelogenous leukemia. *Journal of Clinical Oncology* **5:** 1960–1967.

Chan LC, Sheer D, Drysdale HC et al (1985) Monosomy 7 and multipotential stem cell transformation. *British Journal of Haematology* **61:** 531–539.

Cheson BD (1990) The myelodysplastic syndromes: current approaches to therapy. *Annals of Internal Medicine* **112:** 932–941.

Creutzig U, Cantu-Rajnoldi A, Ritter J et al (1987) Myelodysplastic syndromes in childhood. Report of 21 patients from Italy and West Germany. *American Journal of Pediatric Hematology/Oncology* **9:** 324–330.

De Witte T, Muus P, De Pauw B & Haanen C (1990) Intensive antileukemic treatment of patients younger than 65 years with myelodysplastic syndromes and secondary acute myelogenous leukemia. *Cancer* **66:** 831–837.

De Witte T, Zwaan F, Hermans J et al (1990) Allogeneic bone marrow transplantation for secondary leukaemia and myelodysplastic syndrome: a survey by the Leukaemia Working Party of the European Bone Marrow Transplantation Group (EMBTG). *British Journal of Haematology* **74:** 151–155.

Derbyshire PJ, Shortland DB, Swansbury JG et al (1987) A myeloproliferative disorder in two infants associated with eosinophilia and chromosome t(1;5) translocation. *British Journal of Haematology* **6:** 483–486.

Eguchi M, Sakakibara H, Suda J et al (1989) Ultrastructural and ultracytochemical differences between transient myeloproliferative disorder and megakaryoblastic leukaemia in Down's syndrome. *British Journal of Haematology* **73:** 315–322.

Evans JPM, Czepulkowski B, Gibbons B et al (1988) Childhood monosomy 7 revisited. *British Journal of Haematology* **69:** 41–45.

Festa RS, Shende A & Lanzkowsky P (1990) Juvenile chronic myelocytic leukaemia: experience with intensive combination chemotherapy. *Medical and Pediatric Oncology* **18:** 311–316.

Freedman MH, Estrov Z & Chan HSL (1988) Juvenile chronic myelogenous leukaemia. *American Journal of Pediatric Hematology/Oncology* **10:** 261–267.

Ganesan TS, Rassool F, Guo A-P et al (1986) Rearrangement of the *bcr* gene in Philadelphia chromosome-negative chronic myeloid leukaemia. *Blood* **68:** 957–960.

Gluckman E (1989) Bone marrow transplantation for Fanconi's anaemia. *Clinical Haematology* **2:** 153–162.

Goldman JM (ed.) (1987) *Chronic Myeloid Leukaemia.* London: Baillière Tindall.

Gualtieri RJ, Emanuel PD, Zuckerman KS et al (1989) Granulocyte–macrophage colony-stimulating factor is an endogenous regulator of cell proliferation in juvenile chronic myelogenous leukaemia. *Blood* **74:** 2360–2367.

Guinan EC, Tantravahi R & Weinstein HJ (1989) Bone marrow transplantation for children with myelodysplastic syndromes. *Blood* **73:** 619–622.

Gyger M, Bonny Y & Forest L (1982) Childhood monosomy 7 syndrome. *American Journal of Hematology* **13:** 329–334.

Hardisty RM, Speed DE & Till M (1964) Granulocytic leukaemia in childhood. *British Journal of Haematology* **10:** 551–566.

Hows JM & Bradley BA (1990) The use of unrelated marrow donors for transplantation. *British Journal of Haematology* **76:** 1–6.

Inaba T, Hayashi Y, Hanada R et al (1988) Childhood myelodysplastic syndromes with 11p15 translocation. *Cancer Genetics and Cytogenetics* **34:** 41–46.

Ingram L, Mott MG, Mann JR et al (1987) Second malignancies in children treated for non-Hodgkin's lymphoma and T-cell leukaemia with the UKCCSG regimens. *British Journal of Cancer* **55:** 463–466.

Jacobs A (1989) Oncogenes in the myelodysplastic syndrome. *Blood Reviews* **3:** 105–109.

Kaldor JM, Day NE, Clarke A et al (1990) Leukemia following Hodgkin's disease. *New England Journal of Medicine* **322:** 7–13.

Kaneko Y, Maseki N, Sakurai M et al (1989) Chromosome pattern in juvenile chronic myelogenous leukemia, myelodysplastic syndrome, and acute leukemia associated with neurofibromatosis. *Leukemia* **3:** 36–41.

Kere J, Ruutu T & de la Chapelle A (1987) Monosomy 7 in granulocytes and monocytes in myelodysplastic syndrome. *New England Journal of Medicine* **316:** 499–503.

Le Beau MM, Albain KS, Larson RA et al (1986) Clinical and cytogenetic correlations in 63 patients with therapy related myelodysplastic syndromes and acute non-lymphocytic leukemias: further incidence for characteristic abnormalities of chromosome numbers 5 and 7. *Journal of Clinical Oncology* **4:** 325–345.

Leiper AD, Stanhope R, Lau T et al (1987) The effect of total body irradiation and bone marrow transplantation during childhood and adolescence on growth and endocrine function. *British Journal of Haematology* **67:** 419–426.

Levine EG & Bloomfield CD (1986) Secondary myelodysplastic syndromes and leukaemias. *Clinics in Haematology* **15:** 1037–1080.

Levitt GA, Stiller CA & Chessells JM (1990) Prognosis of Down's syndrome with acute leukaemia. *Archives of Disease in Childhood* **65:** 212–216.

Lilleyman JS, Harrison JF & Black JA (1977) Treatment of juvenile chronic myeloid leukemia with sequential subcutaneous cytarabine and oral mercaptopurine. *Blood* **49:** 559–562.

List AF, Garewal HS & Sandberg AA (1990) The myelodysplastic syndromes: biology and implications for management. *Journal of Clinical Oncology* **8:** 1424–1441.

McGlave PB, Beatty P, Ash R & Hows JM (1990) Therapy for chronic myelogenous leukemia with unrelated donor bone marrow transplantation: results in 102 cases. *Blood* 1728–1732.

Mays JA, Neerhout RC, Bagby GC & Koler RD (1980) Juvenile chronic granulocytic leukemia. *American Journal of Disease in Childhood* **134:** 654–658.

Mufti GJ & Galton DAG (1986) Myelodysplastic syndromes: natural history and features of prognostic importance. *Clinics in Haematology* **15:** 953–971.

Mufti GJ, Stevens JR, Oscier DG et al (1985) Myelodysplastic syndromes: a scoring system with prognostic significance. *British Journal of Haematology* **59:** 425–433.

Nix WL & Fernbach DJ (1981) Myeloproliferative diseases in childhood. *American Journal of Pediatric Hematology/Oncology* **3:** 397–407.

Nowell P, Bergman G, Besa E et al (1984) Progressive preleukemia with a chromosomally abnormal clone in a kindred with the Estren–Dameshek variant of Fanconi's anemia. *Blood* **64:** 1135–1138.

Paul B, Reid MM, Davison EV et al (1987) Familial myelodysplasia: progressive disease associated with emergence of monosomy 7. *British Journal of Haematology* **65:** 321–323.

Phillips M, Richards S & Chessells JM (1991) Acute myeloid leukaemia in childhood: the costs and benefits of intensive treatment. *British Journal of Haematology* **77:** 473–477.

Pugh WC, Pearson M, Vardiman JW & Rowley JD (1985) Philadelphia chromosome-negative chronic myelogenous leukaemia: a morphological reassessment. *British Journal of Haematology* **60:** 457–467.

Pui CH, Behm FG, Raimondi SC et al (1989) Secondary acute myeloid leukemia in children treated for acute lymphoid leukemia. *New England Journal of Medicine* **321:** 136–142.

Randall DL, Reiquam CW, Githens JH & Robinson A (1965) Familial myeloproliferative disease. *American Journal of Disease in Childhood* **110:** 479–490.

Ruutu P, Ruutu T, Vuopio P et al (1977) Defective chemotaxis in monosomy 7. *Nature* **265:** 146–147.

Sanders JE, Pritchard S, Mahoney P et al (1986) Growth and development following marrow transplantation for leukemia. *Blood* **68:** 1129–1135.

Sanders JE, Buckner CD, Thomas ED et al (1988) Allogeneic marrow transplantation for children with juvenile chronic myelogenous leukemia. *Blood* **71:** 1144–1146.

Schwartz CL & Cohen HJ (1988) Preleukaemic syndromes and other syndromes predisposing to leukemia. *Pediatric Clinics of North America* **35:** 853–871.

Shannon K, Nunez G, Dow LW et al (1986) Juvenile chronic myelogenous leukemia: surface antigen phenotyping by monoclonal antibodies and cytogenetic studies. *Pediatrics* **77:** 330–335.

Sieff CA, Chessells JM, Harvey BAM et al (1981) Monosomy 7 in childhood: a myelo-proliferative disorder. *British Journal of Haematology* **49:** 235–249.

Sutherland GR, Baker E, Callen DF et al (1988) Interleukin-5 is at 5q31 and is deleted in the 5q syndrome. *Blood* **71:** 1150–1152.

Teasdale JM, Worth AJ & Corey MJ (1970) A missing group C chromosome in the bone marrow cells of three children with myeloproliferative disease. *Cancer* **25:** 1468–1477.

Tefferi A, Thibodeau SN & Solberg LA Jr (1990) Clonal studies in the myelodysplastic syndrome using X-linked restriction fragment length polymorphisms. *Blood* **75:** 1770–1773.

Third MIC Cooperative Study Group (1988) Recommendations for a morphologic, immuno-logic, and cytogenetic (MIC) working classification of the primary and therapy-related myelodysplastic disorders. *Cancer Genetics and Cytogenetics* **32:** 1–10.

Travis SF (1983) Fetal erythropoiesis in juvenile chronic myelocytic leukemia. *Blood* **62:** 602–605.

Tutschka PJ, Copelan EA & Klein JP (1987) Bone marrow transplantation for leukemia following a new busulfan and cyclophosphamide regimen. *Blood* **70:** 1382–1388.

Urban C, Schwinger W, Slavc I et al (1990) Busulfan/cyclophosphamide plus bone marrow transplantation is not sufficient to eradicate the malignant clone in juvenile chronic myelogenous leukemia. *Bone Marrow Transplantation* **5:** 353–356.

Weatherall DJ, Edwards JA & Donohoe WTA (1968) Haemoglobin and red cell enzyme changes in juvenile chronic myeloid leukaemia. *British Medical Journal* **1:** 679–681.

Wegelius R (1986) Preleukaemic states in children. *Scandinavian Journal of Haematology* **36:** 133–139.

Weinberg RS, Leibowitz D, Weinblatt ME et al (1990) Juvenile chronic myelogenous leukaemia: the only example of truly fetal (not fetal-like) erythropoiesis. *British Journal of Haematology* **76:** 307–310.

Weiss K, Stass S, Williams D et al (1987) Childhood monosomy 7 syndrome: clinical and in vitro studies. *Leukemia* **1:** 97–104.

Woods WG, Roloff JS, Lukens JN & Krivit W (1981) The occurrence of leukemia in patients with the Schwachman syndrome. *Journal of Pediatrics* **99:** 425–428.

Woods WG, Nesbit ME, Buckley J et al (1985) Correlation of chromosome abnormalities with patient characteristics, histologic subtype, and induction success in children with acute nonlymphocytic leukemia. *Journal of Clinical Oncology* **3:** 3–11.

8

Bone marrow transplant for acute leukaemia

NORMA K. C. RAMSAY
STELLA DAVIES

Improvement in chemotherapy protocols for the treatment of childhood leukaemias has made the cure of these previously lethal diseases possible. However, some children with acute lymphoblastic leukaemia (ALL), and most children with acute non-lymphoblastic leukaemia (ANLL), relapse after chemotherapy. For these children bone marrow transplantation (BMT) offers the possibility of cure.

The first successful bone marrow transplants for acute leukaemia were reported in the 1970s, and though results were poor some patients with very advanced disease achieved long-term survival. Since this time, accumulation of experience and development of new techniques has greatly improved outcome.

Substantial research is currently directed towards further improving the results of BMT. Conditioning regimens are being developed to decrease the incidence of post-BMT leukaemic relapse, the major cause of transplant failure. Numerous studies seek new strategies for prevention of graft-versus-host disease (GVHD), another cause of adverse outcomes. Improved techniques are being developed for histocompatibility testing, in order to increase success of transplantation from unrelated donors. Recombinantly produced cytokines, recently available for clinical use, are starting to be applied to BMT and may significantly hasten engraftment and reduce relapse, although this latter claim requires verification.

This chapter will discuss BMT as therapy for acute leukaemias, including donor selection, BMT procedures, results and complications. The emphasis will be on recent developments and future directions.

INDICATIONS FOR BMT

The indications for BMT in leukaemia remain controversial. The debate has been rendered more complex by the ongoing development of new BMT techniques.

ALL in remission

Most children with ALL can be cured with chemotherapy and BMT is not

Baillière's Clinical Haematology—
Vol. 4, No. 2, April 1991
ISBN 0–7020–1532–6

required in first remission. ALL is, however, an extremely heterogeneous disease, and some patients (e.g., those with acquired clonal chromosomal abnormalities including t(4;11) and Philadelphia chromosome positive ALL and infants with leukaemias) are at high risk of relapse when treated with chemotherapy alone (Blume et al, 1987; Buckner et al, 1987; McCarthy et al, 1988a; Bordigoni et al, 1989). BMT has been used successfully in first remission in these groups. Studies of high-risk patients necessarily contain small numbers of patients and results can rarely be compared with the results of chemotherapy. It seems likely, however, that BMT is appropriate in first remission for some patients with ALL.

Relapsed ALL

The prognosis for children with ALL who relapse is poor with conventional chemotherapy. It has been proposed, however, that BMT is limited in its ability to improve survival in relapsed ALL, and the interpretation of data comparing BMT with chemotherapy has been difficult. Studies comparing BMT with chemotherapy are hard to control because many variables (e.g. age, risk factors at diagnosis, initial treatment, duration of first remission, timing of relapse) must be considered. In addition, patients who survive long enough to reach BMT all have achieved second remission, so they probably comprise a better risk group than patients undergoing chemotherapy alone, who may never achieve a remission.

Review of published series by Butturini et al (1987) does indicate that BMT is superior to chemotherapy in patients who relapse within 18 months of diagnosis whilst receiving maintenance chemotherapy. If a donor is available, these patients probably should receive BMT. This conclusion is supported by data showing improved survival after BMT in second remission compared with chemotherapy (Sanders et al, 1987). BMT was not clearly superior to chemotherapy in patients who relapse more than 18 months after the start of first remission and these patients may become long-term survivors with chemotherapy alone (Rivera et al, 1986). There is a need for careful studies of comparable groups of patients to answer this question clearly.

ANLL

Patients with ANLL are less likely than patients with ALL to achieve cure with chemotherapy. For these patients the best results are obtained with allogeneic transplant in first remission if a related HLA-matched donor is available. Disease-free survival of 40–60% is reported (Feig et al, 1987; Helenglass et al, 1988; McGlave et al, 1988; Geller et al, 1989; Niethammer et al, 1990). For patients without a suitable allogeneic donor autografting is possible. There are no current data comparing results of autografting with those of chemotherapy, although studies are under way to address this issue.

DONOR SELECTION

Related donors

Allogeneic BMT is, in most cases, performed with bone marrow from a sibling who is matched at the major histocompatibility complex (MHC). MHC is a family of genes located on chromosome 6, normally inherited as a single group or haplotype. The products of these genes are membrane-associated glyco-proteins called human leukocyte-associated (HLA) antigens. HLA antigens play a central role in immune recognition and in presentation of foreign antigen. HLA antigens must be matched to reduce the incidence of GVHD and immune-mediated graft rejection. The likelihood of a sibling match (one in four) and current family sizes indicate that at most one third of patients will have an HLA-matched sibling donor. For this reason, donor programmes using unrelated HLA-matched donors and autologous BMT are being developed in many centres.

HLA antigens are divided into class I molecules (HLA A, B and C) and class II molecules (HLA DR, DP and DQ). The MHC locus is extremely polymorphic and a total of 79 alleles for class I loci and 18 DR, 9 DQ and 6 DP alleles for class II loci have been described (reviewed in Kaminski, 1989). MHC genes are co-dominant, so both alleles are significant.

Traditionally, HLA has been typed using serological techniques that define the HLA phenotype at the A, B, C and some D loci. Specificity is improving as monoclonal antibodies are replacing polyclonal sera in tissue-typing panels.

Typing of class II antigens is often more problematic than the typing of class I antigens. Serology may give equivocal results due to a lack of appropriate monospecific sera or may be impossible due to low circulating numbers of B cells, on which class II molecules are expressed, in leukaemic patients. Thus, another technique for demonstrating tissue compatibility, mixed lymphocyte culture (MLC), is often used. In MLC, donor and recipient cells are exposed to each other in varying ratios and lymphocyte proliferation is measured. The ideal bone marrow donor is both HLA-identical and MLC non-reactive.

Unrelated donors

Because the MHC genes are closely linked and recombination is rare, a phenotypically identical sibling is likely to also be genotypically identical. Thus when typing siblings who are HLA A and B identical, there is a 95% chance that they will be identical at all loci and MLC non-reactive. This is not the case for unrelated donors, who may be phenotypically identical at all major loci, but genotypically quite different. Increased use of unrelated donors has led to much work on improving HLA-typing techniques, particularly for class II genes.

DNA hybridization techniques, or restriction fragment length poly-morphisms (RFLP), represent one such improvement. In this procedure, probes for class II genes are radiolabelled and hybridized with DNA immobilized by Southern blotting. This produces a series of characteristic banding patterns that can be used to compare genotypes. However, some loci cannot be distinguished by RFLP, and while mismatched RFLP reliably predict a positive MLC reaction, matched RFLP do not reliably predict a negative MLC reaction (Clay et al, 1989).

Some class II differences not detected by RFLP analysis can be detected by oligotyping which hybridizes highly specific oligonucleotide probes to DNA (Angelini et al, 1986). Oligonucleotide probes are available for many class II antigens and more may be developed as this region is further characterized. This technique may be suitable for large-scale donor typing since many oligonucleotide probes can be used simultaneously and the procedure is less time consuming than MLC.

Another predictor of histocompatibility is the cytotoxic lymphocyte precursor (CTL-P) assay which involves priming donor lymphocytes against patient lymphocytes and testing for cytotoxicity. The in vitro frequency of alloreactive cytotoxic lymphocytes in the donor's peripheral blood is then estimated. This is related to the degree of HLA mismatch and the probability of GVHD after transplant (Kaminski et al, 1989).

In addition to the well-characterized HLA antigens others, termed minor histocompatibility antigens, exist and may be the reason for GVHD or occasional graft rejection in what appear to be well-matched donor–recipient pairs (Voogt et al, 1990).

Increased use of unrelated bone marrow donors has resulted in the establishment of registries of typed potential donors. The probability of matching is sigmoidally related to registry size (Sonnenberg et al, 1989). An important determinant of required registry size is the heterogeneity between the recipient and the donor pools. It has been calculated that a registry size of 100 000 donors offers a probability of 58% of finding a match and that further increases in registry size offer little increase in likelihood of finding a match because of current limitations in HLA typing.

Mismatched donors

Although the ideal bone marrow donor is fully HLA-matched and MLC non-reactive, successful transplants have been performed with donors with varying degrees of mismatch and with haploidentical donors (Trigg et al, 1989). However, GVHD and graft rejection occur at higher rates than those seen with well-matched donors.

Autologous BMT

For patients without an allogeneic donor, autologous transplantation is an option. In this process, the patient's own bone marrow is harvested and cryopreserved, then ablative chemotherapy is administered to the patient. The procedure is well tolerated, generally with rapid engraftment, low mortality and no GVHD. Various purging techniques have been used to try to eliminate leukaemic cells from the re-infused marrow, including chemotherapy and treatment with monoclonal antibodies and immunotoxins, but there remains a high rate of post-transplant relapse.

Autologous engraftment has been achieved using peripheral blood stem cells harvested by leukapheresis. Theoretically this reduces the chance of reseeding the donor marrow with tumour, though this remains to be proven in clinical practice (Lasky et al, 1990).

CONDITIONING AND BONE MARROW PURGING

Conditioning

A successful BMT for leukaemia requires conditioning to eradicate all leukaemic cells from the recipient. Conditioning regimens consist of ablative doses of chemotherapy with or without radiotherapy. The most widely used conditioning regimen is cyclophosphamide plus total body irradiation (TBI).

Initially, TBI was given as a single dose, but more recently fractionated radiotherapy regimens have been developed. In vitro data suggest that this reduces radiation-induced toxicity, a major cause of post-transplant morbidity and mortality. Hyperfractionated TBI, administered in 11 fractions three times daily, may give further protection from radiation-induced toxicity, particularly interstitial pneumonitis (Brochstein et al, 1987).

Leukaemic relapse after allogeneic BMT most likely reflects failure of the conditioning regimen to eradicate all remaining leukaemic cells from the body. A significant proportion of morbidity and mortality secondary to bone marrow transplant is due to conditioning therapy, so less toxic and more effective regimens are needed.

Many different drugs, with or without radiation, have been used for conditioning in an attempt to find a superior regimen. Although conditioning regimens which include epipodophyllotoxins (VP16) or cytarabine are encouraging in some situations, animal studies suggest that these agents are less immunosuppressive, and so inferior in preventing graft rejection, than cyclophosphamide (Gassman et al, 1988). This is supported by early clinical data (Schmitz et al, 1988) and should be considered when selecting conditioning for patients at high risk of rejection (e.g., HLA-mismatched transplants).

Marrow purging

It has been suggested that the high rate of leukaemic relapse after autologous BMT is due to reinfusion of leukaemic cells with the bone marrow. Various strategies have been employed to remove these cells, including ex vivo treatment of marrow with drugs, with monoclonal antibodies directed at leukaemic cells, with antibodies conjugated to toxins and with combinations of these (DeFabritiis et al, 1985; Uckun et al, 1987; Ball et al, 1990).

The drugs 4-hydroperoxycyclophosphamide (4HC) and mafosfamide, analogues of cyclophosphamide that do not require hepatic activation, have received the most clinical attention. Studies in rats indicate that ex vivo

Table 1. Allogeneic BMT in patients with ALL.

Reference	Centre/group	Patient no's and remission status	Conditioning	Follow-up (months) median or range	Age (yr) median or range	Leukaemia-free survival	
						Patient no's	Actuarial (%)
Barrett et al (1989)	IBMTR*	56 CR1 218 CR2	TBI ± CTX ± Ara-C ± other	21	13 CR1 15 CR2	37/56 NA	56 CR1 26 CR2
Doney et al (1987)	Seattle	46 CR1	TBI/CTX ± other	12–108	22	15/46	28
Sanders et al (1987)	Seattle	57 CR2	TBI/CTX	17–124	3–17	22/57	40
Weisdorf et al (1987)	Minnesota	14 CR1 26 CR2 + 3	TBI/CTX	42	14.2	13/40	29
Brochstein et al (1987)	Memorial Sloan Kettering	31 CR2 12 CR3 16 CR4 R	TBI/CTX	61 64 74	8.1 9.8 9.0	20/31 5/12 4/16	64 CR2 42 CR3 23 CR4 R
Niethammer et al (1990)	Federal Republic of Germany	8 CR1 121 CR2 + 36 R, NR	TBI ± CTX ± VP16 ± BCNU/Ara-C, Bu/CTX, BU VP16	NA	>18	NA	33
Bordigoni et al (1989)	France	32 CR1	TBI ± CTX ± other	30	13.5	27/32	84.4
Coccia et al (1988)	Case Western Reserve	20 CR2,3	TBI/Ara-C	12–78	7.2	8/20	NA
Blume et al (1987)	City of Hope	5 CR2,3 8 R	TBI/VP16	101 days–387 days	15.8	7/13	NA

* IBMTR, International Bone Marrow Transplant Registry; NA, not available; CTX, cyclophosphamide; Bu, busulphan; R, relapse; NR, non-responder; CR, complete remission; TBI, total body irradiation; BCNU, 1,3-bis(2-chloroethyl)-1-nitrosourea.

incubation with 4HC depletes leukaemic cells without destroying bone marrow stem cells (Sharkis et al, 1980). Clinical trials of 4HC have shown good engraftment with doses up to 100 μg ml^{-1} (Kaizer et al, 1985). In vitro studies of various other drugs have found none to be superior to 4HC, although some benefit might be gained from the addition of vincristine to the protocol (Auber et al, 1988).

Various monoclonal antibodies directed against T- and B-cell surface antigens have been used to purge bone marrow (reviewed in Ramsay and Kersey, 1988). Cell lysis by antibody can be achieved by adding complement or conjugating antibody to a toxin such as ricin-A or pokeweed antiviral protein (Simonsson et al, 1988; Preijers et al, 1989; Ball et al, 1990).

Despite extensive interest in marrow purging, there are no conclusive data showing that it improves leukaemia-free survival. The finding that syngeneic twin transplants relapse at a rate similar to that of autografts, and mathematical models of minimal residual disease (Schultz et al, 1989) suggest that re-infusion of leukaemic cells does not play a major role in post-transplant relapse. However, review of 263 ANLL patients treated with autologous BMT, 69 of whom received marrow purged with mafosfamide, suggest an advantage for the purging procedure (Gorin et al, 1990a). Further randomized study is required if the value of bone marrow purging is to be proven.

OUTCOME OF BMT

ALL/allogeneic BMT

Recent results of allogeneic transplant in patients with ALL are shown in Table 1. Long-term survival for children transplanted in first remission is generally better than 50%; Bordigoni et al (1989) reported 5-year actuarial survival of 84%. Leukaemia-free survival in patients in second remission is much poorer, around 20–40%, though Brochstein et al (1987) reported actuarial survival of 64%.

ALL/autologous BMT

Autologous BMT for ALL carries a significantly lower procedure-related mortality than allogeneic BMT; 6% compared with 24% in the series of Weisdorf et al (1987); due largely to more rapid engraftment and to the absence of GVHD. Despite these advantages, leukaemia-free survival remains poor, particularly in patients in second and higher remissions (Table 2). Most deaths are due to leukaemic relapse in patients with highly resistant disease. Such patients require new approaches to their disease such as the use of biological response modifiers or allogeneic transplant from an unrelated donor to gain the benefit of the graft-versus-leukaemia effect.

ANLL/allogeneic BMT

Results of allogeneic BMT in patients with ANLL in first remission are good

Table 2. Autologous BMT in patients with ALL.

Reference	Centre/group	Patient no's and remission status	Conditioning	Purging agent	Follow-up (months) median or range	Age (yr) median or range	Leukaemia-free survival Patient no's	Leukaemia-free survival Actuarial (%)
Gorin et al (1990b)	EBMTR*	160 CR1 SR 73 CR1 HR 167 CR2 SR 38 CR2 HR	NA	Chemotherapy and/or Mabs + C or no purge	30	15	NA	42 CR1 SR 41 CR1 HR 31 CR2 SR 23 CR2 HR 18
Weisdorf et al (1990)	Minnesota	9 CR1 103 CR2+	TBI/CTX, TBI/ Ara-C	Anti CD24, CD10 + C ± 4HC T-lineage: immunotoxin ± 4HC	NA	9	NA	18
Sallan et al (1989)	Boston	1 CR1 43 CR2,3+	TBI/Ara-C/ VM26 ± L-Asp	Anti CD10± Anti CD9 + C	NA	7.5	15/44	29
Simonsson et al (1989)	Uppsala/ Glasgow London	21 CR1 32 CR2,3 1 R	TBI ± CTX ± Ara-C ± Pred/ VM26/Dauno/ VCR ± Melphalan	Anti CD10, 1987 + C	16 CR1 18.5 CR2,3 R	27 CR1 9 CR2,3 R	15/21 14/32	65 CR1 32 CR2,3 R
Kaizer et al (1985)	Johns Hopkins	1 CR1 13 CR2 7 PR	TBI/CTX	4HC dose escalation	>24	4-37	2/21	NA
Zintl et al (1990)	Univ. of Jena GDR	6 CR1 9 CR2,3	TBI/CTX or TBI/Bu	NK or Mab + C (n = 1)	NA	7.5	10/15	43
Preijers et al (1989)	Amsterdam	5 CR1 2 CR2,3	TBI/CTX or TBI/ Melphalan	Anti CD7 immunotoxin	NA	21	2/7	NA

* EBMTR, European Bone Marrow Transplant Registry; SR, standard risk; HR, high risk; PR, partial remission; Mab, monoclonal antibody; C, complement; 4HC, 4-hydroxycyclophosphamide; L-ASP, L-asparaginase; VCR, vincristine; Dauno, daunorubicin; CD, cluster designation.

Table 3. Allogeneic BMT in patients with ANLL.

Reference	Centre/group	Patient no's and remission status	Conditioning	Follow-up (months) median or range	Age (yr) median or range	Leukaemia-free survival	
						Patient no's	Actuarial (%)
Feig et al (1987)	CCSG*	67 CR1	TBI/CTX ± Ara-C, Bu/CTX	>1300 days	10	NA	53
McGlave et al (1988)	Minnesota	73 CR1	TBI/CTX	40	16.9	47/73	61
Clift et al (1987)	Seattle	231 CR1 49 CR2 54 R 29 NR	TBI/CTX	NA	1–53	107/231 CR1 13/49 CR2 17/54 R 6/29 NR	46 28 30 21
Helenglass et al (1988)	Royal Marsden Hospital, UK	63 CR1	TBI/CTX or TBI/Melphalan	12–60	25	34/63	NA
Geller et al (1989)	Johns Hopkins	49 CR1 50 CR2,3 R	Bu/CTX	NA	26	NA	45 CR1 31 CR2,3 R
Niethammer et al (1990)	Federal Republic of Germany	18 CR1 27 CR2+	TBI ± CTX ± VP16 ± BCNU/Ara-C, Bu/VP16, Bu/CTX	NA	<18	NA	48 CR1 28 CR2+
Dahl et al (1990)	Memphis/ Sacramento/ Chicago/ Seattle	19 CR1	TBI/CTX	54–79	11.3	9/19	43
Snyder et al (1988)	City of Hope	25 CR1	TBI/CTX	NA	23	13/25	50
Bostrom et al (1990)	Minnesota	2 CR1 11 R	TBI/CTX/VP16	20	3–44	7/13	NA
Johnson et al (1988)	Seattle/Memphis	11 CR1	TBI/CTX	42–165	5 months– 24 months	7/11	NA

* CCSG, Childrens Cancer Study Group. See Tables 1 and 2 for explanation of abbreviations.

with leukaemia-free survival of 61% reported in a series of 73 children and adults (McGlave et al, 1988). Results of recent series are summarized in Table 3. Allogeneic BMT can even cure patients transplanted in relapse, albeit in a minority of patients. Increasingly, patients with ANLL are receiving busulphan and cyclophosphamide conditioning. These regimens may provide the same results as cyclophosphamide and TBI (Tutschka et al, 1987). Further data are needed to evaluate this regimen fully.

Results of BMT in first remission must always be compared with results of chemotherapy alone. Lange et al (1990) showed 5-year event-free survival to be significantly superior for BMT over chemotherapy for treatment of ANLL (47% versus 32%). Hermans et al (1989) compared leukaemia-free survival after chemotherapy, allogeneic BMT and autologous BMT in 871 patients in first complete remission of ANLL. They showed a trend in favour of BMT, particularly allogeneic BMT. However, these data should be interpreted cautiously since they represent retrospective analysis of non-randomized patients treated in many centres on non-standardized protocols.

ANLL/autologous BMT

Autologous BMT results in significantly lower leukaemia-free survival than allogenic BMT for ANLL, but has the advantage of being available to all who achieve remission (Table 4). Studies are currently in progress comparing autologous BMT in first remission ANLL with conventional chemotherapy.

Autologous BMT in second remission ANLL can produce long-term survival in patients who are only rarely cured with chemotherapy. In addition, autologous BMT can produce 'inversions', remissions that are longer than the longest pre-transplant remission (Meloni et al, 1989). Randomized trials currently in progress should clarify the role of autologous BMT in ANLL.

The value of bone marrow purging prior to autografting remains unproven, though there is some data supporting a beneficial effect of purging on leukaemia-free survival in ANLL (Gorin et al, 1990a). Purging with chemotherapy does not appear to delay engraftment (Cahn et al, 1986; Rosenfeld et al, 1989).

Post-BMT relapse and chemotherapy

Patients who relapse after BMT, by definition, have resistant disease. Surprisingly, long remissions can sometimes still be achieved with standard chemotherapy. Bostrom et al (1987) described re-induction with conventional (non-experimental) chemotherapy of 52 patients with ALL who relapsed post-BMT. Complete remission occurred in 56% of patients, and survival ranged up to 4.7 years. Mortimer et al (1989) described 20 of 62 patients with post-BMT relapsed ANLL who achieved complete remission with chemotherapy and had a median survival of 6 months. In the same study, 52 of 94 patients with post-BMT relapsed ALL achieved complete remission and had a median survival of 10.5 months.

Table 4. Autologous BMT in patients with ANLL.

Reference	Centre/group	Patient no's and remission status	Conditioning	Purging agent	Follow-up (months) median or range	Age (yr) median or range	Leukaemia-free survival	
							Patient no's	Actuarial (%)
Gorin et al (1990b)	EBMTR	448 CR1 SR 72 CR1 HR 145 CR2 SR 14 CR2 HR	TBI/CTX; TBI/other; UCH; Bu/CTX; BAVC	29% CR1SR 32% CR1HR 42% CR2SR 64% CR2HR Technique unspecified	NA	1-65	NA	36 CR1SR 33 CR1HR 30 CR2SR 28 CR2HR
Rosenfeld et al (1989)	Pittsburgh/Johns Hopkins	24 CR2,34 R	TBI/CTX; Bu/CTX ± Ara-C	4HC	112-615 days	33	4/24	19
Rowley et al (1989)	Johns Hopkins	8 CR1 37 CR2,3	Bu/CTX	4HC	43-722 days	2-53	13/45	NA
Stewart et al (1985)	Seattle	13 CR1	TBI/CTX	None	26-50	14-37	3/13	22
Carella et al (1988)	Genova, Italy	25 CR1	TBI/CTX	None	25	15-51	13/25	NA
Löwenberg et al (1990)	Netherlands	32 CR1	TBI/CTX	None	NA	15-60	12/32	35
Spinolo et al (1988)	MD Anderson, Texas	19 CR1	CTX/BCNU/VP16	None	30	NA	11/19	58
Cahn et al (1986)	France	18 CR1 6 CR1	6TG/Ara-C/CCNU/CTX; TBI/CTX	Mafostamide (16/18)	2.5-47	23.7	8/18	NA
Ball et al (1990)	Dartmouth, Scripps, San Diego	6 CR1 24 CR2,3	TBI/CTX; BU/CTX; BU/VP-16	Mab's + C	NA	11-57	4/6 CR1 6/24 CR2,3	67 CR1 29 CR2 23 CR3
Michel et al (1988)	Marseilles, France	11 CR1	Melphalan; BMT ×2	None	15-56	10	7/11	NA
Meloni et al (1989, 1990)	Rome, Italy	39 CR1 22 CR2	BAVC or CTX/TBI	None	30-63 24	5-48 24	20/39 15/22	51 67

6TG, 6-thioguanine; BAVC, BCNU, amsacrine, etoposide, and Ara-C; UCH, CTX, BCNU, Ara-C, 6TG, and ADR; SR, standard risk; HR, high risk. See Tables 1 and 2 for explanation of abbreviations.

Second transplants

Second BMT has been used to treat relapse after allogeneic BMT. Sanders et al (1988a) described 26 leukaemic patients who received second transplants at a median of 26 months after first BMT. Five patients (19%) were surviving free of leukaemia at a median of 26 months and two were alive with disease. Six of the seven survivors had received a second transplant more than 2 years after their first; it appeared that patients who relapse within 1 year of BMT gained little benefit from a second transplant.

GRAFT VERSUS HOST DISEASE

Graft-versus-host disease (GVHD) is a major cause of morbidity and mortality after allogeneic BMT. Even in BMT between HLA-matched, MLC non-reactive siblings, acute GVHD occurs in 30–70% of patients, and is a primary or contributing cause of death in 15–40% of cases. Death due to GVHD is most commonly due to infection secondary to GVHD-induced immunosuppression.

GVHD arises when donor cells (generally cytotoxic T-cells) attack recipient cells. It occurs in both acute and chronic forms which appear to be clinically and pathologically distinct entities (reviewed in Snover, 1984).

Acute GVHD

Acute GVHD normally occurs between 20 and 100 days post-BMT and is largely restricted to skin, liver and gastrointestinal tract (Table 5). The chief pathological feature is destruction of epithelium with a scant inflammatory response. The limited tissue involvement of acute GVHD suggests that the process may be more complex than attack by donor cytotoxic T-cells on host

Table 5. Clinical features of graft-versus-host disease in BMT patients. From Ramsay (1989).

System	Acute	Chronic
Skin	Maculopapular rash Erythroderma Desquamation and bullae	Pigmentary changes Thickening of the skin Scleroderma Nail changes
Liver	Jaundice	± Jaundice
Gastrointestinal tract	Diarrhoea Abdominal pain Nausea, vomiting	Dysphagia Weight loss Oral dryness and ulcers
Eye	—	Photophobia Eye pain Dry eyes
Lung	—	Symptoms of obstructive lung disease
Other	—	Myasthenia gravis Vaginal strictures/stenosis

HLA antigens; animal models have demonstrated that histoincompatibility is not a prerequisite for acute GVHD (Elson et al, 1977).

Other mechanisms for the epithelial damage seen in acute GVHD have been proposed. The 'innocent bystander' theory suggests that the epithelial damage is due to release of lymphokines or cytotoxic agents during inter-action between host and donor lymphoid cells, leading to damage of adjacent epithelial surfaces. The 'NK cell' theory attributes epithelial damage to loss of lymphocyte suppressor function, allowing interaction of NK (natural killer) cells with host tissues (Dokhelar et al, 1981). Experi-mental and clinical evidence supports both theories and it is possible that both play a role.

Chronic GVHD

Chronic GVHD involves a much wider range of organs than acute GVHD and a much more marked inflammatory response, perhaps reflecting increased immunocompetence later in the post-BMT course. The more generalized organ involvement of chronic GVHD suggests that histo-incompatibility probably plays a more important role than in acute GVHD.

Acute GVHD is a major risk factor for the development of chronic GVHD; around 60% of chronic GVHD cases are preceded by acute GVHD. However, the determinants of progression from acute to chronic disease is not well understood.

Risk factors

Risk factors for the occurrence of GVHD were analysed in a large series of patients who received marrow from HLA-matched siblings (Bortin, 1987). The highest relative risk was in transplants from female donors to male recipients, suggesting that the male minor histocompatibility antigen H-Y is a major target for GVHD. Other risk factors included failure to receive methotrexate post-transplant, receipt of trimethoprim–sulfamethoxazole in the peri-transplant period, increased receipt of transfusions post-transplant and increasing age. The effect of increasing age was modest in this study, but others have shown this to be a strong predictor of GVHD (Ramsay et al, 1982).

Prophylaxis

Much effort has been directed towards prevention of GVHD. The two techniques used for GVHD prophylaxis are post-BMT immunosuppression with drugs and in vitro depletion of T-cells from the donor marrow. Early work in dogs showed that methotrexate post-BMT reduces GVHD. Lazarus and coworkers (1984) showed no significant difference in GVHD when patients were non-randomly assigned to receive methotrexate or no prophylaxis post-BMT, although the incidence of GVHD was unusually high in both groups. The necessity for post-BMT GVHD prophylaxis was confirmed, however, by a report of hyperacute GVHD in patients given no immunosuppression (Sullivan et al, 1986).

Attempts have been made to improve GVHD prophylaxis with various combinations of cyclosporin A, antithymocyte globulin (ATG) and steroids, with and without methotrexate. The multiple regimens attest to the fact that all are in some way unsatisfactory.

Because GVHD starts with activation of donor lymphocytes by recipient antigens, T-cell depletion was developed as a means of combating GVHD. T-cell depletion can be achieved in a number of ways, including physical ones (e.g. elutriation and E-rosetting) and the more widely-used immune-mediated depletion with antibody plus complement or antibody conjugated to toxin. Refinements in technology mean that T-cell depletion is now very efficient, with three-log depletion easily achievable.

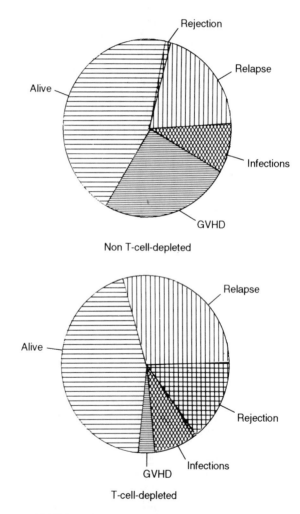

Figure 1. Outcome of BMT in patients receiving T-cell depleted and non T-cell depleted bone marrow. From Poynton (1988) with permission.

Initial experience with T-cell depleted marrow grafts showed an impressive reduction in frequency and severity of GVHD. Franceschini et al (1987) found that in 31 centres using T-cell depletion, moderate to severe GVHD declined from 45 to 11% in well-matched transplants and from 75 to 38% in partially matched transplants. Unfortunately, this reduction in GVHD has not been translated into improved leukaemia-free survival because of increased rates of graft rejection and relapse after T-cell depleted transplants (reviewed in Poynton, 1988). Changes in the pattern of complications seen with T-depleted and non-T-depleted transplants are illustrated in Figure 1.

GVHD and relapses

Leukaemic relapse occurs less frequently in patients with GVHD. This effect has been termed 'graft-versus-leukaemia' (GVL), and it is not clear to what extent this is separable from GVHD. CML patients with or without GVHD who receive T-cell-depleted BMT have a higher probability of relapse than patients with or without GVHD receiving non-T-depleted allogeneic BMT, suggesting an antileukaemic effect independent of GVHD (Horowitz et al, 1990). Truitt et al (1986) found in animal models that it is possible to manipulate GVHD to enhance GVL, raising the hope that it may be possible to retain GVL effects while reducing GVHD.

Treatment

Treatment of acute GVHD requires immunosuppression to control immune-mediated attack on host tissues and to allow development of immunological tolerance. The mainstays of therapy have been corticosteroids, ATG and cyclosporin A. Anti-T-cell monoclonal antibodies and immunotoxins also have been used (Morgan et al, 1987; Kernan et al, 1988).

Analysis of 197 patients with acute GVHD treated with corticosteroids with or without ATG, cyclosporin A and anti-T-cell immunotoxin showed that 41% achieved complete and continuing remission of GVHD (Weisdorf et al, 1990). Of the 197 patients, 70% went on to develop chronic GVHD, but control of GVHD did not appear to affect the risk of leukaemic relapse. Most favourable responses to therapy were seen in patients without liver or skin involvement, patients with ALL, and donor–recipient pairs other than male patients with female donors. The observation that patients with ALL respond better to GVHD treatment requires further study.

Corticosteroids play a major role in the treatment of chronic GVHD, and it appears that early, aggressive treatment is best. Patients not controlled with corticosteroids require additional immunosuppression and improved survival with reduced toxicity has been achieved with an alternating-day regimen of cyclosporin A and prednisone. This regimen is tolerated by patients with GVHD-induced thrombocytopenia, often a limitation for therapy (Sullivan et al, 1988). Treatment of chronic GVHD needs to be prolonged and withdrawn very gradually because the disease frequently recrudesces when treatment stops. Patients with established chronic GVHD suffer a high incidence of infections and antibiotic prophylaxis is required.

A newer approach to treatment of chronic GVHD has been the use of thalidomide, an agent more commonly used for the treatment of leprosy. Vogelsang et al (1986) showed thalidomide to be effective in treatment and prophylaxis of acute and chronic GVHD in animals, and clinical studies in small numbers of patients show responses (Vogelsang et al, 1987; McCarthy et al, 1988b). The mechanism of action is unclear, though various immunological effects have been described. The major toxicity of thalidomide appears to be peripheral neuropathy. Ongoing clinical trials will give more information on this interesting agent.

COMPLICATIONS

Although the major cause of BMT failure is relapse of leukaemia, particularly in ALL, the procedure itself carries a mortality of around 20–25% for allogeneic BMT and 5% for autologous BMT.

Chemoradiotherapy toxicity

Many of the early complications of BMT are secondary to the chemotherapy and radiotherapy used to immunosuppress the patient before transplant. Expected early toxicity includes oral and gastrointestinal mucositis, nausea and vomiting. More problematic is hepatic veno-occlusive disease (VOD), a condition thought to result from endothelial injury leading to fibrous obliteration of small venules. An incidence of around 20% after allogeneic BMT is usually reported, though figures as high as 71% were described by Bearman et al (1990). The reason for a rise in VOD is unclear, but may reflect the use of increasingly toxic conditioning regimens or changing diagnostic criteria.

Risk factors for VOD include pre-existing hepatic disease, higher doses and repeated courses of chemotherapy prior to transplant, therapy with busulphan, older age and possibly GVHD prophylaxis (reviewed in McDonald et al, 1987). The clinical picture of VOD includes fluid retention, ascites, jaundice and right upper quadrant tenderness, usually developing around 1 week after transplant but occasionally as late as 4 weeks. Mortality of VOD is around 30–40% in most published series, with those who recover showing resolution in 3–4 weeks. Recovery is more likely in patients with lower peak enzyme and bilirubin levels, less weight gain and no encephalopathy (McDonald et al, 1985).

Effective prophylaxis for VOD would be of great value. Prostaglandin E_1 (PGE_1), used as a continuous infusion after BMT, shows promise as a preventive agent (Gluckman et al, 1990). Rio et al (1988) have reported that low-dose infusion of heparin may reduce the incidence of VOD, and a pilot study by Bearman et al (1990) has shown that such infusions carry minimal risk of major bleeding in BMT patients. These regimens require further evaluation.

Interstitial pneumonitis (IP), usually occurring within 3 months of BMT, makes a major contribution to procedure-related mortality. The incidence of IP can be as high as 50% after allogeneic BMT and around 14% after autologous BMT (Wingard et al, 1988a). Reported mortality of IP ranges from 24 to over 80%. Clinically IP is characterized by dyspnoea, non-productive cough and hypoxaemia, with diffuse pulmonary infiltrates on chest radiograph. The clinical course is typically one of progressive ventilatory failure and death. Aetiology often is not determined, though some are due to cytomegalovirus (CMV) or *Pneumocystis carinii*. The remainder probably represent toxicity from chemotherapy and/or radio-therapy, a theory supported by the observation that patients with VOD have an increased incidence (relative risk 2.1) of IP (Wingard et al, 1989). Fractionated radiation treatments are now being used to reduce this effect.

Wingard (1988b) and others have identified risk factors for IP overall, including acute and severe GVHD, the diagnosis of leukaemia (as opposed to aplastic anaemia), GVHD prophylaxis with agents other than cyclosporin, high doses of irradiation in patients given methotrexate after transplant, poor performance status prior to transplant and long interval from diagnosis to transplant. Additional risk factors for CMV pneumonitis are pre-transplant seropositivity, CMV excretion and age greater than 10 years.

Reduction in the incidence of chemoradiotherapy-induced IP is unlikely until there is a better understanding of its mechanism. Various approaches have been taken to reduce the incidence of CMV pneumonitis post-BMT, including use of high-dose acyclovir, use of CMV-negative blood products for seronegative recipients and infusion of CMV hyperimmune globulin. Most severe CMV infections are due to reactivation of endogenous virus and 70% of seropositive patients will reactivate virus post-BMT (Meyers et al, 1986).

Seropositive recipients with seropositive donors have an incidence of CMV reactivation similar to those with seronegative donors but a much lower incidence of pneumonitis and lower mortality (Grob et al, 1987). This may be due to adoptive transfer of humoral immunity from donor to recipient, and suggests that active immunization of seronegative donors might benefit seropositive recipients. The incidence of CMV disease after autologous BMT also is high (22.5% in seronegative patients and 61% in seropositive patients) so preventive measures are needed in this setting as well (Reusser et al, 1990).

Infections of all kinds are a continuing problem post-BMT, with the early period dominated by bacterial and fungal infections, and the later period dominated by acquired and endogenous viral infections (reviewed in Winston et al, 1987; Meyers et al, 1987). Patients with severe active GVHD display immune dysregulation with associated lymphoid hypoplasia, result-ing in an extremely high risk of infection.

Graft failure

Graft rejection after well-matched sibling donor allogeneic BMT is un-common, with an incidence of around 2%. Considerable evidence suggests that host immunity plays an important role in graft rejection. First, high rates of graft failure are seen in patients who have been sensitized to the donor prior to BMT. Second, host lymphocytes are found circulating in patients with graft failure, and in some cases these cells have been shown to have the phenotype of cytotoxic T-cells. Voogt et al (1990) demonstrated the presence in patients with graft failure of T-cells that inhibit growth of donor haematopoietic progenitor cells in vitro, confirming their role in graft rejection. Graft rejection usually is immune-mediated, and it has been shown that host lymphocytes can survive standard conditioning regimens (Butturini et al, 1986). Rejection is associated with an increase in circulating host cytotoxic T-cells, which have been shown to be reactive against donor MHC antigens in MHC mismatched patients (Martin, 1988). The observed increase in rejection after T-cell depletion may reflect an alteration in the delicate balance between donor and host immune systems, away from graft-versus-host and towards host-versus-graft.

Antibody-mediated rejection also occurs. Barge et al (1989) reported three patients with erythroid failure associated with persistent host antibodies specific for donor red cell antigens, and one case in which antibodies to a non-shared HLA antigen led to complete marrow failure. These cases illustrate that host antibodies can persist for at least 18 months after transplant and that there may be a number of mechanisms of graft failure.

The incidence of graft rejection seems to be related to the degree of histoincompatibility between donor and recipient. Anasetti et al (1989) showed a graft failure rate of 12.3% among recipients of marrow from a donor with one identical haplotype (one to three antigens disparate), 2% among recipients of marrow from a genotypically identical sibling, and 7% among recipients of marrow from phenotypically HLA-matched, unrelated donors. Donor incompatibility at HLA-B and HLA-D loci appears to be associated with a particularly high risk of graft failure, as has also been observed in recipients of renal allografts (Cicciarelli et al, 1987). This suggests some synergism between the products of these two loci. Reduction in graft failure in patients receiving marrow from donors other than HLA-identical siblings will require conditioning regimens that better remove host lymphocytes. A better understanding of the importance of each of the histocompatibility loci also may allow identification of the most acceptable mismatches.

Techniques such as RFLP identifying the origin of bone marrow cells have demonstrated that stable mixed haematopoietic chimerism (i.e. presence of donor and recipient cells in relatively constant proportions) after BMT does occur and need not herald relapse. Progressive increase in the proportion of host haematopoiesis does, however, indicate imminent relapse (Yam et al, 1987). In a study of 48 recipients of T-cell-depleted marrow, Schattenberg et al (1989) found 32 (67%) to be mixed chimeras at 6 months post-BMT. Mixed chimerism seems to be more common in recipients of T-cell-depleted marrow, supporting a role for donor T-cells in suppressing host haematopoiesis (Bretagne et al, 1987).

LATE EFFECTS OF BMT

The late effects of BMT are assuming increasing importance as the number of BMT survivors increases. Many late effects are related to conditioning therapy.

Growth and development

Routinely used doses of chemoradiotherapy have a profound effect on growth and development, especially in younger children. Bushhouse et al (1989) showed in 28 patients transplanted for leukaemia that TBI is associated with a significant and prospectively increasing loss of relative height. Growth suppression appears to be more marked in the presence of severe, chronic GVHD.

Sanders et al (1986) found growth hormone deficiency in 17 of 25 patients who had received pre-BMT cranial irradiation. However, Dopfer et al (1989) found reduced secretion of growth hormone *per se* to be relatively uncommon (1 of 26). This difference may be due to the use of a more sensitive provocative test by Sanders et al (1986). Dopfer and coworkers found that many more patients (10 of 26) showed low concentrations of insulin-like growth factor I (a somatomedin), and this finding was associated with the presence of GVHD and liver dysfunction. The authors suggested that it may be possible to induce somatomedin production using high-dose exogenous growth hormone and so improve growth.

Study of post-BMT thyroid function has shown that compensated hypothyroidism is the most common abnormality (Sanders et al, 1986; Katsanis et al, 1990). Transient compensated hypothyroidism was found in some patients.

Ovarian failure is a common sequela of TBI. Sanders et al (1988b) showed that 7 years after BMT the probability of normal ovarian function is 92% after conditioning with cyclophosphamide alone and 24% after cyclophosphamide with TBI. Patient age at BMT is inversely associated with probability of normal ovarian function. Successful pregnancy after BMT is uncommon.

Study of 25 boys post-BMT showed elevated luteinizing hormone in ten, elevated follicle stimulating hormone in 23 and normal testosterone in all, suggesting Sertoli cell damage but normal Leydig cell function. Semen analysis in four boys showed all to be azoospermic (Sanders et al, 1986). Most children who are prepubertal at BMT will have a delay in onset and development of secondary sexual characteristics, usually due to hypo-gonadotrophic hypogonadism, which can be corrected with appropriate replacement therapy.

Second malignancies

Second malignant neoplasms have been reported post-BMT, and as the number of survivors increases this is likely to become more common. Deeg et al (1984) identified three groups of post-BMT secondary malignancies: those with recurrence of leukaemia in donor cells, those with lympho-proliferative disorders, and those with solid tumours. Improved DNA technology allowing identification of donor and recipient cells may reassign to recipient cells leukaemic relapse identified as occurring in donor cells by cytogenetics, in at least a proportion of cases (Stein et al, 1989).

The post-BMT occurrence of a peculiar lymphoproliferative disorder appears to be related to immunosuppression and the presence of Epstein–Barr virus (EBV). The disorder generally arises in donor cells, but also can involve host cells and is more common after T-cell-depleted BMT and mismatched BMT and possibly in patients who receive ATG (Shapiro et al, 1988). It may reflect the impaired ability of T-cells to suppress EBV-infected proliferating B-cells. Monoclonal and polyclonal lesions occur and some cases respond well to treatment with α-interferon. Many cases are rapidly fatal, however, despite aggressive therapy.

The post-BMT development of solid tumours may represent the effects of chemoradiotherapy, misfortune or a hereditary predisposition to cancer. The occurrence of solid tumours, particularly brain tumours, after chemoradiotherapy for ALL is well described and may similarly represent toxic effects of therapy.

The late effects of BMT clearly can be profound and it is essential that patients are followed closely as many effects are amenable to therapy.

FUTURE DIRECTIONS

Recent developments in the areas of cytokines and bone marrow biology have exciting possibilities for application to BMT. Cytokines may hasten engraftment and possibly reduce relapse; alternative sources of bone marrow such as long-term culture of autologous marrow, unrelated donors, cadaveric donors or umbilical cord blood may widen the availability of BMT. Induction of lymphokine-activated killer (LAK) activity post-transplant may reduce recurrence of disease. New techniques to control GVHD should allow the use of mismatched donors and improve survival in those with matched donors.

rGM-CSF

One area for progress is in reducing the risk of infection during the period of pancytopenia prior to engraftment. Recombinant human granulocyte–macrophage colony stimulating factor (rGM-CSF) is a cytokine known to increase leukocyte counts in primates. Early studies in autologous BMT recipients with solid tumours showed that rGM-CSF can accelerate myeloid recovery, lessening the period of neutropenia. rGM-CSF and other cytokines such as granulocyte colony stimulating factor (rG-CSF) and interleukin 3 (IL-3) may hasten engraftment, although more clinical studies are required to determine whether these agents are best used in vivo or in vitro prior to marrow re-infusion (Slavin et al, 1989). Myeloid blasts are stimulated in vitro by rGM-CSF, rG-CSF and IL-3, which may limit their usefulness in patients with myeloid leukaemia (Miyauchi et al, 1987).

Blazar et al (1989) used rGM-CSF with variable benefit in patients with lymphoid malignancies receiving autografts. Nemunaitis et al (1990) treated 37 patients with graft failure with rGM-CSF, after allogeneic, autologous and syngeneic BMT. Twenty-seven patients achieved an absolute neutrophil count of $0.5 \times 10^9 l^{-1}$ within 2 weeks, and no patient with myeloid leukaemia relapsed during therapy. rGM-CSF was well tolerated and did not appear to exacerbate GVHD. It is possible that rGM-CSF may simply stimulate differentiation of early stem cells, impairing long-term reconstitution, or that an occasional lymphoid, or myeloid malignancy may express rGM-CSF receptors. Further studies are needed to determine long-term effects, optimum dosage and scheduling to gain maximum benefit from these potentially very powerful agents.

Alternative sources of marrow

Long-term culture of marrow cells has been used to purge leukaemic cells from relapse marrow. Coulombel et al (1985) found that cells grown in long-term culture from patients with relapsed ANLL will, in some cases, show a decline in the leukaemic cell population, which is replaced by apparently normal haematopoietic cells.

Chang et al (1989) described six patients with ANLL in relapse who were conditioned with cyclophosphamide and TBI. Relapse marrow was re-infused after 10 days in culture and two of the six patients engrafted and achieved short complete remissions. Five patients treated similarly in first remission all engrafted and are alive in complete remission, though follow-up is still short.

Stoppa et al (1989) have also described successful engraftment after infusing marrow grown in culture for 7 days and then cryopreserved, but encountered difficulties with the technique. Further work and longer follow up is needed to assess this technique for the ex vivo removal of leukaemic cells. Alternative sources of bone marrow that have been suggested include cadavers (Lucas et al, 1988) and umbilical cord blood (Broxmeyer et al, 1989).

Interleukin-2

Immune response modifiers such as interleukin-2 (IL-2) and lymphokine-activated killer cells (LAK cells) are showing promise in the control of malignancy, even in patients with widespread disease. IL-2 is a glycoprotein molecule that induces the generation of a heterogeneous population of cytotoxic cells (LAK cells). These cells display non-MHC-restricted cytotoxicity and can lyse fresh tumour cells. This raises the possibility of using IL-2 post-BMT to generate autologous LAK cells to remove any residual disease. Though LAK precursor cells are radiosensitive Higuchi et al (1988) showed that LAK precursor activity is measurable post-BMT and increases to normal over 2 to 3 months, suggesting that there is potential for an antitumour effect.

Hauch et al (1990) found lysis of allogeneic CML targets by LAK to be variable in patients with post-BMT CML. The risk of relapse was significantly higher in patients who did not generate lytic activity against host-derived CML targets than in those who did. Clinical trials are needed to assess whether induction of post-BMT LAK activity truly prevents relapse.

Therapy of GVHD

Recent developments in the control of GVHD include the use of a mono-clonal antibody to the IL-2 receptor in vivo. The GVHD reaction is mediated by activated T-cells, which express high affinity to IL-2 receptors. It would be expected that antibody directed specifically at activated T-cells would be less immunosuppressive than polyclonal antithymocyte globulin or pan-T monoclonal antibodies. Herve et al (1990) reported that 65.6% of 32 patients with corticosteroid-resistant GVHD achieved a complete response with infusion of anti-IL-2 receptor antibody. However, 35% of patients relapsed after therapy was discontinued.

Psoralen-UVA (PUVA) therapy, usually used to treat psoriasis, has been used to treat chronic drug-resistant oral and skin GVHD. UV irradiation diminishes the functional capacity of immune system cells and psoralen, a photosensitizer, enhances this effect (Atkinson et al, 1986).

REFERENCES

Anasetti C, Amos D, Beatty PG et al (1989) Effect of HLA compatibility on engraftment of bone marrow transplants in patients with leukemia or lymphoma. *New England Journal of Medicine* **320:** 197–204.

Angelini G, De Preval C, Gorski J & Mach B (1986) High-resolution analysis of the human HLA-DR polymorphism by hybridization with sequence-specific oligonucleotide probes. *Proceedings of the National Academy of Sciences* **83:** 4489–4493.

Atkinson K, Weller P, Ryman W & Biggs J (1986) PUVA therapy for drug-resistant graft-versus-host disease. *Bone Marrow Transplantation* **1:** 227–236.

Auber ML, Horwitz JL, Blaauw A et al (1988) Evaluation of drugs for elimination of leukaemic cells from the bone marrow of patients with acute leukaemia. *Blood* **71:** 166–172.

Ball ED, Mills LE, Cornwell GG et al (1990) Autologous bone marrow transplantation for acute myeloid leukemia using monoclonal antibody-purged bone marrow. *Blood* **75:** 1199–1206.

Barge AJ, Johnson G, Witherspoon R & Torok-Storb B (1989) Antibody-mediated marrow failure after allogeneic bone marrow transplantation. *Blood* **74:** 1477–1480.

Barrett AJ, Horowitz MM, Gale RP et al (1989) Marrow transplantation for acute lympho-blastic leukemia: Factors affecting relapse and survival. *Blood* **74:** 862–871.

Bearman SI, Hinds MS, Wolford JL et al (1990) A pilot study of continuous infusion heparin for the prevention of hepatic veno-occlusive disease after bone marrow transplantation. *Bone Marrow Transplantation* **5:** 407–411.

Blazar BR, Kersey JH, McGlave PB et al (1989) In vivo administration of recombinant human granulocyte/macrophage colony-stimulating factor in acute lymphoblastic leukemia patients receiving purged autografts. *Blood* **73:** 849–857.

Blume KG, Forman SJ, O'Donnell MR et al (1987) Total body irradiation and high dose etoposide: A new preparatory regimen for bone marrow transplantation in patients with advanced hematological malignancies. *Blood* **69:** 1015–1020.

Bordigoni P, Vernant JP, Souillet G et al (1989) Allogeneic bone marrow transplantation for children with acute lymphoblastic leukaemia in first remission: A cooperative study of the group D'Etude de la Greffe de Moelle Osseuse. *Journal of Clinical Oncology* **7:** 747–753.

Bortin MM (1987) Acute graft-versus-host disease following bone marrow transplantation in humans: Prognostic factors. *Transplantation Proceedings XIX:* 2655–2657.

Bostrom B, Woods WG, Nesbit ME et al (1987) Successful reinduction of patients with acute lymphoblastic leukemia who relapse following bone marrow transplantation. *Journal of Clinical Oncology* **5:** 376–381.

Bostrom B, Weisdorf DJ, Kim T et al (1990) Bone marrow transplantation for advanced acute leukemia: A pilot study of high-energy total body irradiation, cyclophosphamide and continuous infusion etoposide. *Bone Marrow Transplantation* **5**: 83–89.

Bretagne S, Vidaud M, Kuentz M et al (1987) Mixed blood chimerism in T-cell depleted bone marrow transplant recipients: Evaluation using DNA polymorphisms. *Blood* **70**: 1692–1695.

Brochstein JA, Kernan NA, Groshen S et al (1987) Allogeneic bone marrow transplantation after hyperfractionated total body irradiation and cyclophosphamide in children with acute leukaemia. *New England Journal of Medicine* **317**: 1618–1624.

Broxmeyer HE, Douglas GW, Hangoc G et al (1989) Human umbilical cord blood as a potential source of transplantable hematopoietic stem/progenitor cells. *Proceedings of the National Academy of Science* **86**: 3828–3832.

Buckner CD, Clift RA, Appelbaum FR et al (1987) Optimal timing of marrow transplantation for patients with acute non-lymphoblastic and acute lymphoblastic leukemia. In Baum SJ, Santos GW & Takaku F (eds) *Recent Advances and Future Directions in Bone Marrow Transplantation*, pp 53–57. Berlin, Heidelberg: Springer-Verlag.

Bushhouse S, Ramsay NKC, Pescovitz OH et al (1989) Growth in children following irradiation for bone marrow transplantation. *American Journal of Pediatric Hematology/Oncology* **11**: 134–140.

Butturini A, Seeger RC & Gale RP (1986) Recipient immune-competent T-lymphocytes can survive intensive conditioning for bone marrow transplantation. *Blood* **68**: 948–956.

Butturini A, Rivera GK, Bortin MM & Gale RP (1987) Which treatment for childhood acute lymphoblastic leukaemia in second remission? *Lancet* **i**: 429–432.

Cahn JY, Herve P, Flesch M et al (1986). Autologous bone marrow transplantation for acute leukemia in complete remission: A pilot study of 33 cases. *British Journal of Haematology* **63**: 457–470.

Carella AM, Gaozza E, Santini G et al (1988) Autologous unpurged bone marrow transplantation for acute non-lymphoblastic leukemia in first complete remission. *Bone Marrow Transplantation* **3**: 537–541.

Chang J, Morgenstern GR, Coutinho LH et al (1989) The use of bone marrow cells grown in long-term culture for autologous bone marrow transplantation in acute myeloid leukemia: An update. *Bone Marrow Transplantation* **4**: 5–9.

Cicciarelli J, Terasaki PI & Mickey MR (1987). The effect of zero HLA class I and II mismatching in cyclosporine-treated kidney transplant patients. *Transplantation* **43**: 636–640.

Clay TM, Jones HP, Bidwell JL et al (1989) A comparison of DNA-RFLP typing with serology and mixed lymphocyte reaction in the selection of matched unrelated bone marrow donors. *Bone Marrow Transplantation* **4**: 493–497.

Clift RA, Buckner CD, Thomas ED et al (1987) The treatment of acute non-lymphoblastic leukemia by allogeneic marrow transplantation. *Bone Marrow Transplantation* **2**: 243–258.

Coccia PF, Strandjord SE, Warkentin PI et al (1988) High dose cytosine arabinoside and fractionated total body irradiation: An improved preparative regimen for bone marrow transplantation of children with acute lymphoblastic leukaemia in remission. *Blood* **71**: 888–893.

Coulombel L, Eaves C, Kalousek D et al (1985) Long-term marrow culture of cells from patients with acute myelogenous leukemia. *Journal of Clinical Investigation* **75**: 961–969.

Dahl GV, Kalwinsky DK & Mirro JA (1990) Allogeneic bone marrow transplantation in a program of intensive sequential chemotherapy for children and young adults with acute non-lymphocytic leukemia in first remission. *Journal of Clinical Oncology* **8**: 295–303.

Deeg HJ, Sanders J, Martin P et al (1984) Secondary malignancies after marrow transplantation. *Experimental Hematology* **12**: 660–666.

DeFabritiis P, Bregni M, Lipton J et al (1985) Elimination of clonogenic Burkitt's cells from human bone marrow using 4-hydroperoxycyclophosphamide in combination with monoclonal antibodies and complement. *Blood* **65**: 1064–1070.

Dokhelar MC, Wiels J, Lipinski M et al (1981) Natural killer cell activity in human bone marrow recipients: Early reappearance of peripheral natural killer activity in graft versus host disease. *Transplantation* **31**: 61.

Doney K, Buckner CD, Kopecky KJ et al (1987) Marrow transplantation for patients with acute lymphoblastic leukaemia in first marrow remission. *Bone Marrow Transplantation* 2: 355–363.

Dopfer R, Ranke M, Blum W et al (1989) Influence of allogeneic bone marrow transplantation on the endocrine system in children. *Transplantation Proceedings* 21: 3070–3073.

Elson CO, Reilly RW & Rosenberg IH (1977) Small intestinal injury in the graft versus host reaction: An innocent bystander phenomenon. *Gastroenterology* 72: 886–889.

Feig SA, Nesbit ME, Buckley J et al (1987) Bone marrow transplantation for acute non-lymphocytic leukemia: A report from the Children's Cancer Study Group of sixty-seven children transplanted in first remission. *Bone Marrow Transplantation* 2: 365–374.

Franceschini F, Butturini A & Gale RP (1987) Clinical trials of T-cell depletion in bone marrow transplantation. In Gale RP & Champlin RE (eds) *Progress in Bone Marrow Transplantation*, 53: 323–335.

Gassman W, Uharek L, Wottge H-U et al (1988) Comparison of cyclophosphamide, cytarabine, and etoposide as immunosuppressive agents before allogeneic bone marrow transplantation. *Blood* 72: 1574–1579.

Geller RB, Saral R, Piantadosi S et al (1989) Allogeneic bone marrow transplantation after high dose busulfan and cyclophosphamide in patients with acute non-lymphocytic leukemia. *Blood* 73: 2209–2218.

Gluckman E, Jocivet I, Scrobohaci ML et al (1990) Use of prostaglandin E_1 for prevention of liver veno-occlusive disease in leukaemic patients treated by allogeneic bone marrow transplantation. *British Journal of Haematology* 74: 277–281.

Gorin NC, Aegerter P, Auvert B et al (1990a) Autologous bone marrow transplantation for acute myelocytic leukemia in first remission: A European survey of the role of marrow purging. *Blood* 75: 1606–1614.

Gorin NC, Aegerter P & Auvert B (1990b) Autologous bone marrow transplantation for acute leukemia in remission: An analysis of 1322 cases. In Buckner T, Schellong G, Hiddeman W & Ritter J (eds) *Acute Leukemia II. Haematology and Blood Transfusion*, pp 660–666. Berlin, Heidelberg: Springer-Verlag.

Grob JP, Prentice HG, Hoffbrand AV et al (1987) Immune donors can protect marrow-transplant recipients from severe cytomegalovirus infections. *Lancet* i: 774–776.

Hauch M, Gazzola MV, Small T et al (1990) Anti-leukemia potential of interleukin-2 activated natural killer cells after bone marrow transplantation for chronic myelogenous leukemia. *Blood* 75: 2250–2262.

Helenglass G, Powles RL, McElwain TJ et al (1988) Melphalan and total body irradiation (TBI) versus cyclophosphamide and TBI as conditioning for allogeneic matched sibling bone marrow transplants for acute myeloblastic leukemia in first remission. *Bone Marrow Transplantation* 3: 21–29.

Hermans J, Suciu S, Stisnen T et al (1989) Treatment of acute myelogenous leukemia. An EBMT-EORTC retrospective analysis of chemotherapy versus allogeneic or autologous bone marrow transplantation. *European Journal of Cancer and Clinical Oncology* 25: 545–550.

Hervé P, Wijdenes J, Bergerat JP et al (1990) Treatment of corticosteroid resistant acute graft-versus-host disease by in vivo administration of anti-interleukin-2 receptor monoclonal antibody (B-BIO) *Blood* 75: 1017–1023.

Higuchi C, Thompson J, Cox T & Fefer A (1988) Lymphokine-activated killer (LAK) function after autologous marrow transplantation. *Proceedings of ASCO* 7: 165.

Horowitz MM, Gale RP, Sondel PM et al (1990) Graft-versus-leukemia reactions after bone marrow transplantation. *Blood* 75: 555–562.

Johnson FL, Sanders JE, Ruggiero M et al (1988) Bone marrow transplantation for the treatment of acute non-lymphoblastic leukemia in children aged less than 2 years. *Blood* 71: 1277–1280.

Kaizer H, Stuart RK, Brookmeyer R et al (1985) Autologous bone marrow transplantation in acute leukaemia: A phase I study of in vitro treatment of marrow with 4-hydroperoxy-cyclophosphamide to purge tumour cells. *Blood* 65: 1504–1510.

Kaminski ER (1989) How important is histocompatibility in bone marrow transplantation? *Bone Marrow Transplantation* 4: 439–444.

Kaminski ER, Hows J, Man S et al (1989) Prediction of graft versus host disease by frequency analysis of cytotoxic T-cells after unrelated donor bone marrow transplantation. *Transplantation* 48: 608–613.

Katsanis E, Shapiro RS, Robison LL et al (1990) Thyroid dysfunction following bone marrow transplantation: Long-term follow-up of 80 pediatric patients. *Bone Marrow Transplantation* **5:** 335–340.

Kernan NA, Byers V, Scannon PJ et al (1988) Treatment of steroid-resistant acute graft-versus-host disease by in vivo administration of an anti-T-cell ricin A chain immunotoxin. *Journal of the American Medical Association* **259:** 3154–3157.

Lange B, Lampkin B, Woods W et al (1990) Childrens Cancer Study Group trials for acute non-lymphoblastic leukemia (ANLL) in children. In Gale RP (ed.) *UCLA Symposia on Molecular Cellular Biology*, Acute Myeloid Leukemia. New York: Wiley-Liss (in press).

Lasky LC, Bostrom B, Smith J et al (1990) Clinical collection and use of peripheral blood stem cells in pediatric patients. *Transplantation* **47:** 613–616.

Lazarus HM, Coccia PF, Herzig RH et al (1984) Incidence of acute graft-versus-host disease with and without methotrexate prophylaxis in allogeneic bone marrow transplant patients. *Blood* **64:** 215–220.

Löwenberg B, Verdonck LS, Dekker AW et al (1990) Autologous bone marrow transplantation in acute myeloid leukemia in first remission: Results of a Dutch prospective study. *Journal of Clinical Oncology* **8:** 287–296.

Lucas PJ, Quinones RR, Moses RD et al (1988) Alternative donor sources in HLA-mismatched marrow transplantation: T-cell depletion of surgically resected cadaveric marrow. *Bone Marrow Transplantation* **3:** 211–220.

McCarthy DM, Barrett AJ, MacDonald D et al (1988a) Bone marrow transplantation for adults and children with poor risk acute lymphoblastic leukaemia in first complete remission. *Bone Marrow Transplantation* **3:** 315–322.

McCarthy DM, Kanfor E, Taylor J & Barrett AJ (1988b) Thalidomide for graft versus host disease. *Lancet* **i:** 1135.

McDonald GB, Sharma P, Matthews DE et al (1985) The clinical course of 53 patients with veno-occlusive disease of the liver after marrow transplantation. *Transplantation* **39:** 603–608.

McDonald GB, Shulman HM, Wolford JL & Spencer GD (1987) Liver disease after human marrow transplantation. *Seminars in Liver Disease* **7:** 210–229.

McGlave PB, Haake RJ, Bostrom BC et al (1988) Allogeneic bone marrow transplantation for acute non-lymphocytic leukemia in first remission. *Blood* **72:** 1512–1517.

Martin PS (1988) Graft failure following T-cell depleted marrow transplantation. *Journal of Cellular Biochemistry* **76 (Suppl. 12c):** abstract K029.

Meloni G, DeFabritiis P, Amadori S et al (1989) Autologous bone marrow transplantation in patients with AML in second complete remission (CR). *Bone Marrow Transplantation* **4:** 207–208.

Meloni G, DeFabritiis P, Carella AM et al (1990) Autologous bone marrow transplantation in patients with AML in first complete remission. Results of two different conditioning regimens after the same induction and consolidation therapy. *Bone Marrow Transplantation* **5:** 29–32.

Meyers JD, Fournoy N & Thomas ED (1986) Risk factors for cytomegalovirus infection after human marrow transplantation. *Journal of Infectious Diseases* **153:** 478–488.

Meyers JD, Petersen FB, Counts GW et al (1987) Bacterial, fungal and protozoan infection after marrow transplantation. In Baum SJ, Santos GW, Takaku F (eds) *Recent Advances and Future Directions in Bone Marrow Transplant*, pp 171–176. Berlin, Heidelberg: Springer-Verlag.

Michel G, Maraninchi D, Demeocq F et al (1988) Repeated courses of high dose melphalan and unpurged autologous bone marrow transplantation in children with acute non-lymphoblastic leukaemia in first complete remission. *Bone Marrow Transplantation* **3:** 105–111.

Miyauchi J, Kelleher CA, Yang Y-C et al (1987) The effects of three recombinant growth factors, K-3, GM-CSF and G-CSF on the blast cells of acute myeloblastic leukemia maintained in short-term suspension culture. *Blood* **70:** 657–663.

Morgan G, Strobel S, Hale G et al (1987) Treatment of acute GVHD with an anti-CD7 monoclonal antibody (Campath-2). *Bone Marrow Transplantation* **1:** 167.

Mortimer J, Blinder MA, Schulman S et al (1989) Relapse of acute leukemia after marrow transplantation: Natural history and results of subsequent therapy. *Journal of Clinical Oncology* **7:** 50–57.

Nemunaitis J, Singer JW, Buckner CD et al (1990) Use of recombinant human granulocyte–macrophage colony-stimulating factor in graft failure after bone marrow transplantation. *Blood* **76:** 245–253.

Niethammer D, Klingebiez TH, Dopfer R et al (1990) Allogeneic bone marrow transplantation in childhood leukemia: Results and strategies in the Federal Republic of Germany. In Buckner T, Schellong G, Hiddmann W & Ritter J (eds) *Acute Leukemia II. Haematology and Blood Transfusion*, pp 638–648. Berlin, Heidelberg: Springer-Verlag.

Poynton CH (1988) T-cell depletion in bone marrow transplantation. *Bone Marrow Transplantation* **3:** 265–279.

Preijers FWMB, DeWitte T, Wessels JMC et al (1989) Autologous transplantation of bone marrow purged in vitro with Anti-CD7-(WT1-) Ricin A immunotoxin in T-cell lymphoblastic leukaemia and lymphomas. *Blood* **74:** 1152–1158.

Ramsay NKC (1989) Bone marrow transplantation in pediatric oncology. In Pizzo PA & Poplack DG *Principles and Practice of Pediatric Oncology*, p 981. Philadelphia: J.B. Lippincott.

Ramsay NKC & Kersey JH (1988) Marrow purging using monoclonal antibodies. *Journal of Clinical Immunology* **8:** 81–88.

Ramsay NKC, Kersey JH, Robison LL et al (1982) A randomized study of the prevention of acute graft-versus-host disease. *New England Journal of Medicine* **306:** 392–397.

Reusser P, Fisher LD, Buckner CD et al (1990) Cytomegalovirus infection after autologous bone marrow transplantation: Occurrence of cytomegalovirus disease and effect on engraftment. *Blood* **75:** 1888–1894.

Rio B, Lamy T & Zittoun R (1988) Preventive role of heparin for liver veno-occlusive disease. *Bone Marrow Transplantation* **3:** 266 (abstract).

Rivera GK, Buchanan G, Boyett JM et al (1986) Intensive retreatment of childhood acute lymphoblastic leukaemia in first bone marrow relapse. *New England Journal of Medicine* **315:** 273–278.

Rosenfeld C, Shadduck RK, Przepiorka D et al (1989) Autologous bone marrow transplantation with 4-hydroperoxycyclophosphamide purged marrows for acute non-lymphocytic leukaemia in late remission or early relapse. *Blood* **74:** 1159–1164.

Rowley SD, Jones RJ, Piantadosi S et al (1989) Efficacy of ex vivo purging for autologous bone marrow transplantation in the treatment of acute nonlymphoblastic leukaemia. *Blood* **74:** 501–506.

Sallan SE, Niemeyer CM, Billett AL et al (1989) Autologous bone marrow transplantation for acute lymphoblastic leukemia. *Journal of Clinical Oncology* **7:** 1594–1601.

Sanders JE, Pritchard S, Mahoney P et al (1986) Growth and development following marrow transplantation for leukemia. *Blood* **68:** 1129–1135.

Sanders JE, Thomas DE, Buckner CD & Doney K (1987) Marrow transplantation for children with acute lymphoblastic leukaemia in second remission. *Blood* **70:** 324–326.

Sanders JE, Buckner CD, Clift RA et al (1988a) Second marrow transplants in patients with leukemia who relapse after allogeneic marrow transplantation. *Bone Marrow Transplantation* **3:** 11–19.

Sanders JE, Buckner CD, Amos D et al (1988b) Ovarian function following marrow transplantation for aplastic anemia or leukemia. *Journal of Clinical Oncology* **6:** 813–818.

Schattenberg A, DeWitte T, Salden M et al (1989) Mixed hematopoietic chimerism after allogeneic transplantation with lymphocyte-depleted bone marrow is not associated with a higher incidence of relapse. *Blood* **5:** 1367–1372.

Schmitz N, Gassmann W, Rister M et al (1988) Fractionated total body irradiation and high-dose VP-16-213 followed by allogeneic bone marrow transplantation in advanced leukaemias. *Blood* **72:** 1567–1573.

Schultz FW, Martens ACM & Hagenbeek A (1989) The contribution of residual leukaemia cells in the graft to leukaemia relapse after autologous bone marrow transplantation: Mathematical considerations. *Leukemia* **3:** 530–534.

Shapiro RS, McClain K, Frizzera G et al (1988) Epstein-Barr virus associated B-cell lymphoproliferative disorders following bone marrow transplantation. *Blood* **71:** 1234–1243.

Sharkis SJ, Santos GW & Colvin M (1980) Elimination of acute myelogenous leukaemic cells from marrow and tumour suspensions in the rat with 4-hydroperoxycyclophosphamide. *Blood* **55:** 521–523.

Simonsson B, Burnett AK, Prentice HG et al (1989) Autologous bone marrow transplantation with monoclonal antibody purged marrow for high risk acute lymphoblastic leukaemia. *Leukaemia* **3**: 631–636.

Slavin S, Mumcuoglu M, Landesberg-Weisz A & Kedar E (1989) The use of recombinant cytokines for enhancing immunohematopoietic reconstitution following bone marrow transplantation. I. Effects of in vitro culturing with K-3 and GM-CSF on human and mouse bone marrow cells purged with mafosfamide (ASTA-Z). *Bone Marrow Transplantation* **4**: 459–464.

Snover DC (1984) Acute and chronic graft versus host disease: Histopathological evidence for two distinct pathogenetic mechanisms. *Human Pathology* **15**: 202–205.

Snyder DS, Findley DO, Forman SJ et al (1988) Fractionated total body irradiation and high dose cyclophosphamide: A preparative regimen for bone marrow transplantation for patients with hematologic malignancies in first complete remission. *Blut* **57**: 7–13.

Sonnenberg FA, Eckman MH & Pauker SG (1989) Bone marrow donor registries: The relation between registry size and probability of finding complete and partial matches. *Blood* **74**: 2569–2578.

Spinolo JA, Dicke KA, Horwitz LJ et al (1988) Autologous bone marrow transplantation (ABMT) for remission intensification in acute myelogenous leukemia (AML): Long-term follow-up. *Experimental Hematology* **16**: 487 (abstract).

Stein J, Zimmerman PA, Kochera M et al (1989) Origin of leukemic relapse after bone marrow transplantation: Comparison of cytogenetic and molecular analysis. *Blood* **73**: 2033–2040.

Stewart P, Buckner CD, Bensinger W et al (1985) Autologous marrow transplantation in patients with acute nonlymphocytic leukemia in first remission. *Experimental Hematology* **13**: 267–272.

Stoppa AM, Maraninchi D, Lafagg M et al (1989) Liquid culture and cryopreservation of marrow cells of leukemic patients prior to autologous bone marrow transplantation. *British Journal of Haematology* **72**: 519–523.

Sullivan KM, Deeg HJ, Sanders J et al (1986) Hyperacute graft-vs-host disease in patients not given immunosuppression after allogeneic marrow transplantation. *Blood* **67**: 1172–1175.

Sullivan KM, Witherspoon RP, Storb R et al (1988) Alternating-day cyclosporine and prednisone for treatment of high-risk chronic graft-versus-host disease. *Blood* **72**: 555–561.

Trigg ME, Gingrich R, Goeken N et al (1989) Low rejection rate when using unrelated to haploidentical donors for children with leukemia undergoing marrow transplantation. *Bone Marrow Transplantation* **4**: 431–437.

Truitt RL, Shih GY, LeFever HV et al (1986) Manipulation of graft versus host disease for a graft versus leukemia effect after bone marrow transplantation in AKR mice with spontaneous leukemia/lymphoma. *Transplantation* **41**: 301–310.

Tutschka PJ, Copelan EA & Klein JP (1987) Bone marrow transplantation for leukaemia following a new busulfan and cyclophosphamide regimen. *Blood* **70**: 1382–1388.

Uckun FM, Gajl-Peczalska K, Meyers DE et al (1987) Marrow purging in autologous bone marrow transplantation for T-lineage acute lymphoblastic leukaemia: Efficacy of ex vivo treatment with immunotoxins and 4-hydroperoxycyclophosphamide against fresh leukaemic marrow progenitor cells. *Blood* **69**: 361–366.

Vogelsang GB, Hess AD & Santos GW (1986) Treatment and prevention of acute graft-versus-host disease with thalidomide in a rat model. *Transplantation* **41**: 644–647.

Vogelsang GB, Hess AD, Ling T et al (1987) Thalidomide therapy of chronic graft versus host disease. *Blood* **70**: 315 (abstract).

Voogt PJ, Fibbe WE, Marijt WAF et al (1990) Rejection of bone marrow graft by recipient-derived cytotoxic T-lymphocytes against minor histocompatibility antigens. *Lancet* **335**: 131–134.

Weisdorf DJ, Nesbit ME, Ramsay NKC et al (1987) Allogeneic bone marrow transplantation for acute lymphoblastic leukaemia in remission: Prolonged survival associated with acute graft-versus-host disease. *Journal of Clinical Oncology* **5**: 1348–1355.

Weisdorf DJ, Ramsay N, LeBien T et al (1990) Allogeneic and autologous bone marrow transplantation for acute lymphoblastic leukaemia. In Büchner T, Schellong G, Hiddemann W & Ritter J (eds), *Acute Leukemia II. Haematology and Blood Transfusion*, pp 679–683. Berlin, Heidelberg: Springer-Verlag.

Wingard JR, Sostrin MB, Vriesendorp HM et al (1988a) Interstitial pneumonitis following autologous bone marrow transplantation. *Transplantation* **46**: 61–65.

Wingard JR, Mellits ED & Sostrin MB (1988b) Interstitial pneumonitis after allogeneic bone marrow transplantation. *Medicine* **67:** 175–186.

Wingard JR, Mellits ED, Jones RJ et al (1989) Association of hepatic veno-occlusive disease with interstitial pneumonitis in bone marrow transplant recipients. *Bone Marrow Transplantation* **4:** 685–689.

Winston DJ, Ho WG, Gale RP & Champlin RE (1987) Prevention and treatment of infections after bone marrow transplant. In Baum SJ, Santos GW & Takaku F (eds) *Recent Advances and Future Directions in Bone Marrow Transplantation*, pp 177–185. Berlin, Heidelberg: Springer-Verlag.

Yam PY, Petz LD, Knowlton RG et al (1987) Use of DNA restriction fragment length polymorphisms to document marrow engraftment and mixed hematopoietic chimerism following bone marrow transplantation. *Transplantation* **43:** 399–407.

Zintl F, Hermann J, Fuchs D et al (1990) Comparison of allogeneic and autologous bone marrow transplantation for treatment of acute lymphocytic leukemia in childhood. In Buchner T, Schellong G, Hiddeman W & Ritter J (eds) *Acute Leukemia II. Haematology and Blood Transfusion*, pp 692–698. Berlin, Heidelberg: Springer-Verlag.

9

Infections in the compromised child

CLAUDIO VISCOLI
ELIO CASTAGNOLA
DAVID ROGERS

SIGNIFICANCE OF INFECTION IN CHILDREN WITH CANCER

Ever since the early trials of combination chemotherapy in childhood acute leukaemia it has been appreciated that control and cure of childhood cancer can only be achieved at the expense of an increased risk of potentially life-threatening infection. The risk–benefit assessment this implies is fundamental not only to the design of protocols, but also in the management of the individual child. Just as modern advances in surgery have been dependent on improvements in anaesthetic technique, so recent advances in paediatric oncology have been made possible only by better understanding of the consequences of different aspects of immunosuppression and improved management of the resulting infections.

An example of the differing immunological consequences of different therapeutic protocols is provided by the report of Rapson and coworkers (1980) which compared the immunological consequences of continuous and intermittent therapy for children with acute lymphoblastic leukaemia in remission. Although neutropenia was more marked in those receiving intermittent therapy, the incidence of infection, particularly with viruses and *Pneumocystis carinii*, was higher in the continuous therapy group, in which all six deaths from infection in children during remission occurred. This high incidence of infection was correlated with an appreciable reduction in total lymphocyte count in the group of children receiving continuous therapy which was not seen in the children receiving intermittent therapy. Final analysis of the trial in which these children were entered showed however that the continuous regimen which caused most immunosuppression was that most likely to control and cure the children's leukaemia. At the same time, improved diagnosis, therapy and in some cases prophylaxis for the infections meant that these no longer needed to be a reason for a less than optimal cytotoxic treatment regimen. Protocols for disease with a high risk of relapse have correspondingly tended to intensify therapy, while for disease with a high chance of cure, for example 'low-risk' acute lymphoblastic leukaemia, protocol design has attempted to reduce the risk of infection, as well as the risk of long-term adverse effects.

Table 1. Relationship between immune defects and most important infecting pathogens in compromised children.

Immune defect	Type of pathogen				
	Viruses	Bacteria	Fungi	Protozoa	Helmints
Phagocytosis	—	Gram-positive cocci Diphtheroids Gram-negative bacilli *Actinomyces* sp.	*Candida* sp. *Aspergillus* sp. Zygomycetes *Fusarium* sp.	—	*Strongyloides stercoralis*
Cell-mediated immunity	Herpesviridae Papovaviridae Paramyxoviridae Enterovirus	Intracellular bacteria (*Myco-bacterium* sp., *Listeria mono-cytogenes*, *Legionella pneumophila*, *Salmonella* sp.) *Nocardia* sp.	*Candida* sp. (muco-cutaneous) *Cryptococcus neoformans* *Histoplasma capsulatum* *Coccidioides immitis*	*Toxoplasma gondii* *Cryptosporidium* *Leishmania* sp. *Pneumocystis carinii**	*Strongyloides stercoralis*
Humoral immunity and spleen function	Enterovirus	Encapsulated bacteria (*Streptococcus pneumoniae*, *Haemophilus influenzae*, *Neisseria meningitidis*)	—	*Giardia lamblia* *Cryptosporidium* *Pneumocystis carinii**	—
Mechanical barriers	—	Gram-positive cocci *Corynebacterium* sp. Gram-negative bacilli	*Candida* sp. *Aspergillus* sp. *Malassezia furfur*	—	—

* *New classification proposed among fungi (Edman, 1989).*

For management of the individual patient, knowledge of the immuno-suppressive consequences of particular therapy has led to dose delay or modification, as for example with the conventional policy of interrupting or delaying cytotoxic therapy until neutropenia has recovered to a specified level. However, increasing confidence in our ability to diagnose and treat infections even in the immunocompromised has led to a reluctance to reduce or delay treatment when the risk of failure to control the underlying disease is known to be high. Risk–benefit questions of such gravity can only be answered rationally on the basis of experience, preferably of controlled clinical trials when such studies have been performed. Day-to-day manage-ment depends on close co-operation with the microbiology laboratories, ideally with the close involvement of a clinical microbiologist or infectious disease specialist, although where the paediatric haematologist does not have the advantage of such a colleague these skills too will be needed as part of the already overstretched armamentarium.

This review will first consider the different patterns of immunosuppres-sion and related infecting pathogens related to childhood malignancies and their management, and then address specific paediatric problems, with particular attention to diagnosis and management of the febrile, granulo-cytopenic child. For reasons of space we are forced to exclude discussion of other important issues, such as for example, the value of prophylactic strategies (bowel decontamination, systemic prophylaxis, environmental procedures and granulocyte transfusions), the management of pneumonia, of the acute abdomen, of hepatic candidiasis and of the syndrome of respiratory distress in patients with streptococcal bacteraemia, and the significance in prophylaxis and/or treatment of some recently developed cytokines (GM-CSF, G-CSF, interleukins). Moreover we will only touch on other important aspects of infections in immunocompromised children, such as viral infections (especially in bone marrow transplant recipients) and management of infections related to central indwelling catheters.

RELATIONSHIP BETWEEN IMMUNE DEFECT AND INFECTING PATHOGEN

The immune system is a complex network of mechanisms targeted at the neutralization of invading foreign organisms. Recognizing that patients with particular types of immune defects are susceptible to invasion by particular types of pathogens may be helpful in the diagnosis and treatment of the infection, as well as in assessing prognosis. Table 1 summarizes the most important immune defects seen in children with cancer and the related pathogenic organisms.

Phagocytosis

Granulocytopenia is common among cancer patients, both because of underlying disease (e.g. acute leukaemia) and because of myelosuppressive cytotoxic or radiation therapy. As shown by Bodey and coworkers several years ago (1966), granulocytopenia is the most important risk factor for bacterial infection, and strong relationships have been shown between total neutrophil count, rate of decline of neutrophil count, duration of neutropenia, and the risk of developing a severe bacterial infection. Granulocytopenic patients also show an increased incidence of fungal infections, especially after prolonged periods of broad-spectrum antibacterial therapy (Khardori, 1989).

In contrast to granulocytes, mononuclear phagocytes are relatively less sensitive to the toxic effects of antineoplastic therapy, thus maintaining a rudimentary defence mechanism in neutropenic patients. Monocytes liberate several cytokines such as interleukin-1 (IL-1), granulocyte–macrophage colony-stimulating factor (GM-CSF), granulocyte colony-stimulating factor (G-CSF) and tumour necrosis factor (TNF) (O'Garra, 1989; Tracey et al, 1989; Weisbart et al, 1989). These are responsible for the development of fever and the synthesis of the so-called acute phase proteins (e.g. C-reactive protein) (Dinarello, 1988a,b). Moreover, these cytokines, by promoting bone marrow recovery (O'Garra, 1989; Weisbart et al, 1989), might be responsible for the relatively rapid granulocytic response seldom observed in some neutropenic patients with severe infection. The dark side of cytokine effects is represented by TNF, which triggers a complex cascade leading to symptoms of septic shock (Parrillo et al, 1990).

Cell-mediated immunity

Patients with abnormalities of cell-mediated immunity tend to develop infections with organisms which differ from those seen in granulocytopenic patients. Impairment of cell-mediated immunity in children with cancer may be due to the underlying disease (e.g. acute lymphoblastic leukaemia or lymphoma), to its treatment or to a combination of both. Prolonged and repeated cycles of antineoplastic chemotherapy impair cell-mediated immunity and predispose patients to develop infection due to intracellular pathogens, such as *Pneumocystis carinii* and cytomegalovirus.

Pneumocystis carinii is one of the major causes of pneumonia in childhood acute lymphocytic leukaemia during the remission maintenance phase and in patients receiving cyclosporin for allogeneic bone marrow transplantation. Masur et al (1989) showed that in adult patients with the acquired immunodeficiency syndrome, the risk of developing this infection seems to be higher when the total number of $CD4^+$ T-lymphocytes falls below $200 \, \text{mm}^{-3}$ ($0.2 \times 10^9 \, \text{l}^{-1}$) or 20% of total lymphocyte count. However, this has not been confirmed in children with the same underlying condition, where pneumocystosis developed with a total $CD4^+$ T-lymphocyte count higher than $0.45 \times 10^9 \, \text{l}^{-1}$ (Leibovitz et al, 1990).

Cytomegalovirus is one of the most important causes of morbidity in patients undergoing allogeneic bone marrow transplantation. Pneumonia is the most important clinical manifestation of CMV infection or reinfection and is strongly associated with acute graft-versus-host disease. The problem has been recently reviewed by Frank and Friedman (1988), who underlined the possible role of an immunopathological mechanism, triggered by the virus, as the basis for pulmonary disease.

Defects of cellular immunity are probably responsible for severe primary infections with varicella-zoster and measles viruses and may explain the high incidence of herpes zoster recurrence in patients after bone marrow transplantation.

Humoral immunity and spleen function

Patients with defects of immunoglobulin synthesis may develop infections with a number of pathogens, especially bacteria and certain types of viruses, mainly enteroviruses (Shearer and Anderson, 1989). Children whose spleens have been removed for staging of Hodgkin's disease are at risk of severe, life-threatening bacteraemias due to encapsulated bacteria requiring opsonization, especially pneumococcal meningitis and septicaemia. Similar infections have been described in children undergoing bone marrow transplantation in the late post-transplant phase (after day 100), possibly related to the patient's inability to make opsonizing antibodies (Meyers and Thomas, 1988). Alternatively, irradiation of the child's spleen may have irreversibly damaged splenic B lymphocytes, thus preventing normal primary humoral response on first encounter with a blood-borne encapsulated organism.

Illustrative case 1

A 2-year-old girl underwent left nephrectomy for Wilms' tumour (completely excised with intact capsule and favourable histology). Subsequently, she was treated with radiotherapy (3080 cGy to the whole abdomen with shielding of the right kidney), and vincristine and actinomicin D, for one year. At age 7 years a renal papillary adenocarcinoma was removed from her right kidney (Breatnach and Androulakis, 1983). She remained well without further therapy for 2 years, and then presented with overwhelming pneumococcal bacteraemia which proved fatal.

Mechanical barriers

Disruption of mechanical barriers is another important cause of increased infectious morbidity in children with cancer. For example, children with leukaemia, lymphoma and solid tumours may experience malignant cellular infiltration of normal tissues facilitating bacterial or fungal superinfections. In other cases tumoral damage affects the mucosal barriers allowing microorganisms to enter the blood stream.

Other defects of mechanical barriers are the result of procedures required for diagnosis (surgery, bone marrow aspirations, biopsies, endoscopy) and therapy (cytotoxic chemotherapy, radiation, parenteral alimentation, presence of indwelling central venous catheters). Of these, indwelling central venous catheters, in particular, present many unresolved issues. On one hand these devices obviate many problems in the management of

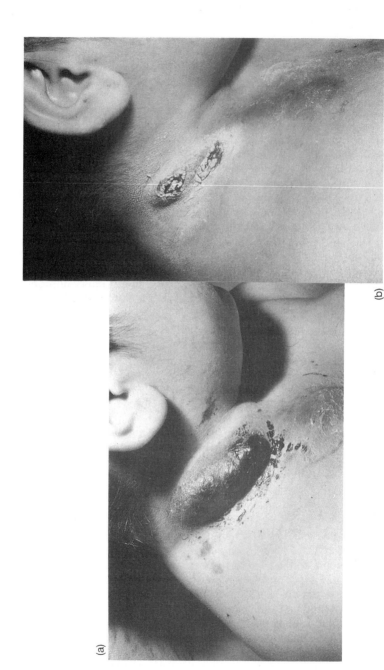

Figure 1. Soft tissue and skin abscess at the entrance of the Broviac catheter into the right jugular vein due to *S. aureus* and *Streptococcus* spp. in a girl with acute lymphoblastic leukaemia. Both organisms were isolated from blood and pus culture. (a) Initial clinical presentation. (b) Clinical picture after catheter removal and 10 days of treatment.

patients with malignancies, because they free the young patient from the discomfort of repeated venipunctures and at the same time allow the administration of medications, blood products and large volumes of fluids, which may be required for the treatment of neoplastic diseases. On the other hand they constitute a well-recognized source of infections (Viscoli et al, 1988) that are sometimes difficult to diagnose and treat (Figure 1). Open questions in the management of catheter-related infections include definition (i.e. clinical or microbiological), optimum catheter care, the optimum management of catheter related infections, and evaluation of the infectious risk inherent in the use of multiple lumen catheters or other intravenous devices such as Port-a-Cath implanted catheters (Maki, 1989).

Others

Patients receiving anticancer therapy are frequently malnourished. Total parenteral alimentation has become common practice, although the results of some controlled trials performed in adults did not show any benefit of this procedure in the outcome of the underlying disease (American College of Physicians, 1989). Both malnutrition (Kensch, 1984) and parenteral alimentation increase the risk of bacterial and fungal infections. For example, candidemias have been related to the use of high-concentration carbohydrate solutions (Crislip and Edwards, 1989), while *Malassezia furfur* and *Staphylococcus epidermidis* have caused severe infections in patients receiving lipid emulsions (Powell DA et al, 1984; Freeman et al, 1990).

Experimental use of cytokines, such as GM-CSF or interleukin-2 (IL-2), has raised new issues in the field of infectious diseases. While GM-CSF may prove to be life-saving in neutropenic patients with severe bacterial (Ganser et al, 1989) and perhaps fungal (Smith et al, 1990) infections, IL-2 has been shown to impair neutrophil function (Klemper et al, 1990) and to cause skin damage with increased risk of staphylococcal colonization and infection (Snydman et al, 1990).

Antibiotic-related alteration of the normal intestinal flora is another important factor in infection in the immunocompromised. It has been shown that approximately 80% of pathogens causing infection in granulocytopenic cancer patients come from the intestinal flora and that half of them were acquired after hospitalization (Schimpff et al, 1972). In an animal model, Steffen et al (1988) demonstrated that bacteria may translocate from the intestinal lumen into mesenteric lymph nodes after the alteration of endogenous flora, after disruptions of the mechanical barriers or in presence of immunodeficiency. When all three of these conditions coexist bacteria may invade the blood stream.

In conclusion, categorization of the infecting pathogens according to the underlying immune defect permits more orderly thinking and facilitates differential diagnosis and microbiological investigation. However, as summarized in Figure 2, the increased risk of infection in cancer patients is multifactorial in origin and more than one immune defect is often present in the individual patient. The importance of the interaction of multiple factors in determining a single infectious event is exemplified by the preliminary

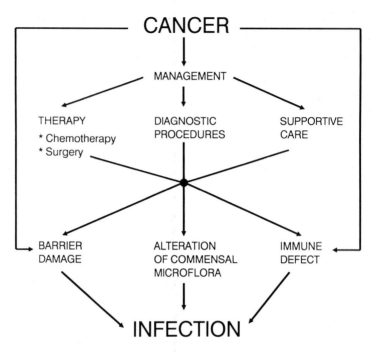

Figure 2. From cancer to infection.

results of a multivariate analysis performed on EORTC data from 834 febrile episodes in neutropenic cancer patients randomized in trial V (EORTC, 1990a). In order to identify clinical and laboratory factors predicting whether or not a febrile, granulocytopenic cancer patient was actually bacteraemic, a backward, stepwise logistic regression analysis of presentation data was performed. The mathematical model identified as influencing the presence of bacteraemia the following factors: bone marrow suppression (duration and severity of neutropenia before fever and platelet count at onset), general clinical condition (highest fever and presence of signs and symptoms of septic shock), presence of an identifiable site of infection (especially if localized at the central catheter), previous administration of antifungals and/or antibacterials as prophylaxis, and the size (i.e. number of patients included in the study) of the randomizing centre.

INITIAL MANAGEMENT OF THE FEBRILE GRANULOCYTOPENIC CHILD

Diagnosis

Diagnosis of infectious complications in immunocompromised and particularly in neutropenic patients is especially challenging because the factors that have decreased the patient's ability to react against offending microorganisms may also have resulted in an impaired inflammatory response, thus masking signs and symptoms of infection. As shown by the studies performed by the EORTC International Antimicrobial Therapy Cooperative Group over the last 10 years, about 20% of febrile granulocytopenic cancer patients who receive empiric antibiotic therapy have bacteraemia. In another 20% a microbiologically-documented infection without bacteraemia is demonstrated and in another 20% an infectious aetiology can be documented on clinical grounds. The remaining febrile episodes, unless unequivocally documented as having a non-infectious cause, are classified as unexplained fevers (fever of unknown origin and possible infection are regarded as synonyms), but are considered as occult bacterial infections and treated accordingly. (EORTC, 1978, 1983, 1986; Pizzo et al, 1982b; Bodey, 1986; Viscoli et al, 1991c).

It has been calculated that 80–90% of first fevers in granulocytopenic cancer patients are bacterial in origin (Hathorn and Pizzo, 1989). Fungal infection is relatively rarely a cause of first fevers, and is far more commonly a cause of secondary infections (Singer et al, 1977; Garaventa et al, 1990). The role played by viruses as cause of first fevers in febrile and granulocytopenic cancer patients has received only limited investigation. Apart from specific clinical situations, such as those involving patients undergoing allogeneic bone marrow transplantation, viruses are not usually considered as primary pathogens in cancer patients but rather as cofactors facilitating both bacterial and fungal infections (Meyers and Thomas, 1988; Morris, 1990). Children are more exposed than adults to the risk of acquiring common respiratory viral pathogens and it is therefore probable that in paediatrics some fevers of unknown origin or clinically documented infections either have a viral aetiology or are polymicrobial in origin. For example, Nachman and Honig (1980) found that 29 of 119 febrile episodes in leukaemic children were caused by viruses, thus suggesting that at least in paediatrics, viruses may be underestimated as cause of fever in neutropenia.

Management of immunocompromised children with cancer may differ somewhat from management of adults. For example, depending on age, children may require anything from mild sedation to general anaesthesia in order to undergo diagnostic procedures, such as bone marrow aspiration, lumbar puncture, percutaneous liver biopsy, CT-scan, MRI or isotope scanning. This may sometimes complicate substantially the investigation of the febrile child.

The following paragraphs discuss some aspects of the initial management of the febrile neutropenic child with cancer with particular attention to bacterial and fungal infections.

Clinical evaluation

Special consideration should be given, in the initial clinical evaluation, to history-taking and physical examination. Signs and symptoms suggestive of an infectious aetiology may be absent and signs of localization misleading. The young child's inability to describe symptoms to physicians and nurses may further complicate diagnosis, as shown in the following case.

Illustrative case 2

A 2-year-old child with acute lymphoblastic leukaemia in relapse developed high fever during severe neutropenia. Several blood cultures yielded *Staphylococcus aureus* and vancomycin was added to the initial empirical treatment, ceftazidime and amikacin, because of lack of clinical response. Despite this pathogen-directed therapy the patient's clinical condition did not improve. There was no objective evidence of secondary infectious localization, but the child was still febrile and was complaining of severe pain apparently localized in the abdomen. Fever and pain continued unmodified, requiring administration of analgesics, in the absence of any signs suggesting an acute abdomen or other localized infections. Because of his age the patient was, of course, unable to describe his symptoms precisely. Eventually it was observed that the patient was particularly distressed complaining in particular during micturition and, even more, during defaecation, and therefore perirectal or perianal cellulitis was suspected. Ceftazidime was then replaced by imipenem–cylastatin, in order to improve coverage against anaerobic bacteria and fecal streptococci, and the child began to improve. Some days later, concomitantly with bone marrow recovery, a perianal abscess was detected and was drained successfully.

In this case the inability of the attending physicians and nurses, as well as of the mother, to communicate fully with the patient, delayed diagnosis and treatment of a potentially fatal infection.

Diagnosis of localized infections

Skin and soft tissue infections (Figure 3) are not infrequent among neutropenic children and their clinical appearance is often altered because of the impaired inflammatory response. A wide variety of pathogens may be involved and therefore microbiological diagnosis is mandatory in order to give appropriate therapy. Biopsy for Gram stain, culture and histology is the method of choice, although good results can also be obtained by thin needle aspiration; this last procedure should probably be preferred in severely thrombocytopenic patients or when general anaesthesia cannot be performed (Bodey and Luna, 1974). Bronchoalveolar lavage or open lung biopsy have been shown to be relatively safe and effective procedures in paediatric patients for the aetiological diagnosis of pulmonary infections, unless they are severely thrombocytopenic (Mason et al, 1982; Frankel et al, 1988). As a general rule, physicians taking care of neutropenic children should not hesitate to try to obtain diagnostic specimens in the presence of signs of localized infections, although the advantage of a microbiological confirmation should always be balanced against the risk of severe procedure-related complications.

Diagnosis of bacteraemia

Other factors may impair diagnosis of infection in the paediatric age group.

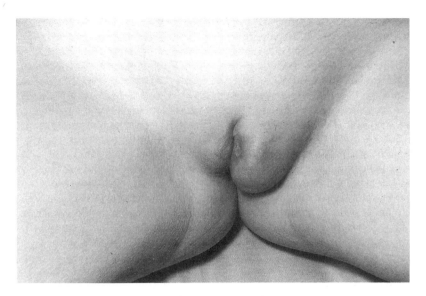

Figure 3. Abscess of the left labium majus due to *Pseudomonas aeruginosa* in a girl with non-Hodgkin's lymphoma. The causative pathogen was isolated from blood and from material obtained by thin needle aspiration.

For example, in febrile and neutropenic children, before starting empiric antibacterial therapy, it is usually recommended that two or three blood cultures should be taken from separate venipuncture sites (Hathorn and Pizzo, 1989). The rationale is to increase the chance of detecting single-agent and polymicrobial bacteraemias, as well as to discriminate between true infection and contamination. However, venous access is frequently poor in children and multiple blood cultures are often impossible to obtain, unless the patient is fitted with an indwelling central catheter. Therefore, in children, physicians and nurses are often forced to draw blood cultures through the catheter, sometimes rendering the results difficult to interpret, because of the increased possibility of contamination. Quantitative cultures from the central catheter and from a peripheral vein may be useful in identifying contaminated intravenous devices (Maki, 1989), although difficulties in venous access may render this procedure impossible. Finally, the amount of blood drawn with each blood culture cannot be as large as in adults, further reducing the possibility of detecting bacteria in blood (Washington, 1990).

Diagnosis by indirect methods

Several indirect methods for the detection of bacterial antigens in blood or cerebrospinal fluid have been shown to be helpful in the diagnosis of bacterial diseases in the normal host (Washington, 1990). Unfortunately, the useful-ness of these methods for the diagnosis of bacterial infections in neutropenic cancer patients is negligible. For fungal infections, the only reliable test currently used in clinical practice is the detection of cryptococcal antigen in serum and cerebrospinal fluid by means of a latex agglutination test (Washington, 1990). However, this test is of limited value in cancer patients, in whom cryptococcosis is not as frequent as other fungal infections (Khardori, 1989; Garaventa et al, 1990). As a general rule, although promising results have been reported in invasive candidiasis and aspergillosis (Bennett, 1987; Armstrong et al, 1990; Walsh et al, 1990), the currently used serodiagnostic methods for the diagnosis of fungal infections should be considered as experimental.

Non-specific diagnostic methods have also been proposed for discriminating between infectious and non-infectious fevers and in assessing the response to treatment. Among these, the quantitative evaluation of the C-reactive protein has been shown to be helpful in clinical practice (Mackie et al, 1979; Pepys, 1981).

Initial clinical manifestation of infection

Fever is the most common clinical manifestation of infection in immuno-compromised children. In the absence of normal bone marrow functions, as is the case in the neutropenic host, the cytokines responsible for the development of fever and of the inflammatory reaction are unable to trigger an effective phagocytic response. Therefore, in neutropenics, fever is often unaccompanied by any other sign of infection. Table 2 reports the clinically detectable sites of infection at initial presentation in children and adults randomized in EORTC trial V, including cases non-evaluable for response to treatment (EORTC, unpublished data). According to these data, fever was the only sign of infection in more than 50% of the infectious episodes. The difference in the distribution of the initial sites of infection between children and adults is statistically significant. It appears that fever is slightly more often the only sign of infection in children than in adults and that a different distribution exists in these two groups concerning the upper and the lower respiratory tract as initial site of infection. The intravenous line was seldom the initial site of infection in children compared to adults, despite that an indwelling device was in situ at the onset of fever in a

Table 2. Initial manifestation of infection in neutropenic children and adults randomized in EORTC trial V.

Initial localization of infection	Children (<14 yr)		Adults (>14 yr)		All patients	
No site (only fever)	99	(63%)	428	(58%)	527	(59%)
Upper respiratory tract	40	(25%)	107	(15%)	147	(16%)
Lungs	5	(3%)	88	(12%)	93	(10%)
Gastrointestinal tract	5	(3%)	18	(2%)	23	(3%)
Intravenous line	0	(0%)	31	(4%)	31	(3%)
Other	9	(6%)	61	(8%)	70	(8%)
Total	158 (100%)		733 (100%)		891 (100%)	

Chi-square overall $p < 0.001$.

comparable proportion of patients in both groups (70 and 71%, respectively). Several important aspects of the initial evaluation of the febrile and neutropenic child need to be underlined. As infectious complications in neutropenic children and adults may develop without clear signs and symptoms, even subtle indications must be considered as suggestive of an infectious process. For example, dyspnoea or tachypnoea with nasal flaring are suggestive of pulmonary infection, even in the absence of clinical or radiological signs. Metabolic acidosis may represent the first sign of bacteraemia and shock, especially if accompanied by skin lesions, hypotension, sudden thrombocytopenia and consumption coagulopathy. Skin redness, with swelling and sometimes serous discharge at the exit site or along the course of a central indwelling catheter may be the harbinger of a catheter-related infection. In our experience (Viscoli et al, 1988) it has proved extremely important when asking parents to describe the onset of fever (with or without chills? accompanied by some pain or other symptoms?) to ascertain if fever was in some way related to catheter flushing or to any other catheter procedure. Often, when the intravenous line is heavily contaminated, catheter flushing may be followed by abrupt onset of fever and chills: blood cultures taken at this time are more likely to yield bacteria. Pain on defaecation and urination with incontinence may herald infection of the perirectal or perianal area, as well as of the urinary tract. In general, any kind of pain, if not otherwise explicable, should raise the suspicion of an infectious complication. The mouth is another common site of infection in paediatric patients. An infectious process initiated in the mouth in the form of dental caries can proceed to periodontitis, ulcerations, oral abscesses and even bacteraemia. Viridans streptococci are a leading cause of bacteraemia related to oral mucositis. Finally, a change in mental status with behavioural abnormalities is suggestive of neurological infectious complications, even in the absence of meningeal signs.

Initial empirical treatment

The appearance of fever in immunocompromised patients should always raise the suspicion of infection and should be followed by an intensive diagnostic evaluation. If the patient is granulocytopenic it has became common practice to start antibacterial treatment even before an infectious aetiology is proved, because delay may result in rapid clinical deterioration and even death. Although this policy goes against the classic teaching of infectious disease, according to which physicians are schooled to know what they treat, and although it has never been verified in controlled trials, it has substantially improved the prognosis of fever and infection in granulocytopenic patients (Schimpff et al, 1971; EORTC, 1978; Love et al, 1980; Klastersky and Zinner, 1982; Schimpff, 1986; Hathorn et al, 1987). Many of these studies were based on mixed populations of patients, including adult and paediatric patients, thus validating this practice in granulocytopenic children, as well. The advantage of the early empirical therapy was demonstrated in patients affected with severe infections due to Gram-negative rods, but the antibiotic regimens were formulated with the intention of providing coverage against both Gram-positive and Gram-negative organisms. The specific composition of the empiric regimen remains controversial. In the following paragraphs the main therapeutic approaches will be reviewed.

Combination therapy

Many studies have shown that combinations of antimicrobial agents should be preferred to single-agent therapy because of the broader antibacterial spectrum achieved, the potential for synergism against Gram-negative rods and the possible reduction in the emergence of resistant strains. The recommended regimens usually consist of an aminoglycoside (usually amikacin) with either an extended spectrum penicillin (e.g. ticarcillin, piperacillin or azlocillin) or an antipseudomonas cephalosporin (e.g. latamoxef disodium (Moxalactam), cefotaxime, cefoperazone or ceftazidime) (De Jongh et al, 1986a; Klastersky, 1986; Young, 1986; Rubin RH, 1988). However, good results with less aminoglycoside-related toxicity have also been reported with double β-lactam combinations (usually piperacillin and ceftazidime), especially in bone marrow transplant recipients (Winston et al, 1984; De Jongh et al, 1986b). Recently there has been increased interest in the new fluoroquinolones, especially for prophylaxis (Karp et al, 1987), but also for treatment of bacterial infections in neutropenic patients (Webster and Gaya, 1988). Unfortunately, these powerful compounds are so far proscribed in children. Whether or not this proscription is justified lies outside the scope of the present article; the problem has been recently reviewed (Chevais et al, 1987; Adam, 1989; Douidar and Snodgrass, 1989).

The 'combination therapy' approach has been verified in the animal model (Johnson, 1985) and has been clinically validated by the first three trials carried out by the EORTC-International Antimicrobial Therapy Group. These studies showed that the response rate of infections due to Gram-negative rods was clearly influenced by the susceptibility of the causative pathogen to the β-lactam rather than to the aminoglycoside component of the antibacterial regimen, but that aminoglycosides increased the bactericidal activity of the combination with improved outcome of Gram-negative bacteraemias (EORTC, 1978, 1983, 1986). However, in recent years, the development and marketing of the new extended-spectrum cephalosporins (in particular ceftazidime) raised increased interest in monotherapy. For this reason, the fourth trial of the EORTC group (EORTC, 1987) was directed to the specific question of whether the so called 'front loading' empirical therapy (Wade, 1989), i.e. ceftazidime combined with a 'loading' initial course (six doses) of amikacin, might be as effective as a prolonged course of both antibiotics. In 129 Gram-negative bacteraemias, front-loading therapy proved to be less effective than traditional therapy, without any advantage in terms of toxicity. Therefore, this study provided evidence against monotherapy, at least in patients with Gram-negative bacteraemia.

In all the EORTC trials amikacin was given every 8 or 12 hours. More recently, however, interest has focused on single daily dosing of aminoglycosides, as these antibiotics have rapid concentration-dependent bactericidal activity in vitro against Gram-negative aerobic bacilli (Vogelman and Craig, 1986) and a significant in vitro post-antibiotic effect, defined as a suppression of bacterial growth that persists after short exposure of organisms to antimicrobial agents (Craig and Vogelman, 1987). These characteristics have been confirmed in the animal model, as well as in an in vitro model of infections; studies have shown that large, intermittent doses result in similar or improved bactericidal effects (Powell et al, 1983; Blaser et al, 1985; Kapusnik et al, 1988; Vogelman et al, 1988; Wood et al, 1988) and less toxicity (Powell et al, 1983; Wood et al, 1988) when compared to continuous infusion or multiple daily dosing. Studies in adults (Powell et al, 1983; Nordstrom et al, 1985; Maller et al, 1988; Sturm, 1989) have demonstrated the safety and efficacy of this approach, which is now being tested by the EORTC group in a large, randomized ongoing study, including patients in the paediatric age group, comparing ceftazidime and amikacin, given three times a day, with ceftriaxone and amikacin given once a day.

In a pilot paediatric study (Viscoli et al, 1991b) febrile, neutropenic children who have undergone bone marrow transplantation were treated with a single daily dose of amikacin in combination with ceftazidime. In this study, a single, large dose of amikacin ($20\,\mathrm{mg\,kg^{-1}}$) resulted in high peak serum concentrations both on day 1 and 4 of therapy (72 and $74\,\mathrm{mg\,l^{-1}}$, respectively), which decreased to approximately half this value 30 minutes later. Amikacin concentrations were below quantifiable limits by 6 hours after infusion in most treatment courses. A modest rise in peak serum concentrations was observed over the duration of therapy, but this was not correlated with changes in serum creatinine and was not associated with any increase in trough concentrations. No auditory toxicity was observed in the ten children undergoing audiometry before and after treatment. Although therapeutic evaluation was not the purpose of the study, the response rate seemed comparable with that usually observed in our paediatric patients.

Further information about the clinical efficacy of single daily dosing of aminoglycosides in combination with a β-lactam should become available from the EORTC trial. Whatever administration schedule is used, monitoring of amikacin serum concentrations seems to be advisable, at least in paediatric cancer patients. This is clearly shown by the results of a recent study carried out in our institution (Viscoli et al, 1991c). In this trial, two antibiotic regimens (ceftazidime plus amikacin and ceftazidime plus vancomycin) were compared in febrile and granulocytopenic children with cancer. In 21 of 84 (25%) febrile episodes treated with amikacin, serum peak concentrations were below the therapeutic range ($15\text{--}25\,\mathrm{mg\,l^{-1}}$): these patients would have received less than the optimal dosage had serum concentrations not been monitored. A similar experience resulted from the study by Prober and coworkers (1981).

Single-drug therapy

In recent years some investigators have claimed that single-agent therapy with a third-generation antipseudomonas cephalosporin or with a carbapenem antibiotic could be as effective as combination therapy, with reduction in cost and side-effects (de Pauw et al, 1985, 1990; Pizzo et al, 1986; Wade et al, 1987). Other investigators reported reduced activity in Gram-negative bacteraemias, increased incidence of Gram-positive super-infections and frequent need to modify treatment by adding other antibiotics in patients receiving ceftazidime alone (Kramer et al, 1986; Wade et al, 1986; EORTC, 1987). Another risk of single-agent empiric therapy in granulocytopenic cancer patients is the possible selection of resistant Gram-negative pathogens. For example, in our experience (Viscoli et al, 1991c) patients receiving ceftazidime and vancomycin had a higher incidence of secondary Gram-negative bacteraemias (4 of 75) than those treated with the same cephalosporin in combination with amikacin (0 of 63).

Supporters of monotherapy rely mainly on the results of a clinical trial published in 1986 by Pizzo and coworkers, in which the efficacy of ceftazidime as single agent was compared with that of a combination of cephalothin, carbenicillin and gentamicin. This study has been criticized on three counts. Firstly, one might ask if the combination of gentamicin, cephalothin and carbenicillin is an appropriate control regimen or if it should not be considered as obsolete, given the entry in use of the new extended spectrum penicillins or third-generation cephalosporins. Secondly, in this study the duration of profound granulocytopenia was relatively short (about 8 days) and the number of documented infections was smaller than would have been expected from such a large trial (only 13 single-agent Gram-negative bacteraemias). Finally, these authors defined treatment as successful if the patient survived the episode of granulocytopenia, regardless of whether this was achieved with the addition of other antibiotics to the initial empiric regimen. When evaluating the same results by means of the classic EORTC definitions, it appeared that patients receiving ceftazidime had required a statistically significantly higher number of modifications (58 of 282, 21%) than those receiving combination therapy (29 of 268, 11%). Two very different approaches have thus been used to evaluate these results. The first approach regards as paramount survival from neutropenia and infection with or without therapeutic modifications. The other approach regards it as inconceivable to accept as equally effective two regimens, one of which has required significantly more treatment modifications than the other in order to obtain the same result.

Studies supporting these different points of view have fuelled several controversies in the recent years. However, most of these studies are not directly comparable, as methodologies and clinical situations (i.e. definitions, underlying diseases, pattern of infecting pathogens, micro-biological facilities, level of care, etc.) vary widely. Moreover, as assessed by Pater and Weir (1986) and Elliot and Pater (1988) and reviewed by Wade (1989), many of the studies are clearly deficient in statistical evaluation and in assessing the limitations (statistical type I and II errors) of the observed results. Many investigators seem not to realize that subgroup analyses are of limited value, because of their low statistical power, unless the sample size was calculated on the basis of the expected number of patients in the specific subgroup under evaluation. Endpoints are often not well-defined and conclusions are not based, as they should be, on a number of criteria, including response to the empirical regimen without modification of the allocated antibiotics, incidence of secondary infections, survival and antibiotic-related toxicity. 'Blinding' of study regimens should also be considered, and interim analyses should be avoided, unless otherwise indicated for ethical reasons. Finally, treatment results should be validated by multivariate analyses of factors likely to influence response to treatment (Hosmer and Lemeshow, 1989).

In order to make methodologies and definitions as uniform as possible the Immunocompromised Host Society (1990) has published a Consensus Report, based on the results of a meeting that was held in the setting of the 5th International Symposium on Infections in the Immunocompromised Host in June 1988. It is to be hoped that from now on all clinical studies in this field will follow these guidelines.

The problem of Gram-positive infections

The pattern of infecting organisms has changed over the past 10 years, and Gram-positive bacteria, which were prevalent in the 1950s and early 1960s, have again become the most common infecting pathogens (Pearson et al, 1977; Ladish and Pizzo, 1978; Pizzo et al, 1978; Kilton et al, 1979; Miser and Miser, 1980; Sotman et al, 1980; Carney et al, 1982; Wade et al, 1982; Winston et al, 1983; Friedman et al, 1984; Langley and Gold, 1988). As shown in Table 3, this has been clearly demonstrated by the results of the five trials performed by the EORTC Group from 1973 to 1988, which showed a statistically significant increase in the proportion of bacteraemias due to Gram-positive bacteria (EORTC 1988, 1990b). This phenomenon was mainly due to an increasing proportion of infections due to Viridans streptococci and coagulase-negative Staphylococci (Pizzo et al, 1978; Wade et al, 1982; EORTC, 1990b). In controlled studies, the increasing role of Gram-positive organisms in neutropenic cancer patients seems even more evident in pediatric populations (Cooper and Sumner, 1970; Kosmidis et al, 1980; Nachman and Honig, 1980; Pizzo et al, 1982b; Viscoli, 1988), support-

Table 3. Distribution of single Gram-positive and single Gram-negative bacteraemia in the five EORTC trials.

Trial	Evaluable cases	Bacteraemia Single agent	Gram-positive	Gram-negative
I (1973–1976)	453	145	42 (29%)	103 (71%)
II (1977–1980)	419	111	37 (33%)	74 (67%)
III (1980–1983)	582	141	58 (41%)	83 (59%)
IV (1983–1985)	872	219	90 (41%)	129 (59%)
V (1986–1988)	747	211	135 (64%)	76 (36%)

Chi-square for trend $p < 0.001$.

ing the suggestion that, in children, Gram-positive cocci are even more likely than in adults to be the leading pathogens of nosocomial infections. The reasons for the increasing role of Gram-positive micro-organisms in causing infection in these patients remain unclear. Cyclical variation over several decades has been recognized in the type of infecting pathogens and may be related to the selective pressure of antibiotics with a modified spectrum of action, such as the cephalosporins. The treatment of cancer has become more intensive and is now associated with more severe mucositis, leading to major damage of mucosal barriers and increasing risk of infection due to the resident oral flora. Herpes simplex oral lesions are increasingly reported in granulocytopenic patients and may further compromise mucous membrane integrity (Corey and Spear, 1986). In addition, patients with cancer, and especially children, are often fitted with indwelling catheters (especially Broviac or Hickman type, or Port-a-Cath); these devices can easily become colonized by skin bacteria and constitute a well-recognized risk factor for Gram-positive infections. For example, in the fourth trial of the EORTC (EORTC, 1990b) there was an increased risk of coagulase-negative staphylococcal infections in patients with an indwelling venous catheter when compared to patients not fitted with any central catheter (36 versus 15%). The exact role of gut decontamination directed against Gram-negative bacilli in selecting Gram-positive cocci is controversial, since a high incidence of Gram-positive infections has also been documented by investigators who do not use oral gut decontamination (Pizzo et al, 1978; Viscoli et al, 1984). Systemic prophylaxis with quinolone antibiotics, which is presently used by several oncology centres in Europe, has been advocated as a major cause of the shifting of the infecting flora (Decker et al, 1987; Karp et al, 1987). Since in the fourth trial of the EORTC International Antimicrobial Therapy Cooperative Group (EORTC, 1990b) only 3 of 90 patients with Gram-positive bacteraemia received a quinolone prophylactically, it seems unlikely that these new antibiotics are the only contributors to the increased frequency of Gram-positive bacteria, at least in the EORTC studies. Concurrently with the increase in Gram-positive infections, a review of the EORTC trials (EORTC, 1990b) shows that the response rate of these infections decreased significantly from 74% (31 of 42) in trial I (comparing carbenicillin plus cephalothin with carbenicillin plus gentamicin and with cephalothin plus gentamicin), to 46% (41 of 90) in trial IV (comparing azlocillin plus amikacin with ceftazidime plus a short course, 6 doses, of amikacin and with ceftazidime plus a full course of amikacin).

However, the decreasing efficacy of the regimens was not accompanied by increased mortality. For example mortality due to *Staphylococcus aureus* bacteraemia remained unchanged from trial I (11%) to trial IV (8%). Indeed, the prognosis of Gram-positive coccal bacteraemia is less severe than that of Gram-negative bacillary bacteraemia, with a mortality of 4% in EORTC trial IV (as compared to a mortality of 12% due to Gram-negative sepsis in the same trial), and none in the study by Pizzo (1986) and in our own experience (Viscoli et al, 1991c). Other paediatric studies confirm the lower mortality rate of Gram-positive bacteraemias as compared to that due to Gram-negative rods (Declerck et al, 1978; Nachman and Honig, 1980).

The impact of Gram-positive infections has led some investigators to suggest the inclusion of a specific anti-Gram-positive antibiotic in the initial empiric antimicrobial regimen. Several studies (Karp et al, 1986; Kramer et al, 1986; Del Favero et al, 1987; Shenep et al, 1988) reported favourable results from the early inclusion of vancomycin or teicoplanin in the empirical regimens, with more rapid resolution of fever and reduction in Gram-positive superinfections, total febrile days and need to use empirical amphotericin B. In contrast, Rubin M et al (1988), the EORTC group (EORTC, 1988; 1990b) and Viscoli et al (1991c) did not find any significant advantage in an early anti-Gram-positive specific coverage and suggested that vancomycin should be added to the early empirical regimen only upon documentation of a Gram-positive infection not responding to the initial empirical treatment. Several factors might explain these discrepancies, including differences in patient characteristics, trial design, antibiotic combinations, spectrum of pathogens and patterns of antibiotic susceptibility. On one hand the early anti-Gram-positive approach might reduce the duration of fever and shorten the interval between antineoplastic treatments. On the other hand the addition of vancomycin upon documentation of a Gram-positive infection in non-responding cases would reduce the number of patients unnecessarily exposed to a potentially toxic antibiotic, as well as reducing hospitalization costs. It is important to remember that the rationale of empirical antimicrobial therapy in neutropenic cancer patients is based on the high mortality rate of Gram-negative bacillary bacteraemias in these patients; since mortality due to Gram-positive bacteraemias appears to be significantly lower, the concept of empirical therapy may not be entirely applicable to Gram-positive infections.

In most of the above-mentioned studies supporting early empirical anti-Gram-positive therapy, the effect of vancomycin was studied in the setting of a triple antibiotic regimen, in combination with both an aminoglycoside and a β-lactam antibiotic. However, vancomycin might not be so effective when used as single anti-Gram-positive drug without aminoglycosides. In the study carried out in our paediatric oncology and infectious disease units (Viscoli et al, 1991c) patients were randomized to receive either ceftazidime plus amikacin or ceftazidime plus vancomycin. The purpose of the study was to evaluate the effect of the replacement of amikacin with vancomycin, in combination with the same cephalosporin. Overall, a difference in the response rate was shown that failed to achieve statistical significance (66% in the amikacin group and 77% in the vancomycin group). Similarly, subgroup analysis (bacteraemias, patients with long-lasting and severe neutropenia, etc.) failed to reveal any appreciable difference between the two regimens. This was also confirmed by the results of the multivariate analysis which showed that factors adversely affecting outcome were the presence of an acute leukaemia (especially a non-lymphoblastic leukaemia) and the presence of a documented infection (especially a clinically documented infection). In conclusion, in this study, despite the high incidence of Gram-positive infections (64%), the early inclusion of vancomycin did not provide the expected advantage. Six out of 12 staphylococcal bacteraemias associated with localized infections, randomized in the vancomycin group, required addition of another antistaphylococcal drug; in three of them failure was documented not only on clinical grounds, but also by persistence of positive cultures. Although definitive conclusions cannot be drawn because of the low statistical power of the study in the subgroup of Gram-positive bacteraemias, this study suggests that the early inclusion of vancomycin in empirical regimens should not be considered as a panacea for all Gram-positive infections; indeed such a policy might give a dangerous feeling of false-security of being protected against any staphylococcal or streptococcal infection.

In conclusion, the choice of the empirical antibiotic regimen should be tailored according to each institution's experience and according to each patient's risk of developing bacteraemia or other severe infection. This choice requires rigorous studies of predisposing factors. As stressed in a recent report from the Infectious Diseases Society of America (1990), a definitive study proving that single-drug treatment is unquestionably as effective as combined therapy is not available at the present time. Therefore, combined therapy including amikacin, at the dosage of $20\,mg\,kg^-$ $q24^{-1}$ or $10\,mg\,kg^{-1}\,q12^{-1}$, and ceftazidime, at the dosage of $25\,mg\,kg$ q.i.d., still remains the 'gold standard' of empirical therapy in febrile granulocytopenic children with cancer. Ceftazidime monotherapy is probably an acceptable therapeutic approach, provided resistance to ceftazidime is infrequent and patients are closely and frequently monitored by experienced staff, with the expectation that modifications in the anti-biotic regimen are likely to be needed because of treatment failures or emergence of secondary infections. Inclusion of an anti-Gram-positive drug in the 'up-front' regimen might be indicated in those patients with signs of infection at the exit site or along the course of a central indwelling catheter or in patients with a history of staphylococcal catheter-related infections.

Subsequent therapeutic modifications in patients with persistent or relapsing fever of unknown origin

While several investigators have proposed different approaches to empirical antibacterial therapy, very few studies have addressed the problem of how to deal with patients with persistent or relapsing fever, in the absence of any microbiological documentation of infection. Algorithms have been proposed (Hathorn and Pizzo, 1989) in order to standardize management of this difficult clinical situation. In our opinion, several options may be acceptable and several pathogens can be involved, sometimes together. Therefore therapeutic management should be altered in the light of each patient's past history and present situation; trying to standardize management for all possible events may in fact prove hazardous. For example, it should be recognized that infection is not the only cause of fever in neutropenic cancer patients. The inflammatory cascade that ultimately leads to the development of fever can also be triggered by pyrogenic antineoplastic medications, blood products, the underlying malignant disease and hypersensitivity reactions. The following case exemplifies this last possibility.

Illustrative case 3

A 12-year-old boy, with acute non-lymphoblastic leukaemia developed high fever and received ceftazidime and amikacin as empirical anti-bacterial treatment. A few days later, because of severe necrotizing stomatitis, therapy was replaced with imipenem–cylastatin and acyclovir, in order to improve antianaerobic and antiviral coverage. The patient showed rapid clinical improvement, but fever persisted, accompanied by a maculopapular, itchy skin rash. This clinical picture was considered to be due to an antibiotic-related reaction and anti-biotics were accordingly discontinued: the fever disappeared. The patient remained in the hospital under close clinical surveillance for 5 more days and was then discharged. This case shows that persistence of fever should not necessarily be considered as due to an infection.

More often, however, persistence or relapse of fever during broad-spectrum antibacterial therapy is actually due to a subsequent occult infection, commonly due to antibiotic-resistant bacteria, filamentous fungi, yeasts or viruses, particularly herpes viruses. These infections are often difficult to diagnose and to treat and are an important cause of morbidity and mortality in patients with neutropenia or just recovering from an episode of neutropenia. The following clinical cases are reported with the aim of giving some examples of how different the infectious localizations can be and how many the pathogens involved.

Illustrative case 4

A 6-year-old girl with acute lymphoblastic leukaemia presented with high fever and seizures during granulocytopenia. The mother reported a 2-week history of behavioural abnormalities. Brain CT-scan and CSF examination were normal. Cultures from blood and CSF were negative. Despite intensive diagnostic evaluation, fever remained unexplained until day 6, when the patient developed neurological signs and under-went lumbar puncture again. This time, CSF examination showed reduced glucose content, with few mononuclear cells. Cultures from blood and CSF yielded *Listeria monocytogenes* and CT-scan showed parenchymal intracerebral localizations. Empirical antibiotic treat-ment was then replaced by pathogen-directed therapy. The patient recovered and 6 months later successfully underwent allogeneic bone marrow transplantation. At the present time she is free of malignant disease and of neurological sequelae.

Viral infections are common complications in patients undergoing bone marrow transplantation, but are regarded as of secondary importance in leukaemic patients receiving first induction chemotherapy. However, the following case demonstrates that viruses may sometimes cause prolonged fevers and life-threatening infections during first induction chemotherapy.

Illustrative case 5

An 11-year-old girl with acute non-lymphoblastic leukaemia during the first course of induction chemotherapy received broad spectrum empiric antibacterial and antifungal therapy for several episodes of fever, in absence of any clinical or microbiological documentation of infection. Almost all episodes were accompanied by abdominal distension, pain and diarrhoea, suggestive of neutropenic enterocolitis. On day 70 of antineoplastic chemotherapy the patient developed clear signs of intestinal perforation, rendering surgery inevitable. Ileostomy with resection was then performed and several samples of the intestinal wall, lymphnodes and liver tissue underwent histological examination. All specimens showed evidence of intranuclear inclusions highly suggestive of cytomegalovirus (CMV) infection (Figure 4). The patient received gancyclovir and recovered. In this case CMV may have played a primary role in the infectious process.

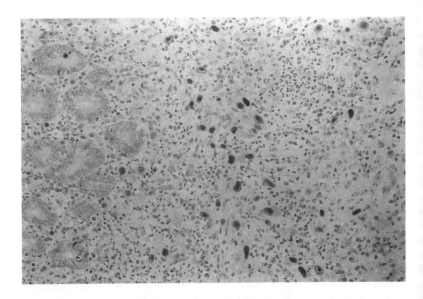

Figure 4. Cytomegalovirus enteritis in a girl affected with acute non-lymphocytic leukaemia and clinical picture of acute abdomen. Immunohistochemical staining shows the presence of cytomegalovirus infected cells in the intestinal wall (400·×, reproduced at 60% of original).

Fungal infections are probably the leading cause of persisting or relapsing fever after prolonged periods of granulocytopenia and antibacterial therapy. The following case underlines a crucial concept: in the absence of bone marrow recovery and remission from the underlying disease invasive fungal infections cannot be controlled and can kill patients despite appropriate therapy.

Illustrative case 6

A 14-year-old boy with acute lymphoblastic leukaemia in first induction, still not responding to multiple courses of anticancer chemotherapy, developed high fever and received broad spectrum antibacterial therapy. Seven days later, a right basal pulmonary infiltrate became evident on his chest X-ray film and amphotericin B was started empirically. Because he had not yet achieved remission, antineoplastic chemotherapy was continued. Despite intensive antibacterial and antifungal therapy, his clinical condition worsened relentlessly, with progression of pneumonia and respiratory failure. The patient died after 30 days of antifungal therapy, with persistent bone marrow aplasia. Autopsy showed diffuse pulmonary infiltration by *Aspergillus fumigatus* (Figure 5).

Empiric antifungal therapy

In recent years many articles have underlined the emerging role of fungal organisms in causing infection in cancer patients. Although the main pathogens still remain *Candida* and *Aspergillus*, there are increasing reports of infections caused by *Mucor* spp, *Pseudallescheria boydii*, *Fusarium* spp and other emerging agents (Rinaldi, 1989). In our paediatric institution from 1980 to 1989 a change in the clinical and aetiological pattern of fungal diseases was observed, with a significant increase both of invasive mycosis, with respect to fungaemias, and of infections due to filamentous fungi and unusual yeasts (Garaventa et al, 1990), with respect to those due to *Candida albicans*. Mortality from fungal infections is high, even if appropriate therapy is promptly instituted. Eradication is difficult if not impossible and relapses are common, especially in patients undergoing repeated cycles of antineoplastic therapy (Robertson and Larson, 1988), unless they are maintained on high-dose intravenous amphotericin B (Karp et al, 1988). Fungal infections may ultimately prevent continuation of the antineoplastic treatment, thus compromising the cure of cancer (Bodey, 1966; Mirsky and Cuttner, 1972; Kirk and Remington, 1976; Fisher et al, 1981; Meunier-Carpentier et al, 1981; Sculier et al, 1981; De Gregorio et al, 1982). Although early treatment is mandatory, early diagnosis is often impossible without invasive procedures and these may be precluded by the risk of bleeding, as well as by the often critical condition of the patient. Fungal colonization at multiple sites has been proposed as a predictor of invasive fungal infection (Martino et al, 1989) and therefore as a justification for empirical or early antifungal coverage. In a multivariate analysis of factors associated with invasive fungal infections Schwartz et al (1984) found that, in fact, the number of sites colonized with fungi on surveillance cultures was one of the factors which distinguished patients who ultimately developed invasive mycosis from those who did not. However, since about 80% of cancer patients undergoing intensive antineoplastic therapy become colonized by *Candida* spp. (Sandiford et al, 1980), one may ask what would be the discriminant power of this analysis had an external validation applied

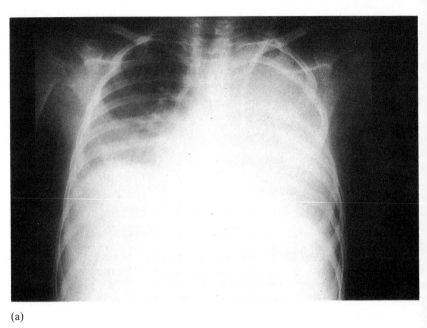

(a)

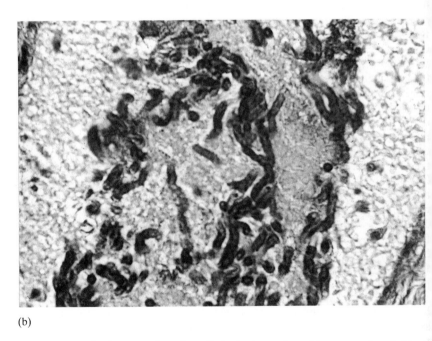

(b)

Figure 5. *Aspergillus fumigatus* disseminated infection in a patient with acute non-lymphoblastic leukaemia. (a) Radiological appearance. (b) Histology at autopsy (PAS stain; 40 ×, reproduced at 68% of original).

to the data. Indeed, other authorities consider surveillance cultures useful for predicting infection due to *Aspergillus* spp. and, perhaps, *Candida tropicalis*, but not reliable for all *Candida* infections (Meunier, 1988). Since surveillance cultures are expensive and time-consuming, it is unlikely that these procedures will become acceptable for routine rather than for research purposes.

In the early 1980s, two articles reported favourable results from the early empirical administration of amphotericin B in the subgroup of cancer patients with persistent or recurrent fever, receiving empirical antibacterial therapy, without any clinical or microbiological documentation of infection (Pizzo et al, 1982a; Stein et al, 1982). The rationale for this approach was based on the recognition that these patients are likely to be affected by an occult fungal infection. The problem has been recently addressed by the EORTC International Antimicrobial Therapy Cooperative Group in an article summarizing the results of two consecutive clinical trials of empiric antibiotic therapy (EORTC, 1989). In both trials patients without a microbiological documentation of infection, remaining febrile after at least 4 days of antibacterial therapy and still severely granulocytopenic, were randomly allocated to receive or not receive amphotericin B in addition to the previous antibacterial regimen. A better response rate was observed only in the subgroups of patients not receiving prior antifungal prophylaxis (78% versus 45%; p 0.04), in patients with a clinically documented infection (75% versus 41%; p 0.03), in those with severe granulocytopenia (69% versus 46%; p 0.06) and in patients older than 15 years of age (67% versus 47%; p 0.06). Patients treated empirically with amphotericin B had a lower number of documented fungal infections than other patients (1 of 68 versus 6 of 64; p 0.1) and no fungal deaths occurred among these patients, as compared to four fungal deaths among patients randomized not to receive empirical amphotericin B (p 0.05). In conclusion, there is some evidence that empirical antifungal therapy with amphotericin B is beneficial for the subgroup of patients with persistent or relapsing fever and granulocytopenia, not responding to empirical antibacterial therapy. Empirical antifungal therapy is widely used in children, too, even though in the EORTC trials a beneficial effect was shown only in patients older than 15 years. How long after initiation of antibacterials one should wait before administering amphotericin B remains controversial. Furthermore, in the light of the recent description of the 'hepatosplenic candidiasis syndrome' (Thaler et al, 1988), which is now increasingly observed in patients who have recovered from neutropenia, persistence of bone marrow failure is not always required for empirical initiation of antifungal therapy, if patients remain persistently febrile, although there are no controlled clinical studies to support such a policy.

Until recently, the choice of the antifungal drug to administer was limited, because amphotericin B was the only active drug in the treatment of systemic mycosis. Adverse effects of this drug, which have been recently reviewed (Koren et al, 1988; Gallis et al, 1990), cause considerable concern in physicians forced to administer the drug empirically. Newer antifungal agents, such as itraconazole and fluconazole, may offer significant options for antifungal treatment in this patient population. Itraconazole has been proposed for long-term treatment of patients recovered from aspergillosis, undergoing anticancer chemotherapy (Denning et al, 1989). Fluconazole is a bis-triazole derivative which has been reported to be effective in vivo against several fungal pathogens, with the possible exception of *Candida krusei* and *Candida glabrata* (Fisher MA et al, 1989). The drug is probably not effective against filamentous fungi, including *Aspergillus* spp., at least at usual dosages. It combines good oral absorption with water solubility, so that it can be administered both orally and intravenously. Experience in adult patients is reasonably large, while there are only anecdotal reports in children (Bunin, 1989; Viscoli et al, 1989). In a pilot study in our centre (Viscoli et al, 1991a) only 4 of 34 (12%) episodes of candidiasis in compromised children (mainly cancer patients and HIV-positive children) failed to respond to treatment. Toxicity was minimal and was represented only by mild transaminase increases. In particular, two *Candida parapsilosis* catheter-related fungaemias were treated successfully, with fluconazole, after increasing the dose up to $12 \, mg \, kg^{-1} \, day^{-1}$, without any increased toxicity. In conclusion, although amphotericin B has a broader spectrum of action and is probably intrinsically more active than fluconazole against *Candida* spp., fluconazole is less toxic and has a better pharmacokinetic profile. These characteristics make fluconazole an attractive therapeutic alternative to amphotericin B in the treatment of candidiasis and, potentially, in empiric antifungal therapy. In order to ascertain if this last indication is valid, we are now conducting a multicentre, comparative clinical study of fluconazole versus amphotericin B in the treatment of persistently febrile and granulocytopenic cancer patients, not responding to empirical antibacterial therapy, without any clinical or microbiological documentation of bacterial or fungal infection and with negative nasal cultures for *Aspergillus* spp.

CONCLUSIONS

This review has drawn attention to a number of controversies and areas of uncertainty in the management of the immunocompromised child. The best regimen for empiric antibacterial therapy, the management of the persistently febrile neutropenic child, the indication and best regimen for empirical antifungal therapy, are all examples of areas of unsettled debate. Paediatric haematologists and oncologists have led the field in submitting therapeutic agents to carefully designed controlled clinical trials. These trials have concentrated primarily on agents for cancer therapy, but the appreciation of the importance of adequate treatment of infection for successful outcome of intensive chemotherapy has prompted the design of additional trials of antimicrobial therapy. Large-scale randomized controlled multicentre trials, running simultaneously with trials of cancer therapy, could answer many of the unanswered questions highlighted by this review.

SUMMARY

Children receiving chemotherapy for malignant diseases show different patterns of infection depending on their underlying disease and its therapy. Granulocytopenia carries the risk of bacterial infection, and also, if prolonged, of fungal infection. Impairment of cell-mediated immunity predisposes to infections with *Pneumocystis carinii* and is thought to be responsible for severe primary infections with varicella and measles, as well as the severe cytomegalovirus infections seen after allogeneic bone marrow transplantation. Absence or impairment of splenic function predisposes to overwhelming septicaemia with encapsulated organisms, while defects in the normal mechanical barriers to infection provide routes for bacterial and fungal invasion.

Despite the lack of physical signs of a normal inflammatory response, clinical evaluation may be critical to the localization of infection in the immunocompromised child. Blood culture and biopsy remain pivotal investigations in the achievement of a microbiological diagnosis. Empirical treatment with a combination of antibiotics has been shown in comparative studies to be effective in initial management of the febrile neutropenic patient: continuing studies are evaluating the role of monotherapy and of different antibiotic combinations, particularly in the light of changing patterns of bacterial infections. Empirical antifungal therapy has been shown to be necessary for persistent or recurrent fever, particularly as persistent fungal infection may compromise the outcome of continuing cytotoxic therapy.

Continuing uncertainties over many aspects of management of the infected immunocompromised child provide scope for clinical trials in parallel with trials evaluating new anticancer regimens. The use of new diagnostic methods, the role of prophylaxis, the most appropriate empirical regimen, the evaluation of new antimicrobial agents, all require careful evaluation for efficacy and safety. Perhaps the greatest dilemma of all is how far results from trials in adults can be extrapolated to paediatric practice.

Acknowledgements

This work has been partially supported by grants of the University of Genova and Consiglio Nazionale delle Ricerche.

REFERENCES

Adam D (1989) Use of quinolones in pediatric patients. *Reviews of Infectious Diseases* **11** (suppl. 5): S1113–S1116.
American College of Physicians (1989) Parenteral nutrition in patients receiving cancer chemotherapy. *Annals of Internal Medicine* **110**: 734–736.
Armstrong D, Yu B, Ferreira R & Niki Y (1990) Tests for antigenuria in aspergillosis and candidiasis. *Abstracts of the 6th International Symposium on Infections in the Immunocompromised Host*, Peebles, 70.
Bennett JE (1987) Rapid diagnosis of candidiasis and aspergillosis. *Reviews of Infectious Diseases* **9**: 398–402.

Blaser J, Stone B & Zinner SH (1985) Efficacy of intermittent versus continuous administration of netilmicin in a two-compartment in vitro model. *Antimicrobial Agents and Chemotherapy* **27**: 343–349.

Bodey G (1966) Fungal infections complicating acute leukemia. *Journal of Chronic Diseases* **19**: 667–687.

Bodey GP (1986) Infection in cancer patients: a continuing association. *The American Journal of Medicine* **81** (suppl. 1A): 11–26.

Bodey GP & Luna M (1974) Skin lesions associated with disseminated candidiasis. *Journal of the American Medical Association* **229**: 1466–1468.

Bodey GP, Buckley M, Sathe YS & Freireich EJ (1966) Quantitative relationship between circulating leukocytes and infection in patients with acute leukemia. *Annals of Internal Medicine* **64**: 328–340.

Breatnach F & Androulakis PA (1983) Renal papillary adenocarcinoma following treatment for Wilms' tumor. *Cancer* **52**: 520–523.

Bunin N (1989) Oral fluconazole for treatment of disseminated fungal infection. *The Pediatric Infectious Disease Journal* **8**: 62.

Carney DN, Fossieck BE, Parker RH & Minna JD (1982) Bacteremia due to *Staphylococcus aureus* in patients with cancer: report of 45 cases in adults and review of the literature. *Reviews of Infectious Diseases* **4**: 1–12.

Chevais M, Reinert P, Rondeau MC et al (1987) Critical risk/benefit analysis of pefloxacin use in children under 15 years—the problem of arthralgy. *International Journal of Clinical Pharmacology* **25**: 306–309.

Cooper RG & Sumner C (1970) Hospital infection data from a children's hospital. *The Medical Journal of Australia* **2**: 1110–1113.

Corey L & Spear PG (1986) Infections with herpes simplex viruses. *The New England Journal of Medicine* **106**: 749–757.

Craig WA & Vogelman B (1987) The post-antibiotic effect. *Annals of Internal Medicine* **106**: 900–902.

Crislip MA & Edwards JE (1989) Candidiasis. *Infectious Disease Clinics of North America* **3**: 103–133.

Decker AW, Rozenberg-Arska M & Verhoef J (1987) Infection prophylaxis in acute leukemia: a comparison of ciprofloxacin with trimethoprim-sulfametoxazole and colistin. *Annals of Internal Medicine* **106**: 7–12.

Declerck Y, Declerck D, Rivaro GE & Benoit P (1978) Septicemia in children with leukemia. *Journal of the Canadian Medical Association* **118**: 1523–1525.

De Gregorio M, Lee W & Ries C (1982) Fungal infections in patients with acute leukemia. *The American Journal of Medicine* **73**: 543–548.

De Jongh CA, Joshi JC, Newman KA et al (1986a) Antibiotic synergism and response in Gram-negative bacteremia in granulocytopenic cancer patients. *The American Journal of Medicine* **80** (suppl. 5C): 96–100.

De Jongh CA, Joshi JH, Thompson BW et al (1986b) A double β-lactam combination versus an aminoglycoside-containing regimen as empiric antibiotic therapy for febrile granulocytopenic cancer patients. *The American Journal of Medicine* **80** (suppl. 5C): 101–111.

Del Favero A, Menichetti F, Guerciolini R et al (1987) Prospective randomized clinical trial of teicoplanin for empiric combined antibiotic therapy in febrile granulocytopenic acute leukemia patient. *Antimicrobial Agents and Chemotherapy* **31**: 1126–1129.

Denning DW, Tucker RM, Hanson LH & Stevens DA (1989) Treatment of invasive aspergillosis with itraconazole. *The American Journal of Medicine* **86**: 791–800.

de Pauw B, Williams K, de Neeff J et al (1985) A randomized prospective study of ceftazidime versus ceftazidime plus flucloxacillin in the empiric treatment of febrile episodes in severely neutropenic patients. *Antimicrobial Agents and Chemotherapy* **28**: 824–828.

de Pauw BE, Feld R & Deresinski S (1990) Multicenter, randomized, comparative study of ceftazidime vs piperacillin + tobramycin as empirical therapy for febrile granulocytopenic patients. *Abstracts of the 6th International Symposium on Infections in the Immunocompromised Host*, Peebles, 116.

Dinarello CA (1988a) Pathogenesis of fever. In Wyngaarden JB & Smith LH (eds) *Cecil textbook of medicine*, pp 1525–1527. Philadelphia: WB Saunders Co.

Dinarello CA (1988b) The acute phase response. In Wyngaarden JB & Smith LH (eds) *Cecil textbook of medicine*, pp 1527–1529. Philadelphia: WB Saunders Co.

Douidar SM & Snodgrass WR (1989) Potential role of fluoroquinolones in pediatric infections. *Reviews of Infectious Diseases* **11:** 878–889.

Edman JC (1989) Molecular biology: future effects on taxonomy, diagnosis, and therapy, pp 822–824. In Masur H, moderator. Pneumocystis pneumonia: from bench to clinic. *Annals of Internal Medicine* **111:** 813–826.

Elliott CR & Pater JL (1988) The effect of different measures of outcome on the results of studies of empiric antibiotic therapy in febrile neutropenic patients. *Clinical and Investigative Medicine* **11:** 327–330.

EORTC-International Antimicrobial Therapy Project Group (1978) Three antibiotic regimens in the treatment of infections in febrile granulocytopenic patients with cancer. *The Journal of Infectious Diseases* **137:** 14–29.

EORTC-International Antimicrobial Therapy Project Group (1983) Combination of amikacin and carbenicillin with or without cefazolin as empirical treatment of febrile neutropenic patients. *The Journal of Clinical Oncology* **1:** 597–603.

EORTC-International Antimicrobial Therapy Project Group (1986) Prospective randomized comparison of three antibiotic regimens for empirical bacteremic infections in febrile granulocytopenic patients. *Antimicrobial Agents and Chemotherapy* **29:** 263–270.

EORTC-International Antimicrobial Therapy Cooperative Group (1987) Ceftazidime combined with a short or long course of amikacin for empirical therapy of Gram-negative bacteremia in cancer patients. *The New England Journal of Medicine* **317:** 1692–1698.

EORTC-International Antimicrobial Therapy Cooperative Group (1988) Vancomycin added to empirical combination antibiotic therapy for fever in granulocytopenic cancer patients. *Abstracts of the 28th Interscience Conference on Antimicrobial Agents and Chemotherapy*, Los Angeles, 18.

EORTC-International Antimicrobial Therapy Cooperative Group (1989) Empiric antifungal therapy in febrile granulocytopenic patients. *The American Journal of Medicine* **86:** 668–672.

EORTC-International Antimicrobial Therapy Cooperative Group (1990a) Factors predicting bacteremia in neutropenic patients. *Abstracts of the 6th International Symposium on Infections in the Immunocompromised Host*, Peebles, 122.

EORTC-International Antimicrobial Therapy Cooperative Group (1990b) Gram-positive bacteraemia in granulocytopenic cancer patients. *European Journal of Cancer* **26:** 569–574.

Fisher BD, Armstrong D, Yu B & Gold JWM (1981) Invasive aspergillosis. Progress in early diagnosis and treatment. *The American Journal of Medicine* **71:** 571–577.

Fisher MA, Shen SH, Jaddad J & Tarry WF (1989) Comparison of in vivo activity of fluconazole with that of amphotericin B against *Candida tropicalis, Candida glabrata* and *Candida krusei. Antimicrobial Agents and Chemotherapy* **33:** 1443–1446.

Frank I & Friedman HM (1988) Progress in the treatment of cytomegalovirus pneumonia. *Annals of Internal Medicine* **109:** 769–771.

Frankel LR, Smith DW & Lewiston NJ (1988) Bronchoalveolar lavage for diagnosis of pneumonia in the immunocompromised child. *Pediatrics* **81:** 785–788.

Freeman J, Goldmann DA, Smith NE et al (1990) Association of intravenous lipid emulsion and coagulase-negative staphylococcal bacteremia in neonatal intensive care unit. *The New England Journal of Medicine* **323:** 301–308.

Friedman LE, Brown AE, Miller DR & Armstrong D (1984) *Staphyloccus epidermidis* septicemia in children with leukemia and lymphoma. *American Journal of Diseases of Children* **138:** 715–719.

Gallis HA, Drew RH & Pickard WW (1990) Amphotericin B 30 years of clinical experience. *Reviews of Infectious Diseases* **12:** 308–329.

Ganser A, Ottmann OG, Erdman H, Schulz G & Hoelzer D (1989) The effect of recombinant human granulocyte–macrophage colony stimulating factor on neutropenia and related morbidity in chronic severe neutropenia. *Annals of Internal Medicine* **11:** 887–892.

Garaventa A, Castagnola E, Fabbri A et al (1990) Fungal infections in children with cancer. *Abstracts of the 6th International Symposium on Infections in the Immunocompromised Host*, Peebles, 73.

Hathorn JW & Pizzo PA (1989) Infectious complications in the pediatric cancer patient. In Pizzo PA & Poplack DG (eds) *Principles and practice of pediatric oncology*, pp 837–867. Philadelphia: JB Lippincott Company.

Hathorn JW, Rubin M & Pizzo PA (1987) Empirical antibiotic therapy in febrile neutropenic cancer patient: clinical efficacy and impact of monotherapy. *Antimicrobial Agents and Chemotherapy* **31**: 971–977.

Hosmer DW & Lemeshow S (1989) *Applied logistic regression*. New York: John Wiley.

Immunocompromised Host Society (1990) Report of a Consensus Panel: The design, analysis, and reporting of clinical trials on the empirical antibiotic management of the neutropenic patient. *The Journal of Infectious Diseases* **161**: 397–401.

Infectious Diseases Society of America (Hughes WT, Armstrong D, Bodey GP et al) (1990) Guidelines for the Use of antimicrobial agents in neutropenic patients with unexplained fever. *The Journal of Infectious Diseases* **161**: 381–396.

Johnson D (1985) Use of discriminative models of *Pseudomonas aeruginosa* bacteremia in granulocytopenic rats for testing antimicrobial efficacy. *European Journal of Clinical Microbiology* **4**: 207–212.

Kupusnik JE, Hackbarth CJ, Chambers HF et al (1988) Single, large, daily dosing versus intermittent dosing of tobramycin for treating experimental pseudomonas pneumonia. *The Journal of Infectious Diseases* **158**: 7–12.

Karp JE, Dick JD, Angelopulos C et al (1986) Empiric use of vancomycin during prolonged treatment induced granulocytopenia. Randomized, double-blind, placebo controlled trial in patients with acute leukemia. *The American Journal of Medicine* **81**: 237–242.

Karp JE, Merz WG, Hendricksen C et al (1987) Oral norfloxacin for prevention of Gram-negative bacterial infections in patients with acute leukemia and granulocytopenia: a randomized, double-blind, placebo-controlled trial. *Annals of Internal Medicine* **106**: 1–7.

Karp JE, Burch PA & Merz WG (1988) An approach to intensive anti-leukemia therapy in patients with previous invasive aspergillosis. *The American Journal of Medicine* **85**: 203–209.

Kensch GT (1984) Nutrition and infection. In Remington JS & Swartz MN (eds) *Current clinical Topics in Infectious Diseases*, pp 106–123. New York: McGraw-Hill.

Khardori N (1989) Host–parasite interaction in fungal infections. *European Journal of Clinical Microbiology and Infectious Diseases* **8**: 331–351.

Kilton LJ, Fossieck BE, Cohen MH & Parker RH (1979) Bacteremia due to Gram-positive cocci in patients with neoplastic disease. *The American Journal of Medicine* **66**: 596–602.

Kirk J & Remington J (1976) Opportunistic invasive fungal infection in patients with leukemia and lymphoma. *Clinics in Haematology* **5**: 249–310.

Klastersky J (1986) Concept of empiric therapy with antibiotic combinations: indications and limits. *The American Journal of Medicine* **80** (Suppl. 5C): 2–12.

Klastersky J & Zinner S (1982) Synergistic combinations of antibiotics in Gram-negative bacillary infections. *Reviews of Infectious Diseases* **4**: 294–301.

Klemper MS, Noring R, Mier JW & Atkins MB (1990) An acquired chemotactic defect in neutrophils from patients receiving interleukin-2 immunotherapy. *The New England Journal of Medicine* **322**: 959–965.

Koren G, Lau A, Golas C et al (1988) Pharmacokinetics and adverse effects of amphotericin B in infants and children. *Journal of Pediatrics* **11**: 559–563.

Kosmidis HV, Lusher JM, Shope TC et al (1980) Infections in leukemic children: a prospective analysis. *Journal of Pediatrics* **96**: 407–412.

Kramer BS, Ramphal R & Rand KH (1986) Randomized comparison between two ceftazidime-containing regimens and cephalothin-gentamicin-carbenicillin in febrile granulocytopenic patients. *Antimicrobial Agents and Chemotherapy* **30**: 64–69.

Ladisch S & Pizzo PA (1978) *Staphylococcus aureus* sepsis in children with cancer. *Pediatrics* **61**: 231–234.

Langley J & Gold R (1988) Sepsis in febrile neutropenic children with cancer. *The Pediatric Infectious Diseases Journal* **7**: 34–37.

Leibovitz E, Rigaud M, Pollack K et al (1990) *Pneumocystis carinii* pneumonia in infants infected with the human immunodeficiency virus with more than 450 CD4 T lymphocytes per cubic millimeter. *The New England Journal of Medicine* **323**: 531–533.

Love JL, Schimpff SC, Schiffer CA & Wiernik PH (1980) Improved prognosis for granulo-cytopenic patients with Gram-negative bacteremia. *The American Journal of Medicine* **68**: 643–648.

Maki DG (1989) Pathogenesis, prevention, and management of infections due to intravascular devices used for infusion therapy. In Bisno AL & Waldvogel FA (eds) *Infections associated with indwelling medical devices*, pp 161–177. Washington, DC: American Society for Microbiology.

Mackie PH, Crockson RA & Stuart J (1979) C-reactive protein for rapid diagnosis of infection in leukaemia. *Journal of Clinical Pathology* **32:** 1253–1256.

Maller R, Isaksson B, Nilsson L & Soren L (1988) A study of amikacin given once versus twice daily in serious infections. *The Journal of Antimicrobial Chemotherapy* **22:** 75–79.

Martino P, Girmenia C, Venditti M et al (1989) *Candida* colonization and systemic infection in neutropenic patients. A retrospective study. *Cancer* **64:** 2030–2034.

Mason WH, Siegel SE & Tucker BL (1982) Diagnostic open lung biopsy for diffuse pulmonary disease in immunocompromised pediatric patients. *The American Journal of Pediatric Hematology and Oncology* **4:** 355–359.

Masur H, Ognibene FP, Yarchoan R et al (1989) CD4 counts as predictors of opportunistic pneumonias in human immunodeficiency virus (HIV) infection. *Annals of Internal Medicine* **11:** 223–231.

Meunier F (1988) Fungal infections in the compromised host. In Rubin RH & Young LS (eds) *Clinical approach to infection in the Compromised Host*, pp 193–220. New York: Plenum Medical.

Meunier-Carpentier F, Kiehn TE & Armstrong D (1981) Fungemia in the immunocompromised host. *The American Journal of Medicine* **71:** 363–370.

Meyers JD & Thomas D (1988) Infection complicating bone marrow transplantation. In Rubin RH & Young LS (eds) *Clinical approach to infection in the compromised host*, pp 525–556. New York: Plenum Medical.

Mirsky S & Cuttner J (1972) Fungal infection in acute leukemia. *Cancer* **30:** 348–352.

Miser JS & Miser AW (1980) *Staphylococcus aureus* sepsis in childhood malignancy. *American Journal of Diseases of Children* **134:** 831–833.

Morris DJ (1990) Virus infections in children with cancer. *Reviews in Medical Microbiology* **1:** 49–57.

Nachman JB & Honig GR (1980) Fever and neutropenia in children with neoplastic diseases. An analysis of 158 episodes. *Cancer* **45:** 407–412.

Nordstrom L, Cronberg S, Rinberg H et al (1985) Prospective, comparative, randomized clinical study of aminoglycosides given once a day versus three times a day in severe infections. In Ishigami J (ed.) *Recent Advances in Chemotherapy*, pp 2653–2654. Tokyo: University of Tokyo Press.

O'Garra A (1989) Interleukins and the immune system. 1. *The Lancet* **i:** 943–947.

Parrillo JE, Parker MM, Natanson C et al (1990) Septic shock in humans: advances in understanding of pathogenesis, cardiovascular disfunction and therapy. *Annals of Internal Medicine* **113:** 227–242.

Pater JL & Weir L (1986) Reporting the results of randomized trials of empiric antibiotics in febrile neutropenic patients: A critical survey. *Journal of Clinical Oncology* **4:** 346–352.

Pearson TA, Braine HG & Rathburn HK (1977) *Corynebacterium* sepsis in oncology patients. Predisposing factors, diagnosis, and treatment. *Journal of the American Medical Association* **238:** 1737–1740.

Pepys MB (1981) C-reactive protein 50 years on. *Lancet* **i:** 653–657.

Pizzo PA, Ladisch S & Witebsky FG (1978) Alpha-hemolitic streptococci: clinical significance in the cancer patient. *Medical and Pediatric Oncology* **4:** 367–370.

Pizzo PA, Robichand KJ, Gill FA & Witebsky FG (1982a) Empiric antibiotic and antifungal therapy for cancer patients with prolonged fever and granulocytopenia. *The American Journal of Medicine* **72:** 101–111.

Pizzo PA, Robichand KJ, Wesley R & Commers JR (1982b) Fever in the pediatric and young adult patient with cancer. A prospective study of 1001 episodes. *Medicine* **61:** 153–165.

Pizzo PA, Hathorn JW, Hiemenz J et al (1986) A randomized trial comparing ceftazidime alone with combination antibiotic therapy in cancer patients with fever and neutropenia. *The New England Journal of Medicine* **315:** 552–558.

Powell DA, Angust J, Snedden S, Hansen B & Brady M (1984) Broviac catheter-related *Malassezia furfur* sepsis in five infants receiving intravenous fat emulsion. *Journal of Pediatrics* **105:** 987–990.

Powell SH, Thompson WL, Luther MA et al (1983) Once-daily vs. continuous aminoglycoside dosing: efficacy and toxicity in animal and clinical studies of gentamicin, netilmicin and tobramycin. *The Journal of Infectious Diseases* **147:** 918–932.

Prober CG, Yeager AS & Arvin A (1981) The effect of chronologic age on the serum concentrations of amikacin in sick term and premature infants. *Journal of Pediatrics* **98:** 636–640.

Rapson NT, Cornbleet MA, Chessells JM et al (1980) Immunosuppression and serious infections in children with acute leukaemia: a comparison of three chemotherapy regimens. *British Journal of Haematology* **45:** 41–52.

Rinaldi MG (1989) Emerging opportunists. *Infectious Disease Clinics of North America* **3:** 65–76.

Robertson MJ & Larson RA (1988) Recurrent fungal pneumonias in patients with acute nonlymphocytic leukemia undergoing multiple courses of intensive chemotherapy. *The American Journal of Medicine* **84:** 233–239.

Rubin M, Hathorn JW, Marshall D et al (1988) Gram-positive infections and the use of vancomycin in 550 episodes of fever and neutropenia. *Annals of Internal Medicine* **108:** 30–35.

Rubin RH (1988) Empiric antibacterial therapy in granulocytopenia induced by cancer chemotherapy. *Annals of Internal Medicine* **108:** 134–136.

Sandiford GR, Merz WG, Wingard JR et al (1980) The value of fungal surveillance cultures as predictors of systemic fungal infections. *The Journal of Infectious Disease* **142:** 503–509.

Schimpff SC (1986) Empiric antibiotic therapy for granulocytopenic cancer patients. *The American Journal of Medicine* **80** (suppl. 5C): 13–20.

Schimpff SC, Saterlee W & Young VM (1971) Empiric therapy with carbenicillin and gentamicin for febrile patients with cancer and granulocytopenia. *The New England Journal of Medicine* **284:** 1061–1065.

Schimpff SC, Young V, Greene E et al (1972) Origin of infection in acute non-lymphocytic leukemia: significance of hospital acquisition of potential pathogens. *Annals of Internal Medicine* **77:** 707–714.

Schwartz RS, Mackintosh FR, Schrier SL & Greenberg PL (1984) Multivariate analysis of factors associated with invasive fungal disease during remission induction therapy for acute myelogenous leukemia. *Cancer* **53:** 411–419.

Sculier JP, Weerts D, Klastersky J (1981) Causes of death in febrile granulocytopenic cancer patients receiving empiric antibiotic therapy. *European Journal of Cancer and Clinical Oncology* **20:** 55–60.

Shearer WT & Anderson DC (1989) The secondary immunodeficiencies. In Stiehm ER (ed.) *Immunologic disorders in infants and children*, pp 400–438. Philadelphia: WB Saunders.

Shenep J, Hughes WT, Roberson PK et al (1988) Vancomycin, ticarcillin, and amikacin compared with ticarcillin-clavulanate and amikacin in the empirical treatment of febrile, neutropenic children with cancer. *The New England Journal of Medicine* **319:** 1053–1058.

Singer C, Kaplan MH & Armstrong D (1977) Bacteremia and fungemia complicating neoplastic disease. A study of 364 cases. *The American Journal of Medicine* **62:** 731–742.

Smith PD, Lamerson CL, Banks SL et al (1990) Granulocyte–macrophage colony-stimulating factor augments human monocyte fungicidal activity for *Candida albicans*. *The Journal of Infectious Diseases* **161:** 999–1005.

Snydman DR, Sullivan B, Gill H et al (1990) Nosocomial sepsis associated with interleukin-2. *Annals of Internal Medicine* **112:** 102–107.

Sotman SB, Schimpff SC & Young VM (1980) *Staphylococcus aureus* bacteremia in patients with acute leukemia. *The American Journal of Medicine* **69:** 814–818.

Steffen EK, Berg D & Deitch EA (1988) Comparison of translocation rates of various indigenous bacteria from the gastrointestinal tract to mesenteric lymph node. *The Journal of Infectious Diseases* **157:** 1032–1038.

Stein RS, Kayser J & Flexner JM (1982) Clinical value of empirical amphotericin B in patients with acute myelogenous leukemia. *Cancer* **50:** 2247–2251.

Sturm AW (1989) Netilmicin in the treatment of Gram-negative bacteremia: single daily versus multiple daily dosage. *The Journal of Infectious Diseases* **159:** 931–937.

Thaler M, Pastakia B, Shawker TH et al (1988) Hepatic candidiasis in cancer patients: the evolving picture of the syndrome. *Annals of Internal Medicine* **108:** 88–100.

Tracey KJ, Vlassara A & Cerami A (1989) Cachectin/tumor necrosis factor. *Lancet* **i:** 1122–1126.

Viscoli C (1988) Aspects of infections in children with cancer. *Recent Results in Cancer Research* **108:** 71–81.

Viscoli C, Perlino GF, Moroni C et al (1984) Gram positive infections in pediatric cancer patients: 84 cases. *Abstracts of the 3rd International Symposium on Infections in the Immunocompromised Host*, Toronto, 136.

Viscoli C, Garaventa A, Boni L et al (1988) Role of Broviac catheters in infections in children with cancer. *The Pediatric Infectious Disease Journal* 7: 556–560.

Viscoli C, Castagnola E, Corsini M et al (1989) Fluconazole therapy in an underweight infant. *European Journal of Clinical Microbiology and Infectious Diseases* 8: 925–926.

Viscoli C, Castagnola E, Fionedda F et al (1991a) Fluconazole in the treatment of candidiasis in immunocompromised children. *Antimicrobial Agents and Chemotherapy* (in press).

Viscoli C, Dudley M, Ferrea G et al (1991b) Serum concentrations and safety of single daily dosing of amikacin in children undergoing bone marrow transplantation. *The Journal of Antimicrobial Chemotherapy* (in press).

Viscoli C, Moroni C, Boni L et al (1991c) Ceftazidime plus amikacin versus ceftazidime plus vancomycin as empiric therapy in febrile neutropenic children with cancer. *Reviews of Infectious Diseases* (in press).

Vogelman B & Craig WA (1986) Kinetics of antimicrobial activity. *Journal of Pediatrics* 198: 835–840.

Vogelman B, Gudmundsson S, Leggett J et al (1988) Correlation of antimicrobial pharmaco-kinetic parameters with therapeutic efficacy in an animal model. *The Journal of Infectious Diseases* 158: 831–847.

Wade JC (1989) Antibiotic therapy for the febrile granulocytopenic cancer patient: combination therapy vs. monotherapy. *Reviews of Infectious Diseases* 11 (suppl. 7): S1572–S1581.

Wade JC, Schimpff SC, Newman KA & Wiernik PH (1982) *Staphylococcus epidermidis*: an increasing cause of infection in patients with granulocytopenia. *Annals of Internal Medicine* 97: 503–508.

Wade J, Johnson D & Bustamante CI (1986) Monotherapy for empiric treatment of fever in granulocytopenic cancer patients. *The American Journal of Medicine* 80 (suppl. 5c): 85–95.

Wade J, Bustamante C, Devlin A et al (1987) Imipenem versus piperacillin plus amikacin, empiric therapy for febrile neutropenic patients: a double-blind trial. *Abstracts of the 27th Interscience Conference on Antimicrobial Agents and Chemotherapy*, New York, 1251, p 315.

Walsh TJ, Hathon J, Crane L et al (1990) Expression of a 48 KD *Candida* cytoplasmic antigen in cancer patients. *Abstracts of the 6th International Symposium on Infections in the Immuno-compromised Host*, Peebles, 91.

Washington JA II (1990) Bacteria, fungi, and parasites. In Mandell GL, Douglas RG Jr & Bennett JE (eds) *Principles and Practice of Infectious Diseases*, pp 160–193. New York: Churchill Livingstone.

Webster A & Gaya H (1988) Quinolones in the treatment of serious infections. *Reviews of Infectious Diseases* 10: S225–S233.

Weisbart RH, Gasson JC & Golde DW (1989) Colony-stimulating factors and host defense. *Annals of Internal Medicine* 110: 297–303.

Winston DJ, Dudnick DV, Chapin M et al (1983) Coagulase-negative staphylococcal bacteremia in patients receiving immunosuppressive therapy. *Archives of Internal Medicine* 143: 32–36.

Winston DJ, Barnes RC, Ho WG et al (1984) Moxalactam plus piperacillin versus moxalactam plus amikacin in febrile, granulocytopenic patients. *The American Journal of Medicine* 77: 442–450.

Wood CA, Norton DR, Kohnen et al (1988) The influence of tobramycin dosage regimens on nephrotoxicity, ototoxicity, and antibacterial efficacy in a rat model subcutaneous abscesses. *The Journal of Infectious Diseases* 158: 13–22.

Young LS (1986) Empirical antimicrobial therapy in neutropenic host. *The New England Journal of Medicine* 315: 580–581.

10

Transfusion and the use of blood products

DEREK JOHN KING

Transfusion practice has evolved from the non-specific use of whole blood to the highly selective use of individual components and plasma fractions, such as coagulation factors and antibodies, with specific activity and indications. The main indications for transfusion of blood and blood products are well established. However there is increasing concern about the complications of transfusion, especially the transmission of infectious agents, and this has made the assessment of alternatives to blood component therapy more relevant in current haematological practice. Simultaneously with the rapid increase in the use of blood and its products there are increasing threats to its supply. This chapter will review new technologies in relation to transfusion medicine, certain indications for transfusion where there is more controversy, and methods of reducing the risks inherent in transfusion. Alternatives to conventional blood products in transfusion practice will also be discussed. A major problem in evaluating new approaches to treatment is the rarity of many of the diseases in children so that it is frequently difficult to find adequate randomized studies to form a critical judgement.

TECHNICAL DEVELOPMENTS

The major clinical development in recent years has been the technique of cannulation of the umbilical vessels of the fetus in utero to permit access to the fetal circulation. This technique is now well established in specialist centres, and reference ranges have been calculated for blood counts, coagulation factors, and red cell enzymes.

In experienced hands the technique has a low complication rate and is efficient (Daffos et al, 1985). When performed on out-patients without sedation, pure fetal blood was obtained at the first attempt in 588 of 606 pregnancies between 17 and 38 weeks of gestation; a second attempt was required in only 18 cases. Based on the results obtained, 58 pregnancies were terminated and in those which continued the complications included premature delivery (5%), intrauterine growth retardation (8%), intrauterine death (1.1%), and spontaneous abortion (0.8%). It seems unlikely that all of these could be directly attributable to the procedure. The same clinicians have outlined their approach to the management of neonatal bleeding disorders, both hereditary and acquired (Daffos et al, 1988). They used the technique to

Baillière's Clinical Haematology—
Vol. 4, No. 2, April 1991
ISBN 0–7020–1532–6

determine platelet counts or coagulation factor levels and to plan therapeutic intervention, such as method of delivery, or to transfuse platelet or coagulation factor concentrates. Based on the fetal blood sample results they suggest algorithms for the management of alloimmune thrombocytopenia and autoimmune thrombocytopenia in pregnancy. Their approach has been adopted by other investigators including Moise et al (1988) who allowed 21 pregnant women with autoimmune thrombocytopenia to deliver vaginally with the knowledge that fetal platelet counts were adequate.

Fetal blood sampling is also helpful in the management of rhesus allo-immunized pregnancies. The fetal blood group and haematocrit are determined and regular monitoring is possible with intrauterine transfusions performed as indicated. Barss et al (1988) managed 22 patients with 23 pregnancies complicated by alloimmunization. Nine patients had a total of 30 fetal blood samples performed without complication. The remaining thirteen mothers had 45 intrauterine intravascular transfusions and 16 intraperitoneal transfusions. The overall fetal survival was 85.7%, with 83.3% for fetuses hydropic at diagnosis. The procedure-related perinatal mortality for intrauterine transfusion was 2.2%. Determination of the fetal blood group and haematocrit allowed individualized treatment and it was suggested that direct intravascular transfusion could be life-saving in hydrops. Blood for intrauterine transfusion should be seronegative for cytomegalovirus (CMV) infection and should be irradiated prior to use. Only a small number of specialized centres have the necessary expertise for intrauterine intravascular transfusion. Because of the advantages of determining the haematocrit to subsequent management and the superiority of intravascular over intraperitoneal transfusion, sensitized mothers at risk of carrying an affected infant should be referred to a centre with the necessary expertise for the optimal management.

The pattern of neonatal transfusion has changed in recent years because of advances in intrauterine transfusion and the delivery of babies at early gestational ages. There has been a marked reduction in exchange trans-fusions performed and the majority of transfusions in the newborn are of small volume and given to replace losses caused by the increased intensity of laboratory monitoring of seriously ill premature neonates. Subdivision of a standard unit of blood into minipacks reduces wastage by providing small volumes of blood for transfusion to the neonate. Wherever possible the blood should be seronegative for CMV. Guidelines for the supply of blood for neonates have been issued (Working Party of the BCSH Blood Trans-fusion Task Force, 1987). If the maternal antibody screen is negative and the baby's direct antiglobulin test is negative, blood of the same ABO and Rhesus D group can be given without cross-matching if the blood groups of the donor units are verified. Infants under 4 months of age do not appear to form alloantibodies even after repeated transfusions.

RED CELL TRANSFUSION

Any patient likely to require regular transfusion, either with red cells or platelets, should receive CMV-negative blood products which have been filtered to remove the white cells. This reduces the risks of infection and alloimmunization, especially if bone marrow transplantation may be a therapeutic option at a later date, for example in children with severe aplastic anaemia.

Thalassaemia major

The benefits of regular transfusion programmes in this disorder are well documented with improved growth, endocrine function and survival, and maintenance of cardiac function (Hoffbrand and Wonke, 1989). However, together with dependence on transfusion, these improvements can only be achieved with the additional inconvenience of iron-chelation therapy. Currently desferrioxamine is the only widely available iron-chelating agent but has the disadvantages of expense and the necessity of parenteral administration, usually by subcutaneous infusion for 12 hours per day.

There are a number of options to alleviate the problems of transfusion and iron overload in thalassaemia major. The first is to reduce the incidence of the disorder and there is evidence that programmes of genetic counselling and antenatal diagnosis can reduce thalassaemia major births by 50–70% (Cao, 1987). This has been demonstrated in countries with a high prevalence of the thalassaemia gene where transfusion-chelation programmes would be more difficult to maintain.

Given that a diagnosis of thalassaemia major has been made bone marrow transplantation offers a chance of 'cure', albeit with the risks of the procedure. In reviewing 222 patients with thalassaemia major undergoing bone marrow transplantation, Lucarelli et al (1990) concluded that patients under 16 years of age without hepatomegaly or portal fibrosis had a high probability of complication-free survival (94% at 3 years). Although the risk of infection from the early blood transfusions would remain, the risks of iron overload are avoided.

In patients with thalassaemia and no compatible sibling a more acceptable option than desferrioxamine would encourage compliance and reduce the risks of iron toxicity. Extensive research has been undertaken into oral iron chelators in the groups of derivatives of pyridoxal isonicotinoyl hydrazone, the phenolic EDTA derivatives and hydroxypyridones. These compounds have improved absorption via the oral route, increased lipid solubility and preferential reaction with parenchymal iron (Hershko et al, 1990). A limiting factor has been the toxicity of these drugs but 1,2-dimethyl-3-hydroxypyrid-4-one (L1) has shown considerable promise (Kontoghiorghes et al, 1987), although there remains debate about its toxicity (Editorial, 1989). Kontoghiorghes and Hoffbrand (1989) reviewed 120 patients treated with L1 for 1 to 15 months and showed no greater toxicity than with desferrioxamine.

Sickle cell disease

The indications for transfusion in this disorder have been reviewed by

Davies and Brozovic (1989) under three types—simple or additive transfusion, exchange transfusion, and hypertransfusion regimens. In addition to
the problems of transfusion discussed elsewhere in the chapter, patients with
sickle cell disease have a higher incidence of alloimmunization to red cell
antigens than other patients having regular transfusions (30% compared
with 5%) and may develop multiple antibodies. This is thought to be related
to racial differences between the patient group and the donor population
which was 90% white in this report (Vichinsky et al, 1990). It is suggested
that the patients should have their red cell phenotype analysed at an early
stage and attempts made to choose appropriate blood.

Experimental work suggests that hydroxyurea therapy can increase fetal
haemoglobin production and reduce the tendency for haemoglobin S
polymerization but at the risk of myelosuppression (Rodgers et al, 1990).
There is a possible role for drugs such as aromatic benzaldehydes that
modify oxygen affinity and improve deformability of red cells (Keidan et al,
1989). Such developments are at an early stage and their ultimate role
remains to be determined.

Recurrence of malignant disease

In adult oncology practice concerns have been expressed about the role of
perioperative blood transfusion in influencing recurrence of solid tumours.
Although not confirmed in all studies (Weiden et al, 1987), there is considerable evidence that blood transfusion can increase the risk of recurrence of
tumours such as colorectal carcinoma (Blumberg and Heal, 1987; Blumberg
et al, 1988) and this may be due to an effect of plasma (March et al, 1990). As
the majority of childhood cancers are quite different from adult solid
tumours in biology and response to treatment, the relevance of these
observations to paediatric practice is not clear but remind us of the possible
risks of unnecessary transfusion.

Autologous blood transfusion

The storage and subsequent transfusion of the patient's own red cells avoids
all the risks of homologous blood transfusion and is an attractive option for
planned surgical procedures which require the transfusion of blood. A
survey between 1982 and 1988 reported a decrease in transfusion of whole
blood, packed red cells and plasma, and a slowing in the growth in platelet
transfusion, together with a tenfold increase in the donation of autologous
blood which was equal to approximately 3% of homologous blood donations
(Surgenor et al, 1990). In adults predepositing autologous blood, physicians
tolerated lower haematocrits on admission and discharge, and had a lower
threshold for transfusion compared with patients who would receive
homologous blood (Wasman and Goodnough, 1987). A national study of
predeposited autologous blood for elective surgery demonstrated that
homologous transfusion was required in 13% of patients with autologous
blood stored, but in 36% without autologous blood available. It was
suggested that the adequate predeposition of autologous blood for certain

procedures could avoid 68–72% of homologous transfusion in those patients who required transfusion (Toy et al, 1987).

The potential for autologous transfusion in paediatric practice has been demonstrated in a group aged 8–18 years undergoing elective orthopaedic and plastic surgery (Silvergleid, 1987). The surgeon predicted the likely requirements and blood was withdrawn at weekly intervals, the volume taken being proportional to the patient's weight. Blood was stored for up to 35 days in citrate–phosphate–dextrose anticoagulant solution. Only 2% had a minor donation reaction and the programme resulted in 88% of children supplying their transfusion requirement from autologous donation. Haughen and Hill (1987) reported similar results in a community hospital programme which included patients in the 10–19 year age group. In this study the blood was stored frozen, adding to the complexity and cost of the procedure. This approach has been confirmed by Novak (1988) with autologous blood supplying 74% of operative transfusion requirements.

PLATELET TRANSFUSION

Haemorrhage is recognized as one of the major causes of death in patients with bone marrow failure due to diseases involving the marrow or myelo-suppressive treatment. The ability to provide temporary replacement therapy in the form of platelet concentrate from individual units of donated blood or as single donor packs obtained by platelet pheresis has led to a marked increase in the use of platelet transfusion. Murphy and Waters (1990) report a three- to fourfold increase in the number of platelet transfusions over a 10-year period in a single hospital unit without a significant change in the number of patients undergoing treatment for acute leukaemia or bone marrow transplant. Between 1980 and 1986 in the United States there was a 191% increase in platelet transfusions compared with a 15% increase in red cell transfusions in the same period (Slichter, 1990). This was attributed to increased numbers of patients receiving chemotherapy, bone marrow transplantation, and the complications of cardiopulmonary bypass operations.

Although prophylactic platelet transfusion is widely practised, there is persistent debate as to its value, mainly due to lack of reliable data. The National Institute of Health Consensus Conference on Platelet Transfusion Therapy (1987) did not clarify matters by stating merely that prophylactic platelet transfusions may benefit patients with severe thrombocytopenia. The potential problems of such a policy were briefly mentioned but no firm recommendations were made.

There are few studies which address the question of prophylactic platelet transfusions in a prospective controlled fashion. In a study of patients with acute non-lymphoblastic leukaemia undergoing induction therapy, Solomon et al (1978) randomized patients to platelet transfusion either at a count of less than 20×10^9 litre^{-1} (17 patients) or if there was clinically significant bleeding (12 patients). Platelet usage was approximately double in the prophylactic group with no difference in the treatment outcome, although the number of patients was small. The arbitrary level of 20×10^9 litre^{-1}, below which prophylactic transfusion was considered to be indicated, was based on old studies and has recently been questioned by Aderka et al (1986). In a retrospective study they assessed the risk of significant bleeding at platelet counts of less than 10×10^9 litre^{-1} and at $10–20 \times 10^9$ litre^{-1}; prophylactic platelet transfusions were given at a platelet count of less than 10×10^9 litre^{-1} only. Bleeding occurred in acute non-lymphoblastic leukaemia on 20.45% of days (severe in 3.8%) at a platelet count of $10–20 \times 10^9$ litre^{-1} and on 51.1% of days when the platelet count was less than 10×10^9 litre^{-1}. There was one death from haemorrhage at this level. Bleeding occurred in acute lymphoblastic leukaemia on 57.75% of days at the higher count and 70.45% of days at the lower count. The authors suggest that administration of platelet transfusions is not simply a matter of choosing a threshold level but consideration has to be given to the type of disease, whether the thrombocytopenia is due to the disease process or to the chemotherapy, the trend of the platelet count, the presence of fever, and the age of the patient.

The problems addressed in this section apply to congenital platelet function abnormalities, such as Bernard–Soulier syndrome and Glanzmann's thrombasthenia, and tend to be magnified because of the long-term requirement for platelet transfusion support.

Refractoriness

A major limiting factor in the use of platelet transfusions is the development of refractoriness as assessed by a poor increment in the platelet count 1 hour after transfusion. Bishop et al (1988) identified a number of factors having a significant influence on the efficacy of platelet transfusions including bone marrow transplantation, disseminated intravascular coagulation, concurrent administration of amphotericin B, splenomegaly and the HLA antibody grade. There was a linear relationship between increasing percentage of HLA antibody grade and decreasing platelet increment. Factors of lesser importance were platelet specific antibodies, concurrent antibacterial antibiotics, clinical bleeding grade, and temperature.

Although other factors have to be considered, HLA-alloimmunization appears to be one of the factors potentially open to manipulation to reduce the problem of refractoriness, despite the observation that only about one third of patients with HLA-antibodies are refractory to random donor platelets. Primary HLA immunization is thought to be a two-signal process requiring both HLA Class I and II antigenic differences, although only Class I antigens are expressed on platelets. It requires intact lymphocytes, and HLA immunization is more efficient if Class II-incompatible dendritic cells (antigen presenting) are present (Lechler and Batchelor, 1982). The latter directly activate the helper T lymphocytes of the recipient but in their absence the alloantigens are processed by the recipient's own dendritic cells in a slower and less efficient response.

Potential options to reduce the incidence of alloimmunization and thus refractoriness include ABO-matching of platelet transfusions, minimizing the white cell contamination of platelet concentrates, minimizing exposure to different HLA antigens by using single donor platelets, and ultraviolet irradiation of the platelet concentrate to inactivate Class II antigens. Although the last is experimental, Andreu et al (1990) have demonstrated that doses of ultraviolet (UV) irradiation sufficient to abolish the ability of mononuclear cells isolated from the platelet concentrate to respond in mixed lymphocyte culture or to phyto-haemagglutinin, or to stimulate allogeneic lymphocytes, failed to impair platelet in vitro aggregatory responses. In volunteers the in vivo recovery and survival of UV-treated platelets was no different from that of untreated platelets.

There is controversy about the need for ABO-matching of platelet transfusions. Carr et al (1990) suggested that ABO-mismatched platelet transfusions resulted in earlier and more frequent development of refractoriness, and a randomized study did indicate that ABO-matching could be important if the patient had either elevated or developed significant rises in anti-A or anti-B isoagglutinins (Lee and Schiffer, 1989). If patients have poor increments to ABO-mismatched platelets a change to ABO-matching might restore responsiveness without the need to resort to more complex methods of providing platelets. The use of filtration techniques to deplete either red cell or platelet concentrates of leukocytes is well established. This has been shown to reduce the incidence of alloimmunization from 31 to 11% (Andreu et al, 1988), and 50 to 15% (Sniecinski et al, 1988) with concomitant reductions in platelet refractoriness from 46 to 11%, and 50 to 15%. Sniecinski et al also demonstrated a marked prolongation in the time to development of refractoriness and an increase in the median number of transfusions to refractoriness, from 8 to 26. An additional benefit of using leukocyte-poor blood products can be the reduction in the transmission of cytomegalovirus infection (de Graan-Hentzen et al, 1989).

When platelet refractoriness is documented both immune and non-immune causes should be investigated and the latter corrected wherever possible. Murphy and Waters (1990) recommend checking for HLA antibodies and, if present, giving HLA-A and -B matched platelets. HLA-matched platelet transfusions should be continued if an adequate response is documented, but as many as 30% of patients may still fail to show an increment. The use of platelet cross-match techniques should rarely be required but, using indirect antiglobulin methods, these tests may identify platelet-specific antibodies and help in the choice of platelet donors. In a randomized study, Kickler et al (1990) found that intravenous immuno-globulin (IVIgG) ($400 \, mg \, kg^{-1} d^{-1}$ for 5 days) could improve the 1-hour platelet recovery in alloimmunized patients but not the 24-hour recovery. They therefore suggested that this was not a suitable substitute for adequate platelet matching. There is evidence (McGrath et al, 1988) that HLA and platelet-specific antibodies can disappear in time even if platelet transfusion continues; thus refractoriness may not always persist.

It is difficult to give precise guidelines for platelet transfusion. The likelihood of marrow recovery and factors predisposing to continued platelet consumption, such as disseminated intravascular coagulation (DIC) and infection, must be taken into consideration. Slichter (1990) advises the following:

1. if platelets less than 5×10^9 litre^{-1} – use prophylactic platelet transfusions;
2. if platelets $5\text{--}10 \times 10^9$ litre^{-1} – use clinical judgement particularly in relation to other factors which may aggravate a bleeding tendency;
3. if platelets over 10×10^9 litre^{-1} – use platelet transfusions if clinically significant bleeding, or if there is evidence of an added platelet function defect;
4. avoid drugs, such as aspirin, which interfere with platelet function; it may be difficult to avoid the semisynthetic penicillins.

The ultimate aim of such rational platelet transfusion therapy would be to minimize alloimmunization and retain efficacy for when incrementation is imperative. However it is recognized that many clinicians would find the levels of platelet count suggested too conservative in their practice.

ALLOIMMUNE THROMBOCYTOPENIA

The incidence of alloimmune thrombocytopenia is probably higher than original estimates and a recent Canadian prospective study of 5000 pregnant women suggested that 1 in 1000 women might be affected by immunization to Pl–A1 antigen, which accounts for approximately 80% of alloimmunization to platelets (Blanchette et al, 1990). Of the 50 Pl–A1-negative women, only three developed anti-Pl–A1 antibodies and only one of their infants was severely thrombocytopenic. All the women who developed antibodies had the HLA-B8, DR3 phenotype. This information can help assess the risk to subsequent pregnancies and guide the choice of therapeutic intervention.

The disorder is not apparent until the first affected baby is born. Management involves the transfusion of compatible platelets, the most convenient source being washed maternal platelets if the blood bank does not have ready access to donors whose Pl–A1 status is known. In subsequent pregnancies the need for invasive procedures to monitor the fetal platelet count depends on an assessment of the risk to the fetus. Mueller-Eckhardt et al (1989) reported intracerebral haemorrhage in 11 out of 88 children affected by alloimmune thrombocytopenia due to Pl–A1 incompatibility, with 5 of the 11 episodes occurring antenatally. The timing of these haemorrhages is unknown although it is suggested that the highest risk period is in the last few weeks of pregnancy or at the onset of labour. Neurological sequelae are found in 10–25% of survivors of intracranial haemorrhage (ICH). The report indicates that transfusion of washed maternal platelets or the administration of IVIgG is effective treatment in the majority of infants with haemorrhagic manifestations.

Two approaches have been advocated for the management of subsequent pregnancies, both aimed at raising the fetal platelet count to levels where vaginal delivery would be considered appropriate. Bussel et al (1988) treated the mothers with intravenous immunoglobulin, with or without dexamethasone, on a weekly basis for up to 17 weeks and documented a rise in the platelet count on fetal blood sampling. The platelet counts at delivery were all substantially higher than previously affected siblings and there were no episodes of haemorrhage. Nicolini et al (1988) reported the successful outcome of in utero platelet transfusion from 26 weeks in an infant with a previously affected sibling. Kaplan et al (1988) monitored nine at risk pregnancies by fetal blood sampling with six requiring in utero platelet transfusion and no adverse effects were seen at follow-up of 6 months to 3 years.

Women who have previously delivered an affected infant should be referred to a centre with facilities for fetal blood sampling and in utero platelet transfusion. If this is not possible, at risk pregnancies are probably best delivered by Caesarean section with washed maternal platelets being available in case the infant has clinical bleeding problems or significant thrombocytopenia develops.

COAGULATION FACTOR THERAPY

Fresh frozen plasma

This is arguably one of the most abused blood products. In the United States of America, a tenfold increase in the use of fresh frozen plasma (FFP) over 10 years prompted the National Institute of Health Consensus Conference (1985) to comment on how few good indications there were. The conference concluded that the valid indications included:

1. therapy of coagulation disorders where specific replacement therapy was not available;
2. reversal of warfarin effect;
3. correction of a documented coagulation defect associated with massive transfusion;
4. thrombotic thrombocytopenic purpura.

In paediatric practice FFP is commonly used to correct a number of coagulation abnormalities, both inherited and acquired. There are anecdotal reports of benefit in the haemolytic–uraemic syndrome. However two randomized studies of the use of FFP in haemolytic–uraemic syndrome have shown no benefit in terms of recovery of platelet count, requirement for red cell transfusion or speed of recovery of renal function, or in the incidence of longer-term sequelae (Loirat et al, 1987; Rizzoni et al, 1988).

Factor VIII concentrates

The provision of replacement therapy for the commonest hereditary coagulation disorder, haemophilia A, has been the major driving force behind the plasma protein fractionation industry. The haemophiliac population has borne the brunt of transfusion-associated HIV infection, although recent developments give some optimism for the future of those not yet infected (Roberts, 1989). Three main initiatives against the HIV problem have increased the safety of standard factor VIII concentrate: (i) discouraging blood donors in high risk groups for HIV infection, (ii) screening all donations for anti-HIV antibody, and (iii) virucidal treatment of the product.

Heat-treated factor VIII concentrate

The various methods of virucidal treatment were reviewed by Mannucci and Colombo (1988). Most involve some form of heating and show clinical efficacy in the prevention of HIV seroconversion, with the additional benefit of reducing the development of non-A, non-B hepatitis (NANBH). In a group of seventeen previously untreated haemophiliacs given the English heat-treated concentrate 8Y for up to 36 months, there was no serological evidence of HIV infection or of NANBH (Pasi and Hill, 1989). A European study (Schimpf et al, 1987) of heat-treated factor VIII concentrate in 26 patients with haemophilia A or von Willebrand's disease showed no evidence of NANBH, and this was confirmed in the United Kingdom (Study Group of UK Haemophilia Centre Directors, 1988) with dry-heat treatment of factor VIII or IX concentrates reducing the risk of NANBH from 90% to a statistically determined 0–9% level.

Highly purified factor VIII concentrate

Highly purified factor VIII concentrate is prepared by using monoclonal antibodies against factor VIII : C or von Willebrand factor in immunoaffinity purification which leads to a purer product with less virus contamination before heat-treatment. Clinical studies have shown this type of product to be effective in controlling bleeding episodes and safe in relation to the transmission of viral infection (Lusher et al, 1990). However, inhibitors to factor VIII developed in 6 out of 38 patients (15.8%) within 4 to 21 months of starting treatment with the product. Although it was a small study this finding is of concern and requires monitoring.

Monoclonally purified concentrate is more expensive and its place in haemophilia therapy remains to be determined. Further investigation of its role in the management of HIV-positive haemophiliacs is required; highly purified concentrate has been reported to stabilise $CD4^+$ lymphocyte counts, reverse cutaneous anergy (Brettler et al, 1987), and possibly slow progression to AIDS.

Recombinant factor VIII

The cloning of the gene for factor VIII : C and its insertion into mammalian cells such as Chinese hamster ovary cells, provides an in vitro method of factor VIII production which has the advantage of avoiding dependence on human blood donations with their inherent risk of transmission of infection. Preliminary reports of the use of recombinant human factor VIII suggest clinical efficacy (White et al, 1989), including use in dental extractions and knee replacement surgery (Harrison et al, 1990). This type of technology opens the possibility of gene replacement therapy in the future.

Other coagulation factors

Highly purified factor IX concentrate is available and appears to have satisfactory pharmacokinetics (Kim et al, 1990) and probable clinical efficacy. The high cost of the monoclonal antibodies to factor IX mean the product is expensive but it may have potential advantages in reduced thrombogenicity compared with standard factor IX concentrates.

Recombinant factor VII is available for the rare patients with hereditary factor VII deficiency. However it may also have a role in the management of haemophiliacs with factor VIII inhibitors after the report of successful synovectomy using this product (Hedner et al, 1988).

Patients with mild haemophilia A and von Willebrand's disease (Type I and IIa) can often be effectively managed with desamino-arginine–vasopressin (DDAVP) together with a fibrinolytic inhibitor, e.g. tranexamic acid, if appropriate (Mannucci, 1988). Clearly alternatives to blood products should be used whenever possible and the safest plasma-derived product transfused where there is no alternative effective therapy. The treatment of von Willebrand's disease requires the replacement of the high molecular weight (HMW) multimers of von Willebrand factor. Virucidally-treated factor VIII concentrates vary greatly in the amount of HMW multimers they contain (Kemball-Cook and Barrowcliffe, 1986) and this determines their efficacy in the treatment of von Willebrand's disease (Mazurier et al, 1989). Non heat-treated cryoprecipitate should only be used if a factor VIII concentrate rich in HMW multimers does not prevent bleeding, because of the risk of transmitting NANBH.

IMMUNOGLOBULIN PREPARATIONS

The major indication for immunoglobulin therapy is replacement in humoral immunodeficiency, but there is increasing exploration of the use of these preparations in disorders such as immune thrombocytopenia, neo-natal infections, Kawasaki disease and haemolytic–uraemic syndrome. Specific antibodies are being used in various infections, such as cytomegalo-virus after bone marrow transplantation, and in the prophylaxis of Rhesus haemolytic disease.

Non-specific immunoglobulin

The use of immunoglobulin is established in antibody deficiency states, in particular X-linked immunodeficiency and common variable immuno-deficiency. Initially the immunoglobulin preparations were only suitable for intramuscular use because of residual impurities which could lead to anaphylaxis if given intravenously. Current preparations are safe for intravenous administration. Initial British studies suggested that the intravenous form was significantly better than the intramuscular in terms of higher serum levels of IgG and reduced incidence of infections with less time off work in adults (Lever et al, 1984). Problems with non-A, non-B hepatitis restricted the studies, but pepsin treatment during the processing of the plasma appears to have greatly reduced or eliminated this complication.

Idiopathic thrombocytopenic purpura (ITP) in children is a relatively benign, self-limiting condition. Mortality from ITP, usually from intracranial haemorrhage, is estimated at less than 1% and is lower in recent series than in older reports, probably because of improved diagnosis of conditions that may mimic ITP. With the low mortality and relatively low morbidity of the condition, many haematologists are reluctant to embark on treatment although a short course of prednisolone has been recommended (Lilleyman, 1986). The use of high-dose IVIgG has been advocated in the treatment of both acute and chronic ITP. However, as the disease is quite rare and the incidence of complications low, it would be difficult to mount even a multinational randomized trial to assess the efficacy of a particular therapy. Thus, most of the studies of the use of IVIgG in childhood ITP have assessed the rapidity of recovery of the platelet count and assumed that a more rapid elevation of the count is beneficial. In a randomized comparison of IVIgG and prednisolone in acute ITP, Imbach et al (1985) demonstrated that IVIgG was associated with a more rapid recovery of the platelet count but failed to show a difference in the overall recovery of the patients; the only death was in the IVIgG group. Because the natural history of acute ITP in children shows a recovery in 80–90%, it has not been possible to assess any effect IVIgG might have on lessening the incidence of chronic ITP.

The use of IVIgG has been advocated in chronic ITP in children but it is prudent to heed the *primum non nocere* (first do no harm) warning of Chessells (1990). The regular use of IVIgG to try to maintain the platelet count at a 'safe' level does not seem rational because of the great variability of clinical manifestations at a given level of platelet count.

The place of IVIgG in acute ITP is likely to be in the emergency treatment of those rare children with evidence of major haemorrhage, including intracranial sites, and who may require urgent splenectomy, and in those children with chronic ITP who require surgery.

IVIgG has been used in haemolytic–uraemic syndrome with apparent benefit compared with historical controls treated with fresh frozen plasma or supportive therapy only (Sheth et al, 1990). However only eight patients were treated with IVIgG and it was not a randomized study.

Neonatal sepsis is defined as bacteraemia occurring within 29 days of birth. Opsonic antibodies are of particular importance in protection against encapsulated bacteria such as *Haemophilus influenzae*, *Streptococcus pneumoniae* and Group B *Streptococcus*, and these, and other types of IgG, do not cross the placenta in significant amounts until after the 34th week of pregnancy. Thus pre-term infants are most susceptible to this type of infection (Hill et al, 1989) and the risk is aggravated by a physiological neutrophil functional defect. Certain studies have suggested a beneficial effect of IVIgG in reducing the incidence of neonatal sepsis and its mortality (Haque et al, 1986), although others have not confirmed this (Stabile et al,

1988). IVIgG was administered to pregnant women at risk of pre-term delivery with chorio-amnionitis. After 32 weeks the pregnant women received either antibiotics or IVIgG plus antibiotics. In the latter group the cord blood IgG levels were significantly higher and the incidence of neonatal sepsis was reduced from 6 out of 16 in controls to 0 out of 7 in those receiving a higher dose of IgG (Sidiropoulos, 1986). In the treatment of neonates with bacterial infection the combination of IVIgG and antibiotics was superior to antibiotics alone with reduction of mortality from 26 to 10%. The difference was particularly noticeable in pre-term infants, who showed a reduction in their mortality rate from 44 to 8% (Sidiropoulos, 1986). In a randomized study, Haque et al (1988) noted a similar improvement in mortality.

Two randomized trials have investigated the use of IVIgG in Kawasaki disease. Newberger et al (1986) found that the combination of IVIgG and aspirin was more effective than aspirin alone in reducing the incidence of coronary artery aneurysms. Similar findings were reported by Nagashima et al (1987) who also suggested that the combination reduced the duration of fever. The dose of aspirin differed between the two trials; the IVIgG was given at a dose of 400 mg kg^{-1} day^{-1} for 3 or 4 days. In Kawasaki disease there is evidence of marked immunological activation with the presence of antibodies lytic for vascular endothelial cells. After IVIgG there is a rise in CD8$^+$ cells, reduction in CD4$^+$ cells and a reduction in spontaneous IgG and IgM synthesis, suggesting that the vasculitis is reduced by suppression of immune activation by the IVIgG (Leung, 1989).

In an attempt to give a degree of passive humoral immunity and limit infections, IVIgG has been used in children with HIV infection (Williams et al, 1988). Five HIV-positive children with failure-to-thrive related to frequent severe infections which were poorly responsive to antibiotics received regular IVIgG with significant reduction in infections and hospital admissions, and weight gain.

Specific immunoglobulins

Immunoglobulin preparations with activity specific for a particular infecting agent or other antigen can be derived from plasma collected by plasma-pheresis from a donor with high titre antibodies. An alternative approach is the development of monoclonal antibodies for this purpose which would avoid much of the potential infective problems.

Varicella-zoster immunoglobulin

Children receiving chemotherapy for malignant disease are at risk from potentially fatal chickenpox infection. The use of Zoster immunoglobulin in children with close contact with chickenpox or shingles reduces the severity of the infection. There are now two possible alternative options. Acyclovir is highly effective against the varicella-zoster virus and trials are in progress assessing its effectiveness in a prophylactic role after exposure to chicken-pox. There are reports of apparently successful immunization against varicella-zoster virus in immunosuppressed patients. In children with acute lymphoblastic leukaemia seroconversion occurred in 98% of those immunized with an attack rate of 14% if there was household exposure to chickenpox (Gershon et al, 1989) and this was lower than historical controls (Ross, 1962). Children with solid tumours can be similarly protected (Heath et al, 1987).

Cytomegalovirus immunoglobulin

Cytomegalovirus (CMV) is the commonest cause of pneumonitis in bone marrow transplant recipients and previously had a high mortality. Screening blood products for anti-CMV antibody and the use of white cell-poor blood products can reduce the incidence of new infection. Winston et al (1987) demonstrated that CMV immunoglobulin used prophylactically decreased the incidence of symptomatic CMV infection and of interstitial pneumonitis. If CMV pneumonitis developed the combination of CMV immunoglobulin and ganciclovir had greater therapeutic efficacy than either modality alone (Emanuel et al, 1988; Reed et al, 1988). However, this remains a controversial finding and there is no proven prophylactic measure.

Anti-rhesus D immunoglobulin

The use of this antibody in the immediate postpartum period in rhesus D negative women delivered of rhesus D positive babies has made a major impact on the incidence of haemolytic disease of the newborn. Clinical trials of postpartum anti-D immunoglobulin have shown a reduction in the incidence of rhesus immunization from 31.4 to 2.3% and 12.3 to 2.8% where the dose of anti-D immunoglobulin was modified on an estimate of the size of the transplacental haemorrhage (Combined Study, 1966) and from 12.9 to 1.3% (Ascari et al, 1969). These trials emphasize the importance of giving anti-D immunoglobulin early in the postpartum period and in adequate dose. As 0.7–1.9% of rhesus immunization may occur during pregnancy anti-D immunoglobulin has been given to rhesus-D negative women during pregnancy and leads to a further reduction in the immunization rate (Bowman and Pollock, 1987).

TRANSMISSION OF INFECTION

The risks of blood transfusion transmitting bacterial, protozoal and viral infections are well recognized. The major concerns remain hepatitis and HIV infection, and CMV in certain groups such as recipients of bone marrow transplants.

Recently the risk of transmission of human T-cell leukaemia virus type I (HTLV I) and the subsequent development of adult T-cell leukaemia/lymphoma has been discussed and the possibility of screening of blood donations for this virus has been raised (Weber, 1990). However, as the seroprevalence in British blood donors is less than 0.01% and knowledge of the natural history of HTLV I infection is lacking, it is too soon to decide on the need for screening.

Hepatitis B

Hepatitis B remains a risk as the use of hepatitis B surface antigen as a screening test cannot exclude all potentially infective units of blood. It is prudent to immunize all patients receiving regular transfusions of blood or blood products against this virus.

Non-A, Non-B hepatitis

Until recently, the screening of donated blood for NANBH has mainly utilized surrogate tests, principally the measurement of serum alanine-aminotransferase (ALT). However, surrogate testing has not been universally adopted and remains controversial. Klein (1990) felt that, despite the low specificity and limited predictive value of the test, it could prevent up to 30% of post-transfusion NANBH and was thus justified. However, Spurling and Saxena (1990) condemned ALT testing with a plea for more informative pre-donation testing, 'otherwise we will be saddled indefinitely with a very non-specific costly test that adversely effects the blood supply but yields uncertain benefit'.

This debate may be rendered sterile with the development of a test for antibody to hepatitis C virus (HCV) infection (Kuo et al, 1989). There has been intensive retrospective and prospective study of post-transfusion NANBH and HCV appears to be the major causative agent (Kuo et al, 1989). In patients following cardiac surgery, Alter et al (1989) demonstrated that all those with histologically-proven chronic NANBH had received blood positive for anti-HCV antibody, compared with 3 out of 6 with transient hepatitis. Studies in haemophiliacs with chronic liver disease indicate that 60–70% of cases are probably due to HCV and are associated with high annual usage of factor concentrates, hepatitis B infection and HIV infection (Brettler et al, 1990; Makris et al, 1990). Haemophiliacs may have anti-HCV antibody present without abnormalities of liver function tests (Rumi et al, 1990) and the significance of this awaits further study.

Twenty-two percent of patients with thalassaemia major who have been multiply-transfused were HCV seropositive; the incidence was higher for patients transfused outside Britain (Wonke et al, 1990). Seropositivity was associated with persistently abnormal liver enzymes and hepatomegaly, but there was no evidence of transmission to sexual partners.

Although there are reports of α-interferon therapy causing some improvement in patients with chronic post-transfusion NANBH there was a high incidence of relapse after stopping treatment (Davis et al, 1989; Di Bisceglie et al, 1989). A more effective method of preventing the disease remains a priority. A retrospective Dutch study (van der Poel et al, 1990) compared the use of anti-HCV antibody and ALT testing in the screening of blood donations and indicated that anti-HCV had greater specificity and positive predictive value. This would have resulted in discarding 0.7% of donations compared with 3.8% using ALT testing with no detrimental effect on patients. The use of 'nested' polymerase chain reaction to detect hepatitis C viral sequences in blood may further improve the prediction of infectivity of blood (Garson et al, 1990). The practical implications of these developments remain to be demonstrated, including the costs of implementing such an additional screening test.

The virucidal treatment of coagulation factor concentrates by a number of methods has resulted in a marked reduction and possibly elimination of the risk of transmission of HCV (Mannucci et al, 1990; Skidmore et al, 1990). This does not preclude the need for a screening test for blood products which are not amenable to virudical treatment.

Human immunodeficiency virus

Although the number of patients with transfusion-derived acquired immunodeficiency syndrome (AIDS) is small in relation to the total numbers, for example 259 out of 3433 in the United Kingdom at the end of June 1990 (Delamothe, 1990), 176 have already died and there is likely to be a larger number infected with HIV and at risk of progression to AIDS. Ward et al (1989) suggested that most recipients of HIV-infected blood became seropositive and the risk of AIDS developing is greater if the donor develops AIDS soon after donation.

The progression from HIV seropositivity to AIDS varies with age in the haemophiliac population, with a mean cumulative incidence at 8 years of 13.3% in the 1–13 year age group and 43.7% in the 35–70 year group (Goedert et al, 1989). These authors suggest that younger patients may have a lower replication rate of the virus and tolerate the immunodeficiency better because they have fewer infections. It has been suggested that monoclonal antibody-purified factor concentrates might have a place in the management of HIV-positive patients as a method of reducing immunological stimulation and possibly slowing progression (Brettler et al, 1987).

The elimination of HIV infection from blood for transfusion necessitates the exclusion of donors in groups at high risk of having HIV infection and in the screening of donations for antibodies to HIV 1, and now HIV 2. Plasma products which have undergone virucidal inactivation with heat, pasteurization, solvent-detergent treatment appear not to transmit HIV infection (Schimpf et al, 1989).

Cytomegalovirus

As with other herpes viruses, CMV causes latent infection of white cells, probably monocytes and lymphocytes. Thus, the degree of white cell contamination of blood or blood products will influence the risk of CMV transmission if the virus is present. There are a number of groups at particular risk of CMV infection including pre-term neonates, children with immunodeficiency whether congenital or acquired, and those receiving bone marrow transplants or transplants of solid organs.

Yeager et al (1981) reported that neonates weighing less than 1200 g or of less than 28 weeks gestation and born of CMV seronegative mothers were particularly at risk of fatal or serious infection. The same study demonstrated the value of using CMV antibody-negative blood products in eliminating CMV infection, especially if transfusion of more than 50 ml of packed red cells was required.

Various methods of reducing CMV infection have been employed in patients undergoing bone marrow transplantation or receiving treatment for haematological malignancy. Bowden et al (1986) showed that the use of CMV seronegative blood products reduced the incidence of CMV infection in seronegative recipients of marrow from a seronegative donor from 32 to 3%. The use of CMV immunoglobulin did not significantly affect the infection rate. In patients with acute leukaemia and non-Hodgkin's lymphoma, the use of red cells and platelets intensively depleted of white cells failed to cause seroconversion at two months after cytoreductive chemotherapy (de Graan-Hentzen et al, 1989). Thus white cell depletion of blood products is an alternative to CMV screening of donors.

HAEMATOPOIETIC GROWTH FACTORS

Extensive in vitro research into the identification and mechanism of action of these glycoprotein hormones has given insight into the control of haematopoiesis (Groopman et al, 1989). The advent of DNA technology has allowed this knowledge to transfer to the clinical setting (Bronchud and Dexter, 1989). This developing area offers a potential mechanism of minimizing the transfusion of blood and blood products and avoidance of their complications.

Erythropoietin

This growth factor is mainly produced by the kidney and has an integral role in the regulation of red cell production. It is now established as an effective method of raising the haemoglobin in patients with the anaemia of end-stage renal failure (Eschbach et al, 1989), resulting in improved exercise tolerance and quality of life (Canadian Erythropoietin Study Group, 1990; Macdougall et al, 1990a). Erythropoietin induces a sustained, dose-dependent rise in haemoglobin but this is accompanied by an increase in whole blood viscosity. Thus, hypertension may be aggravated with an increase in the risk of cardiovascular complications which are already a common cause of death in patients with renal failure (Raine, 1988). While experience with erythropoietin is limited in children with renal failure caution should be shown in relation to these potential complications, particularly as renal transplantation will be actively considered in the majority of patients. It is prudent to consider the algorithm of Macdougall et al (1990b) in the management of patients with the anaemia of end-stage renal failure so that the rise in haemoglobin is optimized and the risk of complications acceptable.

The use of erythropoietin has been assessed in other forms of anaemia. Preliminary data suggest that it may be effective in correcting the anaemia of prematurity although the multifactorial nature of this may limit the benefit (Halperin et al, 1990). In drug-induced anaemia, erythropoietin has reduced the transfusion requirement of patients with AIDS receiving zidovudine therapy (Fischl et al, 1990). Studying a rat model, erythropoietin improved the anaemia induced by the cytotoxic agent cisplatin but not that due to 5-fluorouracil (Matsumoto et al, 1990).

A potential role for erythropoietin may be in improving the collection of blood for autologous transfusion in patients undergoing elective surgery (Goodnough et al, 1989; Graf et al, 1990). This requires further assessment in children in view of the practical problems related to blood volume for the collection of autologous blood.

Granulocyte and granulocyte–macrophage colony stimulating factors

The ability of these growth factors to stimulate an increase in peripheral blood neutrophil counts has been investigated in three main areas— congenital neutropenia, acquired neutropenia and aplastic anaemia, and bone marrow recovery after cancer chemotherapy.

In congenital neutropenia Komiyama et al (1988), using purified human urinary colony stimulating factor, reported a sustained improvement in 5 out of 9 children. The responders lacked mature neutrophils in the bone marrow compared with the non-responders, two of whom had bone marrow hypoplasia and two of whom had maturation arrest at the promyelocyte stage. Bonilla et al (1989) used recombinant human granulocyte colony-stimulating factor (G-CSF) and reported a consistent numerical increase in peripheral blood neutrophil counts and clinical improvement in all five patients treated but continuing maintenance therapy was required. G-CSF appears more effective than granulocyte–macrophage colony-stimulating factor (GM-CSF) in congenital neutropenia (Welte et al, 1990). In cyclic neutropenia G-CSF can reduce the number of days with severe neutropenia and lead to clinical improvement (Hammond et al, 1989).

G-CSF has been effective in acquired neutropenia (Jakubowski et al, 1989) and in severe aplastic anaemia in a child when used in combination with anti-lymphocyte globulin (Potter et al, 1990). Champlin et al (1989) reported GM-CSF to improve the neutrophil, monocyte and eosinophil counts in 10 out of 11 patients with severe aplastic anaemia although only whilst treatment was continued, and the platelet counts were not influenced.

One of the limiting factors in the administration of cancer chemotherapy is myelosuppression which can reduce the ability to deliver an adequate drug dose and intensity, and produce infective and haemorrhagic complications. While platelet transfusion is readily available and usually effective, manage-ment of infections relies on antibiotic therapy because granulocyte trans-fusions have been shown to have a very limited role. G-CSF can improve recovery of neutrophil counts in patients receiving chemotherapy for small cell carcinoma of bronchus (Bronchud et al, 1987) and both G-CSF and GM-CSF can accelerate neutrophil recovery after high-dose chemotherapy and autologous bone marrow transplantation (Brandt et al, 1988; Nemunaitis et al, 1988; Sheridan et al, 1989). Dose-limiting side-effects of this type of growth factor therapy include myalgias and fluid retention (Brandt et al, 1988). In relation to autologous bone marrow transplantation, GM-CSF can increase the number of circulating peripheral blood progenitor cells for harvesting (Gianni et al, 1989; Villeval et al, 1990) which may be valuable as an adjunct to bone marrow harvest or an alternative if the bone marrow is contaminated by malignant cells. Haematopoietic growth factors accelerate recovery of neutrophil counts, reduce febrile days, reduce the requirement for platelet transfusion and lead to shorter hospital stays, but randomized trials are awaited to determine their effect on mortality. There is also the risk that the amelioration of myelosuppression may allow a different dose limiting toxicity to become apparent.

Growth factors used in combination may optimize their effects on marrow recovery and minimize toxicity. Already there is evidence of synergism between interleukin-3 and GM-CSF (Donahue et al, 1988) and interleukin-3 and interleukin-6 (Leary et al, 1988).

SUMMARY

I have reviewed areas of development in the use of blood and blood products, placing emphasis on the complications of transfusion, particularly transmission of infection. Alloimmunization in relation to transfusion of red cells and platelets has been covered and suggestions for reducing this problem assessed. The potential methods of avoiding the infective complications have been discussed including the screening of blood for infective agents, the virucidal treatment of blood products during the manufacturing process and white cell depletion. The use of recombinant DNA technology to produce coagulation factors offers the possibility of further reducing infective risks. An area of clinical promise is the use of haematopoietic growth factors to treat bone marrow failure, either congenital or acquired, such as the myelosuppressive effects of cancer chemotherapy, and reduce reliance on blood products.

The aim of the chapter is to encourage the rational use of a limited resource by considering the risks inherent in transfusion and alternative strategies. In doing this it is important to audit current and future practice, and it is suggested that reference is made to the suggestions of Hume (1989) for quality assessment and assurance in paediatric transfusion medicine.

REFERENCES

Aderka D, Praff G, Santo M et al (1986) Bleeding due to thrombocytopenia in acute leukaemias and re-evaluation of the prophylactic platelet transfusion policy. *American Journal of Medical Sciences* 291: 147–151.

Alter HJ, Purcell RH, Shih JW et al (1989) Detection of antibody to hepatitis C virus in prospectively followed transfusion recipients with acute and chronic non-A, non-B hepatitis. *New England Journal of Medicine* 321: 1494–1500.

Andreu G, Dewailly J, Leberre C et al (1988) Prevention of HLA-immunisation with leukocyte-poor packed red cells and platelet concentrates prepared by filtration. *Blood* 72: 964–969.

Andreu G, Bonaccio C, Lecrubier C et al (1990) Ultraviolet irradiation of platelet concentrates: feasibility in transfusion practice. *Transfusion* 30: 401–406.

Ascari WQ, Levine P & Pollack W (1969) Incidence of maternal Rh immunisation by ABO compatible and incompatible pregnancies. *British Medical Journal* 1: 399–401.

Barss VA, Benacerraf BR, Frigoletto FD et al (1988) Management of isoimmunized pregnancy by use of intravascular techniques. *American Journal of Obstetrics and Gynecology* **159:** 932–937.

Bishop JF, McGrath K, Wolff MM et al (1988) Clinical factors influencing the efficacy of pooled platelet transfusions. *Blood* **71:** 383–387.

Blanchette VS, Chen L, Salomonde Friedberg Z et al (1990) Alloimmunization to the PlA1 platelet antigen: results of a prospective study. *British Journal of Haematology* **74:** 209–215.

Blumberg N & Heal JM (1987) Perioperative blood transfusion and solid tumour recurrence. *Blood Reviews* **1:** 219–229.

Blumberg N, Heal J, Chuang C et al (1988) Further evidence supporting a cause and effect relationship between blood transfusion and early cancer recurrence. *Annals of Surgery* **207:** 410–415.

Bonilla MA, Gillio AP, Ruggeiro M et al (1989) Effects of human granulocyte colony-stimulating factor on neutropenia in patients with congenital agranulocytosis. *New England Journal of Medicine* **320:** 1574–1580.

Bowden RA, Sayers M, Flournoy N et al (1986) Cytomegalovirus immune globulin and seronegative blood products to prevent primary cytomegalovirus infections after marrow transplantation. *New England Journal of Medicine* **314:** 1006–1010.

Bowman JM & Pollock JM (1987) Failures of intravenous Rh immune globulin prophylaxis: An analysis of the reasons for such failures. *Transfusion Medicine Reviews* **1:** 101–112.

Brandt SJ, Peters WP, Atwater SK et al (1988) Effect of recombinant human granulocyte–macrophage colony-stimulating factor on hematopoietic reconstitution after high-dose chemotherapy and autologous bone marrow transplantation. *New England Journal of Medicine* **318:** 869–876.

Brettler DB, Forsburg A, Levine PH et al (1987) Factor VIII:C purified from plasma via monoclonal antibodies: human studies. *Blood* **70**(Suppl.): 327 (abstract).

Brettler DB, Alter HJ, Dienstag JL et al (1990) Prevalence of hepatitis C virus antibody in a cohort of hemophilia patients. *Blood* **76:** 254–256.

Bronchud MH & Dexter TM (1989) Clinical use of haematopoietic growth factors. *Blood Reviews* **3:** 66–70.

Bronchud MH, Scarffe JH, Thatcher N et al (1987) Phase I/II study of recombinant human granulocyte colony-stimulating factor in patients receiving intensive chemotherapy for small cell lung cancer. *British Journal of Cancer* **56:** 809–813.

Bussel JB, Berkowitz RL, McFarland JG et al (1988) Antenatal treatment of neonatal alloimmune thrombocytopenia. *New England Journal of Medicine* **319:** 1374–1378.

Canadian Erythropoietin Study Group (1990) Association between recombinant human erythropoietin and quality of life and exercise capacity of patients receiving haemodialysis. *British Medical Journal* **300:** 573–578.

Cao A (1987) Results of programmes for antenatal detection of thalassaemia in reducing the incidence of the disorder. *Blood Reviews* **1:** 169–176.

Carr R, Hutton JL, Jenkins JA et al (1990) Transfusion of ABO-mismatched platelets leads to early platelet refractoriness. *British Journal of Haematology* **75:** 408–413.

Champlin RE, Nimer SD, Ireland P et al (1989) Treatment of refractory aplastic anaemia with recombinant granulocyte–macrophage colony-stimulating factor. *Blood* **73:** 694–699.

Chessells J (1989) Chronic idiopathic thrombocytopenic purpura: primum non nocere. *Archives of Disease in Childhood* **64:** 1326–1328.

Combined Study (1966) Prevention of Rh-haemolytic disease: Results of the clinical trial. A combined study from centres in England and Baltimore. *British Medical Journal* **2:** 907–914.

Daffos F, Capella-Pavlovsky M & Forestier F (1985) Fetal blood sampling during pregnancy with use of a needle guided by ultrasound. A study of 606 consecutive cases. *American Journal of Obstetrics and Gynecology* **153:** 655–660.

Daffos F, Forestier F, Kaplan C & Cox W (1988) Prenatal diagnosis and management of bleeding disorders with fetal blood sampling. *American Journal of Obstetrics and Gynecology* **158:** 939–946.

Davies SC & Brozovic M (1989) The presentation, management and prophylaxis of sickle cell disease. *Blood Reviews* **3:** 29–44.

Davis GL, Balart LA, Schiff ER et al (1989) Treatment of chronic hepatitis C with recombinant interferon alpha. A multicenter randomised controlled trial. *New England Journal of Medicine* **321:** 1501–1506.

de Graan-Hentzen YCE, Gratama JW, Mudde GC et al (1989) Prevention of primary cyto-megalovirus infection in patients with hematologic malignancies by intensive white cell depletion of blood products. *Transfusion* **29:** 757–760.

Delamothe T (1990) AIDS and 'ordinary heterosexual people'. *British Medical Journal* **301:** 138.

Di Bisceglie AM, Martin P, Kassianides C et al (1989) Recombinant interferon alpha therapy for chronic hepatitis C. A randomized, double-blind, placebo-controlled trial. *New England Journal of Medicine* **321:** 1506–1510.

Donahue RE, Seehra J, Metzger M et al (1988) Human IL-3 and GM-CSF act synergistically in stimulating hematopoiesis in primates. *Science* **241:** 1820–1823.

Editorial (1989) Oral iron chelators. *Lancet* **ii:** 1016–1017.

Emanuel D, Cunningham I, Jules-Elysee K et al (1988) Cytomegalovirus pneumonia after bone marrow transplantation successfully treated with a combination of ganciclovir and high-dose intravenous immune globulin. *Annals of Internal Medicine* **109:** 777–782.

Eschbach JW, Kelly MR, Haley NR et al (1989) Treatment of the anaemia of progressive renal failure with recombinant human erythropoietin. *New England Journal of Medicine* **321:** 158–163.

Fischl M, Galpin JE, Levine JD et al (1990) Recombinant human erythropoietin for patients with AIDS treated with Zidovudine. *New England Journal of Medicine* **322:** 1488–1493.

Garson JA, Tedder RS, Briggs M et al (1990) Detection of hepatitis C viral sequences in blood donations by 'nested' polymerase chain reaction and prediction of infectivity. *Lancet* **335:** 1419–1422.

Gershon AA, Steinberg SP and the Varicella Vaccine Collaborative Study Group of the National Institute of Allergy and Infectious Diseases (1989) Persistence of immunity to varicella in children with leukaemia immunized with live attenuated varicella vaccine. *New England Journal of Medicine* **320:** 892–897.

Gianni AM, Siena S, Bregni M et al (1989) Granulocyte–macrophage colony-stimulating factor to harvest circulating haemopoietic stem cells for autotransplantation. *Lancet* **ii:** 580–585.

Goedert JJ, Kessler CM, Aledort LM et al (1989) A prospective study of human immuno-deficiency virus type 1 infection and the development of AIDS in subjects with hemophilia. *New England Journal of Medicine* **321:** 1141–1148.

Goodnough LT, Rudnick S, Price TH et al (1989) Increased preoperative collection of autologous blood with recombinant erythropoietin therapy. *New England Journal of Medicine* **321:** 1163–1168.

Graf H, Watzinger U, Ludvik B et al (1990) Recombinant human erythropoietin as adjuvant treatment for autologous blood donation. *British Medical Journal* **300:** 1627–1628.

Groopman JE, Molina J-M & Scadden DT (1989) Hematopoietic growth factors. Biology and clinical application. *New England Journal of Medicine* **321:** 1449–1459.

Halperin DS, Wacker P, Lacourt G et al (1990) Effects of recombinant human erythropoietin in infants with the anemia of prematurity: a pilot study. *Journal of Pediatrics* **116:** 779–796.

Hammond WP, Price TH, Souza LM & Dale DC (1989) Treatment of cyclic neutropenia with granulocyte colony-stimulating factor. *New England Journal of Medicine* **320:** 1306–1311.

Haque KN, Zaidi MH, Haque SK et al (1986) Intravenous immunoglobulin for prevention of sepsis in preterm and low birth weight infants. *Pediatric Infectious Diseases Journal* **5:** 622–625.

Haque KN, Zaidi MH & Bahakim H (1988) IgM-enriched intravenous immunoglobulin therapy in neonatal sepsis. *American Journal of Diseases in Childhood* **142:** 1293–1296.

Harrison JFM, Bloom AL & Peake IR (1990) In vivo and in vitro studies of recombinant FVIII. *British Journal of Haematology* **74:** (Suppl. 1): 7 (abstract).

Haugen RK & Hill GE (1987) A large scale autologous blood program in a community hospital. *Journal of the American Medical Association* **257:** 1211–1214.

Heath RB, Malpas JS, Kangro HO et al (1987) Efficacy of varicella vaccine in patients with solid tumours. *Archives of Disease in Childhood* **62:** 569–572.

Hedner U, Glaser S, Pingel K, et al (1988) Successful use of recombinant factor VIIa in a patient with severe haemophilia A during synovectomy. *Lancet* **ii:** 1193.

Hershko C, Pinson A & Link G (1990) Iron Chelation. *Blood Reviews* **4:** 1–8.

Hill HR, Shigeoka AO, Gonzales LA & Christensen RD (1989) Intravenous immunoglobulin use in newborns. *Journal of Allergy and Clinical Immunology* **84:** 617–624.

Hoffbrand AV & Wonke B (1989) Results of long-term subcutaneous desferrioxamine therapy. *Clinical Haematology* **2:** 345–362.

Hume H (1989) Pediatric transfusions: quality assessment and assurance. In Sacher RA & Strauss R (eds) *Contemporary Issues in Pediatric Transfusion Medicine*, pp 55–80. Arlington VA: American Association of Blood Banks.

Imbach P, Wagner HP, Berchtold W et al (1985) Intravenous immunoglobulin versus oral corticosteroids in acute immune thrombocytopenic purpura in childhood. *Lancet* **ii:** 464–468.

Jakubowski AA, Souza L, Kelly F et al (1989) Effects of human granulocyte colony-stimulating factor in a patient with idiopathic neutropenia. *New England Journal of Medicine* **320:** 38–42.

Kaplan C, Daffos F, Forestier F et al (1988) Management of alloimmune thrombocytopenia: antenatal diagnosis and in-utero transfusion of maternal platelets. *Blood* **72:** 340–343.

Keiden AJ, Sowter MC, Johnson CS et al (1989) Pharmacological modification of oxygen affinity improves deformability of deoxygenated sickle erythrocytes: a possible therapeutic approach to sickle cell disease. *Clinical Science* **76:** 357–362.

Kemball-Cook G & Barrowcliffe TW (1986) Factor VIII Concentrates contain factor VIII procoagulant antigen bound to phospholipid. *British Journal of Haematology* **63:** 425–434.

Kickler T, Braine HG, Piantadosi S et al (1990) A randomized, placebo-controlled trial of intravenous gammaglobulin in alloimmunized thrombocytopenic patients. *Blood* **75:** 313–316.

Kim HC, McMillan CW, White GC et al (1990) Clinical experience of a new monoclonal antibody purified factor IX: half-life, recovery, and safety in patients with hemophilia B. *Seminars in Hematology* **27** (Suppl. 2): 30–35.

Klein HG (1990) Controversies in transfusion medicine. Alanine aminotransferase screening of blood donors: Pro. *Transfusion* **30:** 365–367.

Komiyama A, Ishiguro A, Kubo T et al (1988) Increases in neutrophil counts by purified human urinary colony-stimulating factor in chronic neutropenia of childhood. *Blood* **71:** 41–45.

Kontoghiorghes GJ & Hoffbrand AV (1989) Clinical trials with oral iron chelator L1. *Lancet* **ii:** 1516–1517.

Kontoghiorghes GJ, Aldouri MA, Hoffbrand AV et al (1987) Effective chelation of iron in beta thalassaemia with the oral iron chelator 1,2-dimethyl-3-hydroxypyrid-4-one. *British Medical Journal* **295:** 1509–1512.

Kuo G, Choo Q-L, Alter HJ et al (1989) An assay for circulating antibodies to a major etiologic virus of human non-A, non-B hepatitis. *Science* **244:** 362–364.

Leary AG, Ikebuchi K, Hirai Y et al (1988) Synergism between IL-6 and IL-3 in supporting proliferation of human hematopoietic stem cells: comparison with Interleukin-1alpha. *Blood* **71:** 1759–1763.

Lechler RI & Batchelor JR (1982) Restoration of immunogenicity to passenger cell-depleted kidney allografts by the addition of donor strain dendritic cells. *Journal of Experimental Medicine* **155:** 31–41.

Lee EJ & Schiffer CA (1989) ABO compatibility can influence the results of platelet transfusion. Results of a randomized trial. *Transfusion* **29:** 384–389.

Leung DYM (1989) Immunomodulation by intravenous immune globulin in Kawasaki disease. *Journal of Allergy and Clinical Immunology* **84:** 588–594.

Lever AML, Webster ADB, Brown D & Thomas HC (1984) Non-A, non-B hepatitis occurring in agammaglobulinaemic patients after intravenous immunoglobulin. *Lancet* **ii:** 1062–1064.

Lilleyman JS (1986) Changing perspectives in idiopathic thrombocytopenic purpura. In Meadow R (ed.) *Recent Advances in Paediatrics 8*, pp 239–258. Edinburgh: Churchill Livingstone.

Loirat C, Sonsino R, Hinglais N et al (1987) Treatment of hemolytic–uremic syndrome (HUS) with fresh frozen plasma (FFP)—a prospective trial from the French Society of Pediatric Nephrology. *Pediatric Nephrology* **1:** C52 (abstract).

Lucarelli G, Galimberti M, Polchi P et al (1990) Bone marrow transplantation in patients with thalassemia. *New England Journal of Medicine* **322:** 417–421.

Lusher JM, Salzman PM & the Monoclate Study Group (1990) Viral safety and inhibitor development associated with factor VIIIC ultra-purified from plasma in hemophiliacs previously unexposed to factor VIIIC concentrates. *Seminars in Hematology* **27** (Suppl. 2): 1–7.

Macdougall IC, Lewis NP, Saunders MJ et al (1990a) Long-term cardiorespiratory effects of amelioration of renal anaemia by erythropoietin. *Lancet* 335: 489–493.

Macdougall IC, Hutton RD, Cavill I et al (1990b) Treatment renal anaemia with recombinant human erythropoietin: practical guidelines and a clinical algorithm. *British Medical Journal* 300: 655–659.

McGrath K, Wolf M, Bishop J et al (1988) Transient platelet and HLA-antibody formation in multitransfused patients with malignancy. *British Journal of Haematology* 68: 345–350.

Makris M, Preston FE, Triger DR et al (1990) Hepatitis C antibody and chronic liver disease in haemophilia. *Lancet* 335: 1117–1119.

Mannucci PM (1988) Desmopressin: a nontransfusional form of treatment for congenital and acquired bleeding disorders. *Blood* 72: 1449–1455.

Mannucci PM & Colombo M (1988) Virucidal treatment of clotting factor concentrates. *Lancet* i: 782–786.

Mannucci PM, Schimpf K, Brettler DB et al (1990) Low risk of hepatitis C in hemophiliacs given a high purity, pasteurised factor VIII concentrate. *Annals of Internal Medicine* 113: 27–32.

March J, Donnan PT & Hamer-Hodges DW (1990) Association between transfusion with plasma and the recurrence of colorectal carcinoma. *British Journal of Surgery* 77: 623–626.

Matsumoto T, Endoh K, Kamisango K et al (1990) Effect of recombinant human erythropoietin on anticancer drug-induced anaemia. *British Journal of Haematology* 75: 463–468.

Mazurier C, de Roheuf C, Parquet-Gernez A & Goudemand M (1989) In vitro and in vivo characterization of a high purity, solvent/detergent-treated factor VIII concentrate: evidence of its therapeutic efficacy in von Willebrand's disease. *European Journal of Haematology* 43: 7–14.

Moise KJ, Carpenter RJ, Cotton DB et al (1988) Percutaneous umbilical cord blood sampling in the evaluation of fetal platelet counts in pregnant patients with autoimmune thrombo-cytopenic purpura. *Obstetrics and Gynecology* 72: 346–350.

Mueller-Eckhardt C, Kiefel V, Grubert A et al (1989) 348 cases of suspected neonatal alloimmune thrombocytopenia. *Lancet* i: 363–366.

Murphy MF & Waters AH (1990) Platelet transfusions: the problem of refractoriness. *Blood Reviews* 4: 16–24.

Nagashima M, Matsushima M, Matsuoka H et al (1987) High-dose gamma globulin therapy for Kawasaki disease. *Journal of Pediatrics* 110: 710–712.

National Institute of Health Consensus Conference (1985) Fresh frozen plasma. Indications and risks. *Journal of the American Medical Association* 253: 551–553.

National Institute of Health Consensus Conference (1987) Platelet Transfusion Therapy. *Journal of the American Medical Association* 257: 1777–1780.

Nemunaitis J, Singer JW, Buckner CD et al (1988) Use of recombinant human granulocyte–macrophage colony-stimulating factor in autologous marrow transplantation for lymphoid malignancies. *Blood* 72: 834–836.

Newburger JW, Takahashi M, Burns JC et al (1986) The treatment of Kawasaki syndrome with intravenous gamma globulin. *New England Journal of Medicine* 315: 341–347.

Nicolini U, Rodeck CH, Kochenour NK et al (1988) In utero platelet transfusion for allo-immune thrombocytopenia. *Lancet* ii: 506.

Novak RW (1988) Autologous blood transfusion in a pediatric population. *Clinical Pediatrics* 27: 184–187.

Pasi KJ & Hill FGH (1989) The safety trial of heated factor VIII concentrate (8Y). *Archives of Disease in Childhood* 64: 1463–1467.

Potter MN, Mott MG & Oakhill A (1990) The successful treatment of a case of very severe aplastic anaemia with granulocyte–macrophage colony stimulating factor and anti-lymphocyte globulin. *British Journal of Haematology* 75: 618–619.

Raine AEG (1988) Hypertension, blood viscosity, and cardiovascular morbidity in renal failure: implications of erythropoietin therapy. *Lancet* i: 97–100.

Reed EC, Bowden RA, Dandiker PS et al (1988) Treatment of cytomegalovirus pneumonia with ganciclovir and intravenous cytomegalovirus immunoglobulin in patients with bone marrow transplants. *Annals of Internal Medicine* 109: 783–788.

Rizzoni G, Claris-Appiani A, Edefonti A et al (1988) Plasma infusion for hemolytic–uremic syndrome in children: results of a multicentre controlled trial. *Journal of Pediatrics* 112: 284–290.

Roberts HR (1989) The treatment of hemophilia. Past tragedy and future promise. *New England Journal of Medicine* **321**: 1188–1190.

Rodgers GP, Dover GJ, Noguchi T et al (1990) Hematologic responses of patients with sickle cell disease to treatment with hydroxyurea. *New England Journal of Medicine* **322**: 1037–1045.

Ross AH (1962) Modification of chickenpox in family contacts by administration of gamma globulin. *New England Journal of Medicine* **267**: 369–376.

Rumi MG, Colombo M, Gringeri A & Mannucci PM (1990) High prevalence of antibody to hepatitis C virus in multitransfused hemophiliacs with normal transaminases. *Annals of Internal Medicine* **112**: 379–380.

Schimpf K, Mannucci PM, Kreutz W et al (1987) Absence of hepatitis after treatment with a pasteurized factor VIII concentrate in patients with hemophilia and no previous transfusion. *New England Journal of Medicine* **316**: 918–922.

Schimpf K, Brachman HH, Kreuz W et al (1989) Absence of anti-human immunodeficiency virus types 1 and 2 seroconversion after the treatment of hemophilia A or von Willebrand's disease with pasteurized factor VIII concentrate. *New England Journal of Medicine* **321**: 1148–1152.

Sheridan WP, Morstyn G, Wolf M et al (1989) Granulocyte colony-stimulating factor and neutrophil recovery after high-dose chemotherapy and autologous bone marrow transplant. *Lancet* **ii**: 891–895.

Sheth KJ, Gill JC & Leichter HE (1990) High-dose intravenous gammaglobulin infusions in hemolytic-uremic syndrome: a preliminary study. *American Journal of Diseases in Childhood* **144**: 268–270.

Sidiropoulos D (1986) Immunoglobulin therapy in preterm neonates with perinatal infections. In Morell A & Nydegger (eds) *Clinical Uses of Intravenous Immunoglobulins*, pp 159–168. London: Academic Press.

Silvergleid AJ (1987) Safety and effectiveness of predeposit autologous transfusions in preteen and adolescent children. *Journal of the American Medical Association* **257**: 3403–3404.

Skidmore SJ, Pasi KJ, Mawson SJ et al (1990) Serological evidence that dry heating of clotting factor concentrates prevents transmission of non-A, non-B hepatitis. *Journal of Medical Virology* **30**: 50–52.

Slichter SJ (1990) Platelet transfusion therapy. *Hematology/Oncology Clinics of North America* **4**: 291–311.

Sniecinski I, O'Donnell MR, Nowicki B & Hill LR (1988) Prevention of refractoriness and HLA-immunization using filtered blood products. *Blood* **71**: 1402–1407.

Solomon J, Bokefkamp T, Fahey JL et al (1978) Platelet prophylaxis in acute non-lymphoblastic leukaemia. *Lancet* **i**: 267.

Spurling CL & Saxena S (1990) Controversies in transfusion medicine. Alanine aminotransferase screening of blood donors: Con. *Transfusion* **30**: 368–373.

Stabile A, Miceli Sopo S, Romanelli V et al (1988) Intravenous immunoglobulin for prophylaxis of neonatal sepsis in premature infants. *Archives of Disease in Childhood* **63**: 441–443.

Study Group of UK Haemophilia Centre Directors on Surveillance of Virus Transmission by Concentrates (1988) Effect of dry-heating of coagulation factor concentrates at 80°C for 72 hours on transmission of non-A, non-B hepatitis. *Lancet* **ii**: 814–816.

Surgenor DM, Wallace EL, Hao SHS & Chapman RH (1990) Collection and transfusion of blood in the United States, 1982–1988. *New England Journal of Medicine* **322**: 1646–1651.

Toy PTCY, Strauss RG, Stehling LC et al (1987) Predeposited autologous blood for elective surgery: a National Multicenter Study. *New England Journal of Medicine* **316**: 517–520.

van der Poel CL, Reesink HW, Schaasberg W et al (1990) Infectivity of blood seropositive for hepatitis C virus antibodies. *Lancet* **335**: 558–560.

Vichinsky EP, Earles A, Johnson RA et al (1990) Alloimmunization in sickle cell anemia and transfusion of racially unmatched blood. *New England Journal of Medicine* **322**: 1617–1621.

Villeval J-L, Duhrson U, Morstyn G & Metcalf D (1990) Effect of recombinant human granulocyte–macrophage colony-stimulating factor on progenitor cells in patients with advanced malignancies. *British Journal of Haematology* **74**: 36–44.

Ward JW, Bush TJ, Perkins HA et al (1989) The natural history of transfusion-associated infection with human immunodeficiency virus. Factors influencing the rate of progression to disease. *New England Journal of Medicine* **321:** 947–952.

Wasman J & Goodnough LT (1987) Autologous blood donation for elective surgery. *Journal of the American Medical Association* **258:** 3135–3137.

Weber J (1990) HTLV-I infection in Britain. Official recognition of the need for surveillance is overdue. *British Medical Journal* **301:** 71–72.

Weiden PL, Bean MA & Schultz P (1987) Perioperative blood transfusion does not increase the risk of colorectal cancer recurrence. *Cancer* **60:** 870–874.

Welte K, Zeidler C, Reiter A et al (1990) Differential effects of granulocyte–macrophage colony-stimulating factor and granulocyte colony-stimulating factor in children with severe congenital neutropenia. *Blood* **75:** 1056–1063.

White GC, McMillan CW, Kingdom HS & Shoemaker CB (1989) Use of recombinant anti-hemophiliac factor in the treatment of two patients with classic hemophilia. *New England Journal of Medicine* **320:** 166–170.

Williams PE, Hague RA, Yap PL et al (1988) Treatment of human immunodeficiency virus antibody positive children with intravenous immunoglobulin. *Journal of Hospital Infection* **12** (Suppl. D): 67–73.

Winston DJ, Ho WG, Lin C-H et al (1987) Intravenous immune globulin for prevention of cytomegalovirus infection and interstitial pneumonia after bone marrow transplantation. *Annals of Internal Medicine* **106:** 12–18.

Wonke B, Hoffbrand AV, Brown D & Dusheiko G (1990) Antibodies to hepatitis-C virus (anti-HCV) in multiple transfused thalassaemia major patients, their relatives and sexual partners. *British Journal of Haematology* **74** (Suppl. 1): 19 (abstract).

Working Party of BCSH Blood Transfusion Task Force (1987) Guidelines for compatibility testing in hospital blood banks. *Clinical and Laboratory Haematology* **9:** 333–341.

Yeager AS, Grumat FC, Hafleigh EB et al (1981) Prevention of transfusion-acquired cytomegalovirus infections in newborn infants. *Journal of Pediatrics* **98:** 281–287.

Index

Note: Page numbers of article titles are in **bold** type.

571